CARDIOLOGY RESEARCH AND CLINICAL DEVELOPMENTS

HEMODYNAMICS

MONITORING, THEORY AND APPLICATIONS

CARDIOLOGY RESEARCH AND CLINICAL DEVELOPMENTS

Additional books in this series can be found on Nova's website under the Series tab.

Additional e-books in this series can be found on Nova's website under the e-books tab.

CARDIOLOGY RESEARCH AND CLINICAL DEVELOPMENTS

HEMODYNAMICS

MONITORING, THEORY AND APPLICATIONS

HIDEAKI SENZAKI
EDITOR

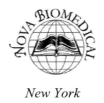

New York

Copyright © 2013 by Nova Science Publishers, Inc.

All rights reserved. No part of this book may be reproduced, stored in a retrieval system or transmitted in any form or by any means: electronic, electrostatic, magnetic, tape, mechanical photocopying, recording or otherwise without the written permission of the Publisher.

For permission to use material from this book please contact us:
Telephone 631-231-7269; Fax 631-231-8175
Web Site: http://www.novapublishers.com

NOTICE TO THE READER

The Publisher has taken reasonable care in the preparation of this book, but makes no expressed or implied warranty of any kind and assumes no responsibility for any errors or omissions. No liability is assumed for incidental or consequential damages in connection with or arising out of information contained in this book. The Publisher shall not be liable for any special, consequential, or exemplary damages resulting, in whole or in part, from the readers' use of, or reliance upon, this material. Any parts of this book based on government reports are so indicated and copyright is claimed for those parts to the extent applicable to compilations of such works.

Independent verification should be sought for any data, advice or recommendations contained in this book. In addition, no responsibility is assumed by the publisher for any injury and/or damage to persons or property arising from any methods, products, instructions, ideas or otherwise contained in this publication.

This publication is designed to provide accurate and authoritative information with regard to the subject matter covered herein. It is sold with the clear understanding that the Publisher is not engaged in rendering legal or any other professional services. If legal or any other expert assistance is required, the services of a competent person should be sought. FROM A DECLARATION OF PARTICIPANTS JOINTLY ADOPTED BY A COMMITTEE OF THE AMERICAN BAR ASSOCIATION AND A COMMITTEE OF PUBLISHERS.

Additional color graphics may be available in the e-book version of this book.

Library of Congress Cataloging-in-Publication Data

ISBN: 978-1-62257-361-5

LCCN: 2012941274

Published by Nova Science Publishers, Inc. † New York

Contents

Preface vii

Chapter 1   Arterial Impedance   1
Hirotaka Ishido, Akiko Tamai and Hideaki Senzaki

Chapter 2   Pressure-Volume Relationships   9
Satoshi Masutani and Hideaki Senzaki

Chapter 3   Murine Cardiac Hemodynamics:
The Development and Use of Invasive Catheters,
and the Emergence of New Methodologies   25
Christakis Constantinides

Chapter 4   Analysis of Arterial Waveform: Noninvasive
Estimation of Ventricular Contractility
Using Arterial Pressure Waveform   49
Hidenori Kawasaki and Hideaki Senzaki

Chapter 5   Assessment of Arterial Stiffness in Children   55
Ryo Nakagawa, Akiko Tamai and Hideaki Senzaki

Chapter 6   Wave Intensity Analysis   69
Mitsuru Seki and Hideaki Senzaki

Chapter 7   Hemodynamic Assessment by Echocardiographic
Tissue Imaging   77
Hirofumi Saiki and Hideaki Senzaki

Chapter 8   Atrial Function   101
Clara Kurishima and Hideaki Senzaki

Chapter 9   Noninvasive Estimation of Central Venous Pressure
by Measuring the Inferior Vena Cava
Diameter Using Echography   113
Yoichi Iwamoto and Hideaki Senzaki

Chapter 10   Serological Monitoring of Hemodynamics   121
Masaya Sugimoto and Hideaki Senzaki

Chapter 11	Red Blood Cell Distribution Width as a Monitoring Tool for Cardiovascular Diseases *Takuro Kojima and Hideaki Senzaki*	137
Chapter 12	Computer Simulation of Hemodynamics in Children with Congenital Heart Disease *Ryo Inuzuka and Hideaki Senzaki*	143
Chapter 13	Applications of Computational Fluid Dynamics in Abdominal Aortic Aneurysms *Zhonghua Sun*	153
Chapter 14	Echocardiographic Evaluation of Fetal Hemodynamics *Mio Taketazu and Hideaki Senzaki*	179
Chapter 15	Contribution of Renal or Glomerular Hemodynamic in Evaluating Renal Diseases and Drug Effects in the Kidney *Ana D. O. Paixão, Bruna R. M. Sant'Helena and Leucio D. Vieira-Filho*	195
Chapter 16	The Hemodynamics of Esophageal Varices *Takahiro Sato*	207
Chapter 17	The Modulation of Portal Venous Hemodynamics in Living Donor Liver Transplantation *Hiroshi Sadamori, Yuzo Umeda, Takahito Yagi and Toshiyoshi Fujiwara*	217
Chapter 18	Optimizing Hemodynamic Performance after Heart Surgery, the Role of Cardiac Resynchronization Therapy *F. Straka and D. Schornik*	231
Index		249

Preface

In humans, hemodynamic stability is essential to maintain homeostasis. In order to achieve this, atrial, ventricular, and vascular properties and their interactions are rigorously and, in a sense, elegantly controlled. Cardiovascular diseases are associated with impairments of one or more such properties and interactions, and they often lead to end-organ damage, including damage to the liver, kidney, and gastrointestinal system.

Impairments of such organs can, in turn, influence the cardiovascular system and overall hemodynamics. Therefore, to better understand the underlying pathophysiology of several diseases and conditions of hemodynamic instability, each of the cardiovascular properties together with the organ functions other than those of the cardiovascular system should be precisely assessed. For this purpose, many researchers all over the world have put in efforts to develop the theory and applications of monitoring tools for hemodynamics.

This book, entitled *"Hemodynamics: Monitoring, Theory and Applications"* contains essential information regarding hemodynamic monitoring, encompassing issues from fetuses to adults, including experimental and clinical findings and data on invasive and non-invasive methodologies.

In chapters 1 to 9, monitoring parameters for the cardiovascular system, including impedance, wave intensity, and pressure-volume relationships, as well as the recent innovative technique of echocardiography are introduced. In chapters 10 and 11, the authors summarize the serological methods useful for hemodynamic monitoring. Computer simulation also provides a powerful tool to easily assess the rather complicated hemodynamics in a living human body, and it has been described in chapters 12 and 13. Chapter 14 introduces important aspects of fetal hemodynamics.

In chapters 15 to 17, important findings regarding hemodynamics of the portal venous system and renal system are summarized. Lastly, surgery-related hemodynamics, with special focus on the role of cardiac resynchronizing therapy, is well presented in chapter 18. The editor believes that this book provides comprehensive information on hemodynamic monitoring and would improve the readers' understanding of hemodynamic assessment.

The impetus for this book arose from the members of my clinical and research team who have devoted themselves to curing and caring patients with cardiovascular diseases, all of whom I sincerely appreciate. Each of the members has contributed in writing a book chapter. There have also been substantial contributions from members outside my team, from around the world.

Finally, I express my gratitude to my wife, Chizu, and children, Hikaru, Hinako and Choco, for their understanding and support throughout my life as well as for this project.

02/14/2012
Hideaki Senzaki

In: Hemodynamics: Monitoring, Theory and Applications
Editor: Hideaki Senzaki
ISBN: 978-1-62257-361-5
© 2013 Nova Science Publishers, Inc.

Chapter 1

Arterial Impedance

Hirotaka Ishido, Akiko Tamai and Hideaki Senzaki
Department of Pediatric Cardiology, Saitama Medical University, Saitama, Japan

Introduction

Circulatory status and overall hemodynamics, as represented by blood pressure and cardiac output, are determined by the complex interaction between cardiac properties and loading conditions, including preload and afterload. Therefore, it is a prerequisite to precisely evaluate each property and their interaction to better understand human cardiovascular dynamics. This is especially true for congenital heart disease, because congenital heart disease is associated with a variety of loading abnormalities, due to the diversity in anatomy, surgical procedure, and procedural-associated cardiovascular lesions.

Because the ventricle ejects blood intermittently into a distensible arterial system with a finite length, a comprehensive measure of ventricular afterload should include not only nonpulsatile components (resistive) but also pulsatile components (compliance and wave reflection). [1] Impedance analysis provides such information and can be easily obtained by simultaneous measurements of arterial pressure and flow and mathematical transformation of pressure and flow data, using Fourier analysis. [1, 2]

In this chapter, methodological and theoretical issues related to both impedance measurements will be discussed.

Measurement of Vascular Impedance

Arterial resistance is the most commonly used index of vascular property based on the relationship between mean blood pressure and mean blood flow. [3] However, this measure only represents the opposition to nonpulsatile flow; blood pressure and flow in the human arterial system have pulsatility and travel along the finite arterial bed that can produce wave reflection. Therefore, measurement of resistance alone does not provide a complete picture of vascular physiology. Input impedance can provide information of vascular physiology incorporating the nature of "pulsatility" and "wave reflection." [4] Impedance can be calculated using a Fourier analysis for simultaneously measured pressure and flow at any site of the arterial system. Pressure (P[t]) and flow (F[t]) waveforms can be described as the sum of a trigonometric function with multiples of fundamental frequency (frequency at heart rate = HR/60) as below [5,6]:

$P(t) = P_o + \sum P_n \sin(2\pi f_n t + \theta_n)$

$F(t) = F_o + \sum F_n \sin(2\pi f_n t + \varphi_n)$

where P_n, F_n = pressure and flow amplitude of nth harmonic, respectively:

f_n = n HR/60 (frequency of nth harmonic);

θ_n, φ_n = pressure and flow phase angle of nth harmonic

t = time.

Information Conveyed by Impedance Spectra

The ratio of pressure and flow amplitude for each harmonic (P_n/F_n) yields the input impedance of the nth harmonic (Figure 1). The ratio at n = 0 (P_o/F_o) corresponds to vascular resistance, which represents the nonpulsatile (0 frequency) component of impedance. The phase angle of the nth harmonic is estimated by subtracting the flow phase from the pressure phase ($\theta_n - \varphi_n$), and its negative value indicates that flow harmonics lead pressure harmonics and vice versa.

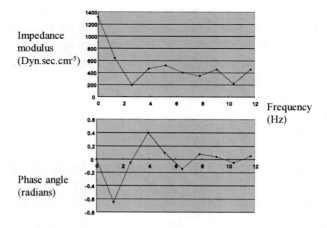

Figure 1. Typical impedance spectra. Impedance modulus values decline from a high value at 0 Hz (resistance) to a minimum around at 3 to 4 Hz, and then oscillate thereafter. The impedance phase generally goes to negative values from 0 radians at 0 Hz, then crosses zero at around the frequency of impedance minimum.

Impedance moduli at low frequency ranges are predominantly influenced by wave reflection and peripheral arterial compliance in a way that increased wave reflection and decreased compliance increase low frequency impedance. [7] Impedance at the first harmonic impedance comprehensively incorporates such information and, thus, is very useful to represent a pulsatile load. [8] Arterial compliance can also directly be estimated from the aortic pressure trajectory. Those methods are generally based on the windkessel model of the arterial tree, and the method proposed by Liu et al., [9] which uses the area under the diastolic pressure waveform, is one of the most commonly used methods. The summarized equation for calculating compliance (C_A) by Liu's method is as follows:

$$C_A = SVI/K(P_s - P_d)$$

where:

P_s = aortic pressure at the incisura;

P_d = aortic diastolic pressure;

K = an area index obtained by dividing the total area under the aortic pressure curve by the area under the diastolic pressure waveform.

More recently, Stergiopulos et al. [10] have proposed another approach to estimate compliance, the pulse pressure method. This method requires the measurements of pressure and flow and is based on fitting the pulse pressure predicted by the two-element windkessel model to the measured pulse pressure. Advantage of their method over others, including the area method by Liu et al., is that the calculation is relatively independent of the wave reflection intensity, providing the most consistent method for estimating total arterial compliance. [10] However, the applicability and validity of this method in the field of pediatric cardiovascular disease have yet to be determined.

At higher frequencies, input impedance approaches characteristic impedance, which represents impedance when there is no wave reflection. [11] The characteristic impedance is therefore approximated by the average of high-frequency impedances (usually above 2 Hz). [12] Because the characteristic impedance is predominantly determined by the stiffness of proximal arteries, it has been extensively used as an index of proximal arterial stiffness and provided important findings in both experimental and clinical settings. [13-15]

The transmission velocities of pressure/flow pulse in the arterial tree (pulse wave velocity: PWV) increase when arterial wall stiffness increases, and thus, PWV and characteristic impedance are closely related [13]:

Characteristic impedance = $\rho PWV/\pi r^2$

where:

ρ = blood density

r = arterial lumen radius

Because PWV is much easier to measure compared to the characteristic impedance, PWV has often been used as a useful index of arterial wall stiffness and found to provide important information in several clinical settings. [16,17]

Oscillation of impedance moduli at high frequencies around the characteristic impedance occurs due to wave reflection. When the wave reflection increases, the oscillation also increases. Therefore, we can evaluate the magnitude of wave reflection by using several indexes denoting the magnitude of oscillation. [4] In addition, an impedance minimum, approximately at which the frequency phase crosses zero, provides information about the major reflection site. [4] Because the wavelength (λ) of the first impedance minima is determined as:

$\lambda = PWV/f$

where:

PWV = pulse wave velocity

f = frequency at first impedance minima

and because the reflection site of this wave is a quarter of the wavelength (as a rule of physics), the distance (d) from the site of measurement to the major reflection site is given by:

$d = PWV/4f$

Therefore, at a constant PWV, a shift in the frequency at the impedance minima and at the point where the phase crosses zero degree to the right (higher frequency) indicate a shift in the major reflection site to a more proximal part of the arterial bed. [18] Conversely, without any change in the reflection site, increased PWV also induces a shift in the frequency at the impedance minima and at the point where the phase crosses zero degree to the right. These conditions have important clinical implications as to the afterload faced by the ventricle. [19-21]

Reflected pressure and flow waveform can also be directly obtained from impedance analysis. [22,23] The measured pressure wave (Pm) is equal to the sum of forward (Pf) and reflected (Pr) pressure waves. The measured flow wave (Fm) is also equal to the sum of forward (Ff) and reflected (Fr) flow waves. The forward and reflected pressure and flow are related to the characteristic impedance of the aorta as follows:

Pf = Zo Ff

Pr = -Zo Fr

where:

Zo = characteristic impedance

Thus, by combining these equations, we can yield the forward and reflected pressure and flow waves:

Pf = (Pm + Zo Fm)/2

Pr = (Pm - Zo Fm)/2

With this approach, the timing and magnitude of wave reflections can be identified more clearly, and the relative contribution of wave reflection as a pulsatile load on the ventricle can be understood easily.

Conclusion

Impedance analysis provides detailed information about vascular physiology and, thus, ventricular afterload, including arterial resistance, compliance, characteristic impedance, and wave reflection. The method to obtain impedance only requires measurement of simultaneous pressure and flow and, thus, can be applied in a noninvasive way. Although the methodology is rather traditional, the information obtained can provide novel findings for cardiovascular hemodynamics in various diseases and conditions.

References

[1] Milnor W. R. (1972) Pulsatile blood flow. *N. Engl. J. Med.* 287:27-34.
[2] Nichols W., O'Rourke M. *Age-related changes in left ventricular/arterial coupling.* New York: Springer-Verlag; 1987: pp. 79-114.
[3] Senzaki H., Isoda T., Ishizawa A., Hishi T. (1994) Reconsideration of criteria for the Fontan operation. Influence of pulmonary artery size on postoperative hemodynamics of the Fontan operation. *Circulation* 89:266-271.
[4] Nichols W. W., McDonald D. A. (1972) Wave-velocity in the proximal aorta. *Med. Biol. Eng.* 10:327-335.
[5] Westerhof N., Elzinga G., Sipkema P. (1971) An artificial arterial system for pumping hearts. *J. Appl. Physiol.* 31:776-781.
[6] Senzaki H., Chen C. H., Ishido H., Masutani S., Matsunaga T., Taketazu M., Kobayashi T., Sasaki N., Kyo S., Yokote Y. (2005) Arterial hemodynamics in patients after Kawasaki disease. *Circulation* 111:2119-2125.
[7] Maughan W. L., Sunagawa K., Burkhoff D., Sagawa K. (1984) Effect of arterial impedance changes on the end-systolic pressure-volume relation. *Circ. Res.* 54:595-602.
[8] Kussmaul W. G., 3rd, Altschuler J. A., Matthai W. H., Laskey W. K. (1993) Right ventricular-vascular interaction in congestive heart failure. Importance of low-frequency impedance. *Circulation* 88:1010-1015.

[9] Liu Z., Brin K. P., Yin F. C. (1986) Estimation of total arterial compliance: an improved method and evaluation of current methods. *Am. J. Physiol.* 251:H588-600.

[10] Stergiopulos N., Meister J. J., Westerhof N. (1994) Simple and accurate way for estimating total and segmental arterial compliance: the pulse pressure method. *Ann. Biomed. Eng.* 22:392-397.

[11] Senzaki H., Iwamoto Y., Ishido H., Matsunaga T., Taketazu M., Kobayashi T., Asano H., Katogi T., Kyo S. (2008) Arterial haemodynamics in patients after repair of tetralogy of Fallot: influence on left ventricular after load and aortic dilatation. *Heart* 94:70-74.

[12] Senzaki H. Ventricular-Vascular Pathophysiology in Children with Cardiovascular Disease:Basic Concepts of Ventricular and Vascular Physiology. In: *Congenital Heart Disease*; 2009.

[13] Mitchell G. F., Lacourciere Y., Ouellet J. P., Izzo J. L., Jr., Neutel J., Kerwin L. J., Block A. J., Pfeffer M. A. (2003) Determinants of elevated pulse pressure in middle-aged and older subjects with uncomplicated systolic hypertension: the role of proximal aortic diameter and the aortic pressure-flow relationship. *Circulation* 108:1592-1598.

[14] Mitchell G. F., Arnold J. M., Dunlap M. E., O'Brien T. X., Marchiori G., Warner E., Granger C. B., Desai S. S., Pfeffer M. A. (2006) Pulsatile hemodynamic effects of candesartan in patients with chronic heart failure: the CHARM Program. *Eur. J. Heart Fail* 8:191-197.

[15] Senzaki H., Masutani S., Kobayashi J., Kobayashi T., Sasaki N., Asano H., Kyo S., Yokote Y., Ishizawa A. (2002) Ventricular afterload and ventricular work in fontan circulation: comparison with normal two-ventricle circulation and single-ventricle circulation with blalock-taussig shunts. *Circulation* 105:2885-2892.

[16] Saiki H., Kojima T., Seki M., Masutani S., Senzaki H. (2012) Marked disparity in mechanical wall properties between ascending and descending aorta in patients with tetralogy of Fallot. *Eur. J. Cardiothorac. Surg.* 41:570-573.

[17] Seki M., Kurishima C., Kawasaki H., Masutani S., Senzaki H. (2012) Aortic stiffness and aortic dilation in infants and children with tetralogy of Fallot before corrective surgery: evidence for intrinsically abnormal aortic mechanical property. *Eur. J. Cardiothorac. Surg.* 41:277-282.

[18] Westerhof B. E., van den Wijngaard J. P., Murgo J. P., Westerhof N. (2008) Location of a reflection site is elusive: consequences for the calculation of aortic pulse wave velocity. *Hypertension* 52:478-483.

[19] Blacher J., Asmar R., Djane S., London G. M., Safar M. E. (1999) Aortic pulse wave velocity as a marker of cardiovascular risk in hypertensive patients. *Hypertension* 33:1111-1117.

[20] Blacher J., Guerin A. P., Pannier B., Marchais S. J., Safar M. E., London G. M. (1999) Impact of aortic stiffness on survival in end-stage renal disease. *Circulation* 99:2434-2439.

[21] Blacher J., Pannier B., Guerin A. P., Marchais S. J., Safar M. E., London G. M. (1998) Carotid arterial stiffness as a predictor of cardiovascular and all-cause mortality in end-stage renal disease. *Hypertension* 32:570-574.

[22] Murgo J. P., Westerhof N., Giolma J. P., Altobelli S. A. (1980) Aortic input impedance in normal man: relationship to pressure wave forms. *Circulation* 62:105-116.

[23] Murgo J. P., Westerhof N., Giolma J. P., Altobelli S. A. (1981) Manipulation of ascending aortic pressure and flow wave reflections with the Valsalva maneuver: relationship to input impedance. *Circulation* 63:122-132.

Chapter 2

Pressure-Volume Relationships

Satoshi Masutani and Hideaki Senzaki
Department of Pediatric Cardiology,
Saitama Medical University, Saitama, Japan

Introduction

Hemodynamic abnormalities in heart disease are caused by complex interactions between the heart and vessels, both of which are affected by hormonal systems. Hemodynamic conditions can change drastically in response to medical therapy, cardiac or noncardiac events, and surgical or catheter interventions. Cardiac systolic and diastolic functions are intrinsic to the heart itself and independent of loading conditions (preload and afterload) and heart rate. The performance of the cardiovascular system depends on the interactions of its components [1]. Moreover, these elements affect each other in complex ways. Thus, to better understand the pathophysiology of each patient with heart disease, it is crucial to assess their cardiac function that is independent of and integrated with loading conditions. The pathophysiology in each patient, as well as in each disease, can be more clearly understood by pressure-volume relationships. Therefore, an understanding of the concepts of pressure-volume relationships [2] is needed for all who participate in circulatory management. This chapter will concentrate on the physiological and clinical bases of left ventricular (LV) pressure-volume loop analyses.

A Pressure-Volume Loop is a Loop of 1 Cardiac Cycle

A single pressure-volume loop represents 1 cardiac cycle (Figure 1). The simultaneous measurement of LV pressure and volume is needed to construct a pressure-volume loop. When volume is on the x axis and pressure is on the y axis, 1 cardiac cycle is displayed as 1 loop (counter-clockwise loop).

One cardiac cycle consists of 4 elements, which correspond to each side of the loop rectangle. The starting point of the QRS complex in an electrocardiographic recording indicates the end of diastole and the beginning of systole, which is indicated by point A in Figure 1. In systole, LV pressure first increases straight up to point B without a change in LV volume because both of the mitral and aortic valves are closed during the isovolumic contraction. When the LV pressure becomes greater than the aortic pressure, the aortic valve opens and the ejection of blood from the LV to the aorta starts.

During this ejection phase (between points B and C), LV volume decreases, and the pressure-volume curve is convex upward. The blood stream from the LV to the aorta ceases when the aortic valve closes (Point C; the upper left-hand corner of the LV pressure-volume loop) after the LV pressure becomes less than the aortic pressure.

Then, the LV pressure decreases without a change in LV volume (isovolumic relaxation: between points C and D). When the LV pressure decreases to the level of the left atrial (LA) pressure (Point D), the mitral valve opens (MVO), LV filling starts, and the LV volume begins to increase. Figure 2 shows the LV and LA pressures and LV filling [3]. LV relaxation persists after the MVO, and, thus, the LV pressure continues to decrease, even with an increase of LV volume. After the LV minimum pressure point (Point E in Figure 1) is reached, LV pressure and volume increase up to the end of diastole when the filling by atrial contractions ceases (Point A).

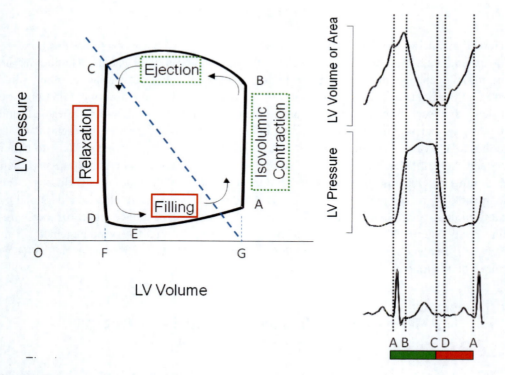

Figure 1. Pressure-volume loops during one cardiac cycle. See text for details.

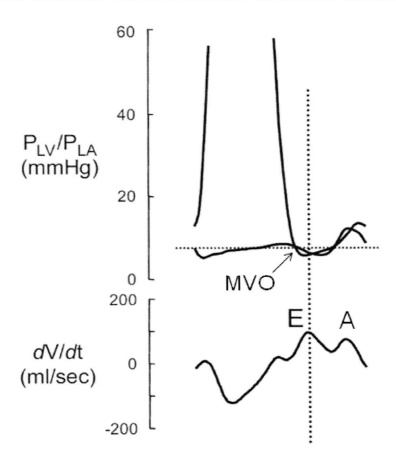

Figure 2. Relationship between pressures in the left ventricle (LV), left atrium (LA), and filling. LV and LA pressure and the rate of LV volume (dV/dt) were obtained in conscious chronically instrumented dogs. The dV/dt shows LV filling and LV ejection in each phase. See text for details. Reprinted with permission from Masutani et al. [3].

The pressure-volume loop of 1 cardiac cycle provides useful and important hemodynamic information. The x-axis of Points C and D represent the end-systolic volume (OF), and the x-axis of Points A and B represent the end-diastolic volume (OG; preload). FG represents the stroke volume (SV), while FG/OG represents the ejection fraction (EF). In contrast, when we noninvasively determine the LV end-systolic and end-diastolic volumes, the relative position of the pressure-volume loop on the x-axis can be determined. The y axis of C and A represent the end-systolic and end-diastolic pressures, respectively. The slope of CG (thick-dashed line in Figure 1) represents the effective arterial elastance (Ea) [4], which indicates the relationship between the SV and the end-systolic pressure (Pes). Ea is an integrated measure of LV afterload [5,6]. The slope of the line between Points E and A, which is calculated by dividing the change in the pressure from the time of minimal LV pressure to end-diastolic pressure by the change in the volume during this period, is defined as the LV chamber stiffness [7,8].

Model

Here, we return to the basic model upon which the pressure-volume relationship stands. Suga developed a time-varying elastance model [9] in which the elastance of the ventricle changes with time during the cardiac cycle. Figure 3 illustrates the concept of the time-varying elastance model (A and B) of the ventricle. This model is analogous to the elastic energy stored in a stretched spring; mechanical energy must be increased within the time-varying elastance when the elastance increases within the ventricular wall according to the following equation:

$$E(t) = P(t)/(V(t) - V_0),$$

where V_0 is almost equal to the volume axis intercept of the end-systolic pressure-volume relationship (ESPVR). This analogy is symbolically displayed in Panel C during a cardiac cycle: the increasing slope of the pressure-volume relationship and, hence, the increasing elastance during systole is analogous to a thickening spring within the ventricular wall. When it is the end of systole, the elastance generally reaches the maximum, Emax [9].

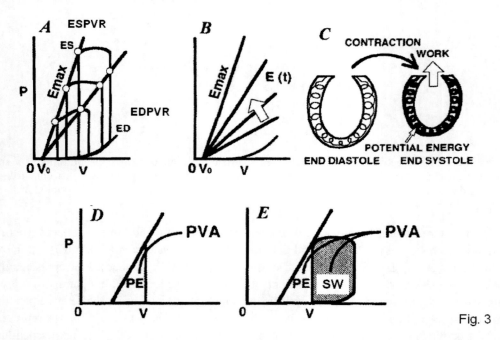

Fig. 3

Figure 3. The time-varying pressure-volume relationship and time-varying elastance model of the ventricle and relationship to energy efficiency. The time-varying pressure-volume relationship of the ventricle (A and B). The linear end-systolic pressure-volume relationship (ESPVR) and curvilinear end-diastolic pressure-volume relationship (EDPVR) are shown in A. The increasing elastance during systole are symbolized by a thickening spring within the ventricular wall (time-varying elastance model) in Panel C. Panel D shows the potential energy (PE), which is defined as the area under ESPVR and left of the pressure-volume loop. Panel E shows the pressure-volume area (PVA), which is the sum of PE and stroke work (SW) or external work (EW). Reprinted with permission from Suga et al. [9].

Multiple Loops Obtained by Changing Loads

In order to obtain load-insensitive measures of contractility or ventricular stiffness, variably loaded multiple pressure-volume loops are needed. Variably loaded multiple pressure-volume loops are obtained by changing the preload/afterload. Figure 4A [10] and 5A [11] are examples of such multiple pressure-volume or area loops, respectively, that are obtained by inferior vena cava (IVC) occlusion. As shown in Figure 3A, the trajectory of points C and A in Figure 1 represent the ESPVR and the end-diastolic pressure-volume relationship (EDPVR), respectively. End-systolic elastance (Ees) is defined as the slope of the ESPVR. The position and slope of the ESPVR provide load-insensitive measures of contractility. As shown in Figures 4 and 5, increasing contractility induced by dobutamine causes the position of the ESPVR to shift to the left- and upper-side and the slope of the ESPVR (Ees) to increase. In contrast, decreasing contractility causes the position of the ESPVR to shift to the right- and lower-side and the slope of the ESPVR (Ees) to decrease. Increased ventricular diastolic stiffening causes a steep EDPVR in the physiologically working range regardless of right or left position.

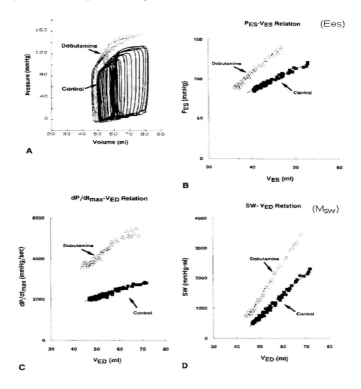

Figure 4. Pressure-volume relationships during vena caval occlusion before and after dobutamine and contractility assessment. Variably loaded pressure-volume loops during vena caval occlusion before and after dobutamine. The left- and upper-corner of each loop is end systole. The line fitted to the end-systolic points is the end-systolic pressure-volume relationship (ESPVR), and the slope of the ESPVR is the end-systolic elastance (Ees). Pes-Ves (B), dP/dt max-Ved (C), and SW-Ved (D) relationships derived from these loops are shown. The slope of each relationship increased after the enhanced contractility by dobutamine and provided load-independent measures of left ventricular contractility. Reprinted with permission from Little et al. [10].

With respect to the nonlinearity of the ESPVR, the value of Ees may differ between preload and afterload manipulations [12]. Thus, the ways to change the load should be noted. More importantly, it cannot be emphasized enough that an understanding of the entire pressure-volume relationship has more strengths compared to knowing just a single value of Ees [12]. Next, the way to change the load will be described.

a) Drug-induced vasoconstriction

To change the afterload, drugs, such as phenylephrine [13], have been sometimes, but not often, used in clinical settings. However, in light of ease, safety, quick recovery to original state, and repeatability, drug-induced modulations have significant disadvantages over transient IVC occlusion, as described in the next section.

b) Transient IVC occlusion

Currently, transient IVC occlusion seems to be the most easily repeatable, and thus suitable, way to change load. In contrast to the use of drugs to change load, IVC occlusion does not take a long time (usually about 5 s of inflation time). During the simultaneous measurement of LV pressure and volume/area at catheterization, transient IVC occlusion can be safely performed in both adults [14] and children [11,15]. Usually, a balloon catheter is introduced from the femoral vein through an appropriately sized sheath and advanced into the right atrium under fluoroscopic guidance. The balloon is inflated with CO_2 gas in the right atrium and then withdrawn toward the IVC, thus obstructing venous inflow [15].

Methodology of Pressure and Volume Measurements

For accurate pressure-volume analyses, LV pressure is preferably and accurately measured by a micromanometer due to the limitations of pressure measurements done by transducers that are connected to heparinized saline-filled lines. For pediatric catheterization, pressure transducers mounted on a 0.014-F guide wire (RADI Medical Systems AB, Uppsala, Sweden), which can be placed in a 3- to 5-F pigtail catheter, are useful for measurements of LV pressure [11].

However, accurate and continuous measurements of LV volume have been challenging. Although the 3 pairs of crystals that are used to measure cardiac dimensions can be placed in experimental animals, this methodology cannot be applied to patients. Volumetry by cineangiograms has been used to construct human pressure-volume loops. However, this method has several limitations. It takes huge amounts of time to measure the LV volume by determining the border of the LV cavity frame by frame. Moreover, the frame rate on cineangiograms is relatively too low for precise pressure-volume analyses. The development of a conductance catheter has overcome these issues and enabled a relatively feasible way to continuously monitor LV volume [14] with simultaneous measurements of LV pressure. This is currently 1 of the most frequently used tools for pressure-volume data acquisition in adult clinical settings. However, in small children, conductance catheters cannot be used due to the limitations in catheter size.

Although volume measurement by magnetic resonance imaging (MRI) is the best methodology as it does not depend on geometrical assumptions, pressure-volume analyses employing MRI [16,17] are currently under development and await further progress in order to overcome a number of technical aspects that limit its broader clinical use.

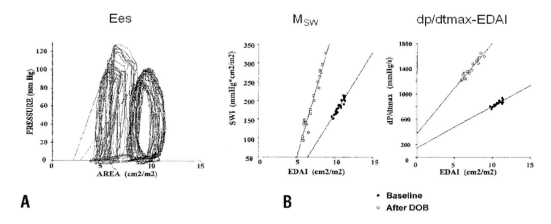

Figure 5. Pressure-area relationships during vena caval occlusion before and after dobutamine and contractility assessment. Similar to the pressure-volume relationship shown in Figure 4, the end-systolic pressure-area relationship, the stroke work-end-diastolic area relationship, and the dp/dt max-end-diastolic area relationship are linear, and their slopes increase with dobutamine. Reprinted with permission from Senzaki et al. [11].

Because of difficulties in continuous volume measurements, LV diameters or areas have sometimes been used in clinical settings to generate pressure-dimension or pressure-area loops, respectively. Although caution should be exercised, pressure-dimension [18] and pressure-area relationships (Figure 5) [11] provide essentially the same physiological evaluations as pressure-volume relationships in the physiological range and have already been validated. Calibrations and adjustments to body size, such as body surface area, have been variously reported.

Assessment of Systolic Function

Previous indices of systolic function or ventricular contraction, such as EF and dp/dt_{max}, are load dependent. In contrast, 3 indices of Ees, M_{SW} (the slope of stroke work [SW] to end-diastolic volume), the slope of dp/dt_{max} and end-diastolic volume relationships [19], are highly load independent and therefore useful for assessing ventricular function independent of loading conditions [19]. Figure 4 displays pressure-volume loops and the aforementioned 3 relationships with transient vena caval occlusions before and after dobutamine infusion in conscious dogs [10]. This figure shows the linearity of these 3 relationships in physiological ranges as well as the increases in slope in response to increased contractility by dobutamine. Similarly, as shown in Figure 4, these 3 relationships have also been obtained in pressure-area relationships in children [11]. Among these 3 relationships, the strong points of M_{SW} are that the dimensions of M_{SW} consist of mmHg in pressure volume, area, or dimension relationships and that adjustment by body size is unnecessary in contrast to the other 2 indices, which need body size corrections. Among the 3 indices, M_{SW} is the most stable but the least sensitive to changes in inotropic states, whereas the slope of dp/dt_{max} and the end-diastolic volume relationship are the most sensitive but most variable measures of the contractile state [10]. Among these, Ees has advantages over the other 2 in that Ees can be used to assess ventricular-arterial coupling and predict systemic pressure responses to afterload or preload reduction therapy [12,20,21]. This issue will be described in the next section.

Assessment of Ventricular-Arterial Coupling

The LV pumps blood into the artery, which then delivers the flow to the tissues. To effectively achieve this, the relationship between the ventricular and arterial system, or ventricular-arterial coupling, is the key determinant. This ventricular-arterial coupling is quantified by the ratio between ventricular and arterial elastance: Ea/Ees (or Ees/Ea). Given the preload, which is defined as end-diastolic volume (OG in Figure 1), the SV and the Pes result from the balance between Ees (describing the ventricle) and Ea (describing the arterial system) [1].

The SW is the external work of the heart during 1 cardiac cycle, which is represented by the shadowed area in Figure 3E. The pressure-volume area (PVA) is defined as the area circumscribed by the ESPVR, the EDPVR, and the systolic segment of the pressure-volume trajectory. The area under ESPVR and to the left of the area of SW is the potential energy (PE), namely,

PVA = SW + PE.

PVA represents the total mechanical energy that is produced by the LV. The efficiency of the conversion of mechanical energy to external work of the heart is calculated as SW/PVA [22]. The mechanical efficiency (SW/MVO_2) of the LV can be expressed as the product of the ratio of PVA to MVO_2 (the conversion of metabolic energy to mechanical energy) and the ratio of SW to PVA (the conversion of mechanical energy to external work), as follows [23]:

SW/MVO_2 = PVA/MVO_2 × SW/PVA,

where SW is approximated by SV × Pes. The efficiency of SW/PVA and ventricular-arterial coupling is a tight relationship, as follows:

SW/PVA = 1/(1 + 0.5 Ea/Ees).

This equation shows the close relationship between ventricular-arterial coupling and efficiency, explaining the importance of ventricular-arterial coupling.

Based on experimental studies, Suga et al. clarified the close relationship between the metabolic energy of the heart (MVO_2) and PVA [9], which established the integrated concept of heart energy in pressure-volume analyses based upon the following time-varying elastance model:

$$MVO_2 = a \times PVA + b = a \times PVA + c \times Emax + d,$$

where a × PVA corresponds to the PVA-dependent VO_2, and b corresponds to the PVA-independent VO_2. Because b changes with Emax, b can be written as the sum of c × Emax + d. Then, a indicates the O2 cost of PVA, and c indicates the O2 cost of Emax, while d indicates basal metabolism [9]. Thus, PVA is a measure of the total mechanical energy that is generated by each contraction of the ventricle. This PVA concept is an important extension of the Emax concept.

The left ventricle and arterial system are optimally coupled to produce SW when Ea/Ees = 1.0. When Ees exceeds Ea (Ea/Ees < 1.0), SW remains nearly optimal, but, when Ea exceeds Ees (Ea/Ees > 1.0), SW falls and the LV becomes less efficient [24]. In normal subjects, the LV and arterial system are optimally coupled both at rest and during exercise [22,25]. In contrast, in patients with systolic heart failure, Ees is reduced, and peripheral vascular resistance and Ea are increased. In this situation, the LV and arterial system are suboptimally coupled (Ea/Ees > 1.0). Because Ea is approximately equal to the peripheral vascular resistance times the heart rate, any increase in heart rate will further increase Ea, making the coupling even worse [26,27].

Prediction of Hemodynamic Changes

By employing pressure-volume planes, changing SV and blood pressure by changing preloads, afterloads, and contractility can be easily predicted. As shown in Figure 6(a), increases in preload (end-diastolic volume, shown in blue) without changes in the other 2 factors would increase SV and blood pressure and vice versa. Increases in afterload (Ea, shown in blue) without changes in the other 2 factors would increase blood pressure but decrease SV (Figure 6B). Increases in contractility (Ees, shown in blue) without changes in the other 2 factors would increase blood pressure and SV (Figure 6C). Although these factors affect each other and real circulation status is much more complex, this is an important model because complex responses are understood as the sum of each factors' response.

Heart failure is a syndrome in which the heart cannot effectively eject blood as the body demands. Thus, the key target in treating heart failure is improving ventricular-arterial coupling under optimal preload. Vasodilator therapy, which lowers Ea, will bring the Ea/Ees ratio back down toward 1.0, or inotropic therapy, which increases Ees, will also improve the Ea/Ees ratio [1]. Which way works more effectively depends on each situation. Compared to normal (Figure 7A), patients with systolic heart failure with LV dilation and poor contractility (Figure 7B) will have an effective increase in SV with minimal pressure decrease with afterload reduction, supporting the usefulness of afterload reduction therapy in such a population. Normotensive or hypotensive patients with reduced EF should have significantly reduced contractility (reduced Ees), and, thus, inotropic therapy may first be indicated if the problem is in a critical phase because vasodilation in this condition may result in hypotension accompanied with hypoperfusion of major organs. However, hypertensive patients with reduced EF should have primarily increased afterload (Ea = Pes/SV), and they will benefit most from vasodilation therapy. In patients with heart failure with preserved EF (Figure 7C) who have ventricular and arterial stiffening [28], afterload reduction results in marked decreases of blood pressure and slight increases of SV. In such patients, we can predict an enhanced blood pressure response to slight changes in preload but minimal changes in SV. We can also predict hypertensive responses to exercise because exercise increases preload and further increases both Ees and Ea in these patients.

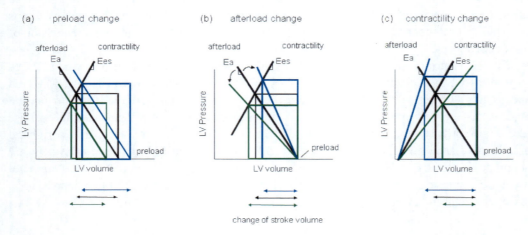

Figure 6. Prediction of stroke volume and blood pressure changes using pressure-volume planes. Among the 3 factors of (a) preload, (b) afterload, and (c) contractility, the change of one factor will make the loop shift as shown. Blue and green indicate increases and decreases in each factor, respectively. See text for details.

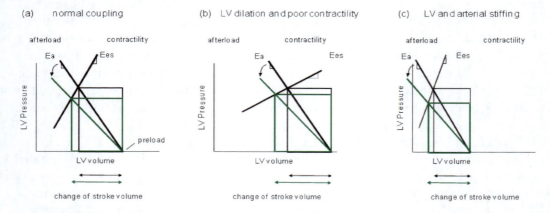

Figure 7. Effects of afterload reduction predicted by the pressure-volume plane. Compared to normal patients (a), in the patients with left ventricular (LV) dilation and poor contractility (b), afterload reduction will cause an effective increase of stroke volume with mild reductions of blood pressure. In contrast, in the patients with LV and arterial stiffening (c), afterload reduction will cause small increases of stroke volume with possibly marked reductions of blood pressure.

Figure 8(b) schematically displays the pressure-volume loops of hypertensive patients with a dilated heart and a poor EF. In such patients, the primary pathophysiology is increased with afterload (Ea = Pes/SV). However, if the decreased EF is focused, one may choose to use catecholamines to increase contractility. In such cases, hypertension will become more severe with trivial increases of SV (Figure 8C). In contrast, when a vasodilator is appropriately used, SV will greatly increase with blood pressure remaining in acceptable ranges (Figure 8D).

These responses to treatment can be easily predicted with an understanding of the concepts of pressure-volume loops, in which the SV and the Pes results from the balance between Ees and Ea with a given preload.

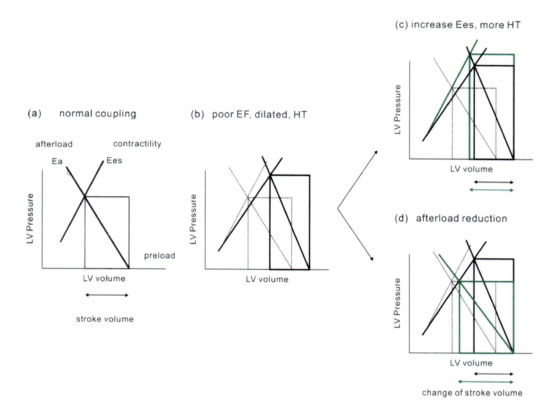

Figure 8. Effects of treatment in the hypertensive patients with a dilated heart and reduced ejection fraction predicted by the pressure-volume plane. In contrast to normal (a), pressure-volume loops of the hypertensive patients with a dilated heart and reduced ejection fraction was show in (b). If catecholamines is applied due to decreased ejection fraction, hypertension will become more severe with trivial increases of stroke volume (c). In contrast, when a vasodilator is appropriately used, stroke will greatly increase with blood pressure remaining in acceptable ranges (d).

Assessment of Diastolic Function

Diastole consists of 2 parts: isovolumic relaxation and filling. Thus, diastolic function is assessed in each phase. Diastolic function in each phase that is related to the pressure-volume plane will be described in this section.

a) Isovolumic relaxation

Early diastolic function is how fast the LV can relax and the LV pressure can decrease (relaxation). Early diastolic relationships can be assessed by the time constants of relaxation. The LV pressure of this phase (from end-systole to MVO) is approximately fitted to a monoexponential curve. Thus, relaxation can be assessed by the time constant (τ) of the monoexponential curve with a zero asymptote and a nonzero asymptote [29]. To better fit the LV pressure, another method, logistic fit, has been developed for an accurate and robust fit [30-32]. If relaxation of the LV is severely impaired, it may develop a characteristic change in the diastolic pressure-volume relationship, as shown in Figure 9A [33]. Although it was shown that a change in relaxation affected the shape of the pressure-volume curve [34], it seems difficult to evaluate an abnormality in relaxation from an actual pressure-volume curve.

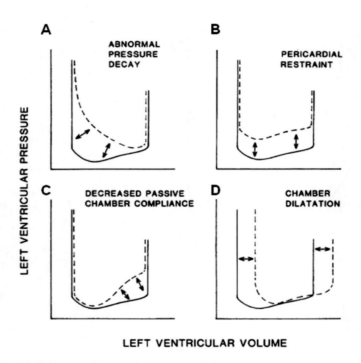

Figure 9. Characteristic pressure-volume loop patterns in diastolic dysfunction. See text for details. Reprinted with permission from Carroll et al. [33]. EF, ejection fraction; HT, hypertension.

b) Filling

Late diastole is the filling phase. Late diastolic function is how the LV can easily receive blood from the left atrium. Such an ability is expressed as compliance ($\Delta V/\Delta P$). Stiffness ($\Delta P/\Delta V$) is the reciprocal of compliance, which indicates how much pressure is needed to increase the unit volume. The slope of the line between Points E and A in Figure 1, which is calculated by dividing the change in the pressure from the time of minimal LV pressure to end-diastolic pressure by the change in the volume during this period, is defined as LV chamber stiffness [7,8]. LV chamber stiffness can be noninvasively assessed by the E-wave deceleration time in echocardiography. LV chamber stiffness may have a greater impact on LV filling than the absolute position of the EDPVR curve [35]. However, chamber stiffness is preload dependent; chamber stiffness becomes higher with more preload. Moreover, in hypertrophic cardiomyopathy, there may be a large disparity between flat pressure-volume relations during filling and steep end-diastolic relationships [36].

The position and slopes of EDPVR indicate the LV stiffness, which can be obtained by multiply loaded pressure-volume loops by IVC occlusion as curvilinear trajectories (Figure 3A) of the end-diastolic point (Point A in Figure 1). The EDPVR is shallow in a compliant LV, while the EDPVR is steep in a stiff LV. Quantification of EDPVR is obtained by calculating the stiffness constant (β) by fitting it to the exponential curve [37,38]. Increased ventricular stiffening causes steep EDPVRs in physiologically working ranges regardless of right or left position.

Diastolic LV-right ventricular interaction (ventricular interaction) [39] is an important factor of LV diastolic pressure-volume relationships because LVs and right ventricles exist in the cavity in the pericardium and share the intraventricular septum and an outside layer of muscle. A substantial proportion of the up and down positions of the diastolic pressure-volume relationship stems from forces that are extrinsic to the LV rather than from diastolic stiffness in the LV itself. This is called pericardial (or external) constraint [39,40], and right-heart filling is one major factor of it. When the resting diastolic pressure was more than 6 mmHg, almost 38% of the pressure was due to external factors [39]. Thus, in patients with high LV end-diastolic pressure, unloading of the right ventricle would decrease the LV diastolic pressure and improve LV filling.

c)   Noninvasive assessment of diastolic pressure-volume relationships

In contrast to the systolic phase in which the blood pressure gives considerable information of the LV pressure, it seems more difficult to noninvasively predict the diastolic LV pressure. Thus, diastolic function has been evaluated from the dynamics of LV filling [41] by evaluating the mitral valve flow velocity that is measured by Doppler echocardiography and mitral annular velocity (LV long-axis lengthening) by tissue Doppler imaging. However, Doppler-derived indexes of ventricular filling may not provide specific information on intrinsic passive diastolic properties, and, thus, abnormal filling dynamics do not necessarily equate with intrinsic myocardial diastolic dysfunction [42].

It is true that all echo-derived indices are not pure measurements of diastolic function, and they are affected by loading conditions. In addition, each index has its own limitations. However, comprehensive echocardiography, including Doppler, 2-dimensional echocardiography [35,43], and chest radiography, physical examinations, and clinical symptoms, such as exertional dyspnea, may help us to predict whether LV end-diastolic pressure (y axis of point A in Figure 1) is high or low or within acceptable ranges.

Conclusion

Pressure-volume loops clearly show loading conditions (preload and afterload) and cardiac function (systolic and diastolic functions) as well as those relationships in one plane. Importantly, stroke volume and end-systolic pressure result from the balance between contractility and afterload, i.e. between end-systolic elastance (Ees) and effective arterial elastance (Ea) in a given preload. While the position and the slope of end-diastolic pressure volume relation provide the information of intrinsic myocardial stiffness, caution needs to be exercised because it is also highly affected by the factors outside the left ventricle (external constraint). Although an invasive measurement is needed to accurately obtain pressure-volume loops, understanding of the concept will make the non-invasive assessment possible with all clinical symptom and history taken into consideration. Such hemodynamic assessment is crucial for all those who manage hemodynamically ill patients to provide optimal therapy in tailor-made manner based upon the evaluation of each factor and those interactions.

References

[1] Little WC, Pu M. Left ventricular-arterial coupling. *J Am Soc Echocardiogr* 2009;22:1246-8.
[2] Suga H. Ventricular energetics. *Physiological reviews* 1990;70:247-77.
[3] Masutani S, Little WC, Hasegawa H, Cheng HJ, Cheng CP. Restrictive left ventricular filling pattern does not result from increased left atrial pressure alone. *Circulation* 2008;117:1550-4.
[4] Sunagawa K, Maughan WL, Sagawa K. Optimal arterial resistance for the maximal stroke work studied in isolated canine left ventricle. *Circulation research* 1985;56:586-95.
[5] Sunagawa K, Maughan WL, Burkhoff D, Sagawa K. Left ventricular interaction with arterial load studied in isolated canine ventricle. *The American journal of physiology* 1983;245:H773-80.
[6] Kelly RP, Ting CT, Yang TM et al. Effective arterial elastance as index of arterial vascular load in humans. *Circulation* 1992;86:513-21.
[7] Little WC, Ohno M, Kitzman DW, Thomas JD, Cheng CP. Determination of left ventricular chamber stiffness from the time for deceleration of early left ventricular filling. *Circulation* 1995;92:1933-1939.
[8] Ohno M, Cheng CP, Little WC. Mechanism of altered patterns of left ventricular filling during the development of congestive heart failure. *Circulation* 1994;89:2241-2250.
[9] Suga H. Paul Dudley White International Lecture: cardiac performance as viewed through the pressure-volume window. *Japanese heart journal* 1994;35:263-80.
[10] Little WC, Cheng CP, Mumma M, Igarashi Y, Vinten-Johansen J, Johnston WE. Comparison of measures of left ventricular contractile performance derived from pressure-volume loops in conscious dogs. *Circulation* 1989;80:1378-87.
[11] Senzaki H, Chen CH, Masutani S et al. Assessment of cardiovascular dynamics by pressure-area relations in pediatric patients with congenital heart disease. *The Journal of thoracic and cardiovascular surgery* 2001;122:535-547.
[12] Kass DA, Maughan WL. From 'Emax' to pressure-volume relations: a broader view. *Circulation* 1988;77:1203-12.
[13] Lim DS, Gutgesell HP, Rocchini AP. Left Ventricular Function by Pressure-Volume Loop Analysis before and after Percutaneous Repair of Large Atrial Septal Defects. *Journal of interventional cardiology* 2008.

[14] Kass DA, Midei M, Graves W, Brinker JA, Maughan WL. Use of a conductance (volume) catheter and transient inferior vena caval occlusion for rapid determination of pressure-volume relationships in man. *Catheterization and cardiovascular diagnosis* 1988;15:192-202.

[15] Senzaki H, Miyagawa K, Kishigami Y et al. Inferior vena cava occlusion catheter for pediatric patients with heart disease: for more detailed cardiovascular assessments. *Catheter Cardiovasc Interv* 2001;53:392-396.

[16] Kuehne T, Yilmaz S, Steendijk P et al. Magnetic resonance imaging analysis of right ventricular pressure-volume loops: in vivo validation and clinical application in patients with pulmonary hypertension. *Circulation* 2004;110:2010-6.

[17] Pattynama PM, de Roos A, Van der Velde ET et al. Magnetic resonance imaging analysis of left ventricular pressure-volume relations: validation with the conductance method at rest and during dobutamine stress. *Magnetic resonance in medicine : official journal of the Society of Magnetic Resonance in Medicine / Society of Magnetic Resonance in Medicine* 1995;34:728-37.

[18] Senzaki H, Isoda T, Paolocci N, Ekelund U, Hare JM, Kass DA. Improved mechanoenergetics and cardiac rest and reserve function of in vivo failing heart by calcium sensitizer EMD-57033. *Circulation* 2000;101:1040-1048.

[19] Little WC. The left ventricular dP/dtmax-end-diastolic volume relation in closed-chest dogs. *Circulation research* 1985;56:808-15.

[20] Chen CH, Fetics B, Nevo E et al. Noninvasive single-beat determination of left ventricular end-systolic elastance in humans. *Journal of the American College of Cardiology* 2001;38:2028-34.

[21] Senzaki H, Iwamoto Y, Ishido H et al. Ventricular-vascular stiffening in patients with repaired coarctation of aorta: integrated pathophysiology of hypertension. *Circulation* 2008;118:S191-8.

[22] Nozawa T, Cheng CP, Noda T, Little WC. Effect of exercise on left ventricular mechanical efficiency in conscious dogs. *Circulation* 1994;90:3047-54.

[23] Nozawa T, Yasumura Y, Futaki S, Tanaka N, Uenishi M, Suga H. Efficiency of energy transfer from pressure-volume area to external mechanical work increases with contractile state and decreases with afterload in the left ventricle of the anesthetized closed-chest dog. *Circulation* 1988;77:1116-24.

[24] Little WC, Cheng CP. Left ventricular-arterial coupling in conscious dogs. *The American journal of physiology* 1991;261:H70-6.

[25] Little WC, Cheng CP. Effect of exercise on left ventricular-arterial coupling assessed in the pressure-volume plane. *The American journal of physiology* 1993;264:H1629-33.

[26] Masutani S, Cheng HJ, Tachibana H, Little WC, Cheng CP. Levosimendan Restores the Positive Force-Frequency Relation in Heart Failure. *American journal of physiology* 2011;301:H488-H496.

[27] Ohte N, Cheng CP, Little WC. Tachycardia exacerbates abnormal left ventricular-arterial coupling in heart failure. *Heart and vessels* 2003;18:136-141.

[28] Kawaguchi M, Hay I, Fetics B, Kass DA. Combined ventricular systolic and arterial stiffening in patients with heart failure and preserved ejection fraction: implications for systolic and diastolic reserve limitations. *Circulation* 2003;107:714-720.

[29] Raff GL, Glantz SA. Volume loading slows left ventricular isovolumic relaxation rate. Evidence of load-dependent relaxation in the intact dog heart. *Circulation research* 1981;48:813-24.

[30] Matsubara H, Takaki M, Yasuhara S, Araki J, Suga H. Logistic time constant of isovolumic relaxation pressure-time curve in the canine left ventricle. Better alternative to exponential time constant. *Circulation* 1995;92:2318-26.

[31] Senzaki H, Kass DA. Analysis of Isovolumic Relaxation in Failing Hearts by Monoexponential Time Constants Overestimates Lusitropic Change and Load-dependence: Mechanisms and Advantages of Alternative Logistic Fit. *Circ Heart Fail* 2010;3:268-76.

[32] Senzaki H, Fetics B, Chen CH, Kass DA. Comparison of ventricular pressure relaxation assessments in human heart failure: quantitative influence on load and drug sensitivity analysis. *Journal of the American College of Cardiology* 1999;34:1529-36.

[33] Carroll JD, Lang RM, Neumann AL, Borow KM, Rajfer SI. The differential effects of positive inotropic and vasodilator therapy on diastolic properties in patients with congestive cardiomyopathy. *Circulation* 1986;74:815-25.

[34] Thomas JD, Weyman AE. Echocardiographic Doppler evaluation of left ventricular diastolic function. Physics and physiology. *Circulation* 1991;84:977-90.

[35] Oh JK, Hatle L, Tajik AJ, Little WC. Diastolic heart failure can be diagnosed by comprehensive two-dimensional and Doppler echocardiography. *Journal of the American College of Cardiology* 2006;47:500-506.

[36] Pak PH, Maughan L, Baughman KL, Kass DA. Marked discordance between dynamic and passive diastolic pressure-volume relations in idiopathic hypertrophic cardiomyopathy. *Circulation* 1996;94:52-60.

[37] Senzaki H, Gluzband YA, Pak PH, Crow MT, Janicki JS, Kass DA. Synergistic exacerbation of diastolic stiffness from short-term tachycardia-induced cardiodepression and angiotensin II. *Circulation research* 1998;82:503-512.

[38] Zile MR, Baicu CF, Gaasch WH. Diastolic heart failure--abnormalities in active relaxation and passive stiffness of the left ventricle. *The New England journal of medicine* 2004;350:1953-9.

[39] Dauterman K, Pak PH, Maughan WL et al. Contribution of external forces to left ventricular diastolic pressure. Implications for the clinical use of the Starling law. *Ann Intern Med* 1995;122:737-42.

[40] Smiseth OA, Frais MA, Kingma I, Smith ER, Tyberg JV. Assessment of pericardial constraint in dogs. *Circulation* 1985;71:158-64.

[41] Nishimura RA, Tajik AJ. Evaluation of diastolic filling of left ventricle in health and disease: Doppler echocardiography is the clinician's Rosetta Stone. *Journal of the American College of Cardiology* 1997;30:8-18.

[42] Maurer MS, Spevack D, Burkhoff D, Kronzon I. Diastolic dysfunction: can it be diagnosed by Doppler echocardiography? *Journal of the American College of Cardiology* 2004;44:1543-1549.

[43] Redfield MM, Jacobsen SJ, Burnett JC, Jr., Mahoney DW, Bailey KR, Rodeheffer RJ. Burden of systolic and diastolic ventricular dysfunction in the community: appreciating the scope of the heart failure epidemic. *JAMA* 2003;289:194-202.

In: Hemodynamics: Monitoring, Theory and Applications
Editor: Hideaki Senzaki

ISBN: 978-1-62257-361-5
© 2013 Nova Science Publishers, Inc.

Chapter 3

Murine Cardiac Hemodynamics: The Development and Use of Invasive Catheters, and the Emergence of New Methodologies

Christakis Constantinides[*]
Department of Mechanical and Manufacturing Engineering,
School of Engineering, University of Cyprus, Nicosia, Cyprus

1. Introduction

More than a century ago the German and British physiologists, Otto Frank [Frank 1899] and Ernest Henry Starling [Starling 1918], independently laid the foundations of a theory based on the pressure-volume (PV) relationship, for understanding and characterization of cardiac mechanics. Conceptualized formulations of such work in large animals became known as Starling's (or Frank-Starling's) law, applicable and useful in Cardiology ever since. Significant additional contributions to cardiac mechanics and the study of PV-derived hemodynamics emerged almost 80 years later from Kirchi Sagawa's groundbreaking work in the period spanning 1970-1989 [Sagawa 1988]. In direct extension to accumulated knowledge on cardiac contractile function, was Hiroyuki Suga's initial establishment and subsequent collaborative work with Sagawa, of the concepts of time-varying ventricular elastance and the PV area, as mechano-energetic hemodynamic indices of contraction, allowing inferences to be drawn on ventricular-vascular coupling and muscle energetics in normal and failing hearts [Suga 1969, Suga 1994]. While such early work employed ex-vivo, isolated perfused systems, pressurized balloon constructions and methodologies to measure and monitor pressure and volume, invasive catheters were not introduced until 1981. Invented by Jaan

---

[*] Correspondence Address:Dr. Christakis Constantinides, Assistant Professor, Laboratory of Physiology and Biomedical Imaging, Department of Mechanical and Manufacturing Engineering, University of Cyprus, 75 Kalipoleos Avenue, Green Park Building, Room 503, 1678 Nicosia, Cyprus, Tel: 357 22 89 2195, Email: constantinides@ucy.ac.cy.

Baan [Baan 1984] as conductance (inverse of electric resistance) measurement catheters, they allowed invasive PV recordings, based on electric field excitation and its interaction with cardiac tissue. Based on Baan's classic equation, conductance volume was related to a constant gain factor α, inherently dependent on stroke volume, geometrical catheter features, blood resistivity, measured muscle conductance, and to the concept of parallel conductance, to address electric field leakage in neighboring organs or other signal-emanating structures. Capitalizing on such pioneering studies was early work by Davis Kass on catheter use in human disease [Kass 1990, Kass 1999], and parallel work in the Kass laboratory with Jim Georgakopoulos [Georgakopoulos 1998] with a modified miniature single-frequency catheter design for in-vivo murine cardiac studies, and proposed dual-frequency versions by the same group [Georgakopoulos 2000] and by Feldman et al. [Feldman 2000]. In view of the completion of the mouse and human genome projects in 2002 and 2003, respectively, scientific interest on mouse and human physiomics and genomics exploded in the early 2000, and led to the widespread use of miniature mouse catheters for a plethora of studies on cardiac physiology [Yang 1999, Reyes 2003, Segers 2005, Joho 2006, Reyes 2006, Patcher 2008, [Constantinides 2011_TBE] and pathology [Oosterlinck 2011, Litwin 1999, McGowan 2001, Shioura 2007], targeted transgenesis [Barbee 1994, Milano 1994, Hoit 2001, Yang 2001], and pharmacologic challenges [Constantinides 2011_ABME, Mercure 2008, Thomas 2009, Sampath 2011], establishing them as a prominent technique to study mechanical function of the intact heart in the modern era of molecular physiology.

This chapter summarizes the theory, instrumentation, and methodologies for catheter calibration, and quantification of in-vivo hemodynamic parameters of systolic and diastolic cardiac function in mice, and discusses new approaches and emerging computational methodologies that ascertain prior findings and identify important technique shortcomings, from a biomedical engineering perspective.

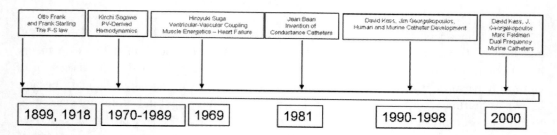

Figure 1.1. Timeline of major findings and breakthroughs in cardiac mechanics and in-vivo cardiac catheterizations in humans and mice during the past century.

2. In-Vivo Catheterizations and Hemodynamics: Instrumentation, Calibration Methodologies, and Quantification

2.1. Catheter Design and Instrumentation

In alignment with concerted efforts for mouse-phenotyping (invasive, telemetric, or image-based) initiated almost a decade ago [Gehrmann 2000, Hoit 2001, Ruff 1998, Epstein

2002, Ross 2002, Leatherbury 2003, Pallares 2008, Auerbach 2010], catheter-based measurements are extensively used nowadays in animals to quantify global cardiac function and intra-ventricular hemodynamics [Georgakopoulos 1998]. While numerous catheter models have emerged over the years, their basic features resemble closely the first prototype developed by Georgakopoulos and Kass in the late 1990s [Georgakopoulos 1998]. Standard commercial products nowadays include catheters approximately 1.2-3.5 Fr in diameter, made of polymide that typically ensheath four ring-sensor electrodes (in two pairs), flanked by a central pressure transducer (Figure 2.1). The outer ring-sensors (emission electrodes) are connected to a driving source (with an internal resistance of approximately 7.5 Ohms) via miniature cables (that run within the polymide sheath catheter encase), driven with a 20 µA current source at a single frequency of excitation, typically 20 kHz. The inner ring electrodes (sensing) also connect to miniature cables that detect induced, through-space voltage differences from within the ventricular chamber (recorded in conductance units). Such induced voltages are reflective of the interaction of the electrical emission field with the existing left ventricular (LV) blood pool and conducting surrounding structures, the latter described by a term known as parallel conductance [Baan 1984]. The primary contributory term to the total recorded conductance signal is the LV blood conductance, followed by the time-varying blood flow signal, the ventricular tissue signal, and emanating recorded signals from fixed-surrounding structures (including large vessels and chambers with flowing blood, and other non-ventricular tissue-structures).

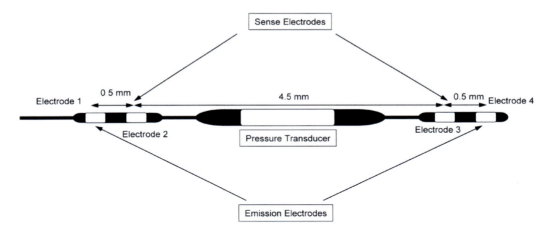

Figure 2.1. Simplified schematic representation showing the transmission (emission) and sensing electrodes of a typical micro-catheter.

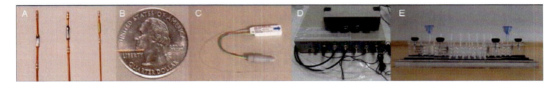

Figure 2.2. (Left to right) [A-B] Typical commercial Millar micro-catheters; [C] dedicated interfacing cable and acquisition hardware (catheter pressure-volume recording device equipped with internal pressure and volume calibration controls, and [D] eight channel recording system); [E] dedicated plexiglass phantoms for ex-vivo catheter volume-conductance calibrations; [Images 2(A-C) courtesy of Millar Instruments Inc. – use with permission].

The catheter is in-turn interfaced via dedicated cabling to a pressure-volume transducer measuring module (equipped with internal calibration pressure and conductance volume devices), and attached (via co-axial cables) to a multi-channel recording system (such as the commercially available eight-channel system from ADI Instruments Inc.) (Figure 2.2). Data acquisition is often conducted at high sampling rates (> 1000 samples/s) in accordance to the Nyquist criterion, and subsequent hemodynamic index analysis is achieved via dedicated software.

2.2. In Vivo Pressure and Volume Recordings

Prior catheterization attempts have focused on targeted pharmacological or transgenetic studies where acquisition protocols span recordings of only a few minutes in duration. Complementary to such efforts, were new strides, based on imaging technology (micro Computer Tomography [CT] and Magnetic Resonance Imaging [MRI]), that have imposed stringent limitations in terms of the temporal window of study (either for concurrent imaging and catheterization, or bench studies complementary to imaging). These latter efforts have led to animal protocol modifications (for invasive catheterizations) to accommodate the increased imaging times for the mouse (typically 30-90 minutes in duration), as well as account for the adverse (moderate to severe) cardio-depressive effects of prolonged inhalational anesthesia (with isoflurane [ISO] being one of the most commonly used inhalational anesthetic for experimental interventions in mice, widely preferred for mouse imaging technologies).

2.2.1 Animal Protocol

While a number of murine surgical approaches have been developed over the years, the closed-chest catheterization approach is adopted in the presented section, which is more physiologically relevant (normal intra-thoracic pressures, no need for intubation procedures) [Shioura 2008, Hoit 2001], in comparison to open chest approaches, including apical stub procedures [Hoit 1997].

Upon induction (approximately 3-5% ISO v/v for 2-3 minutes in an isolation chamber), sex-, age- and weight-matched mice (male, 8-12 weeks, 20-30 g) are maintained with continuous administration of ISO at 1.2-1.5% v/v, with a fractional inspiratory ratio (FiO$_2$) of 50%, complemented with N$_2$O, delivered via a nose cone (with a volume of 1 µl and 0.2 µl dead space) to attain optimal physiological responses [Constantinides 2011_ILAR]. Gas flow rates are optimized to approximately 0.6-0.7 ml/min. Respiratory rates typically range between 80-140 bpm and tidal volumes between 0.1-0.2 ml, in accordance to prior reports [Schwartz 2000, Tankersley 1994]. ECG, respiratory, and thermal probes and sensors are used to monitor vital signs and maintain thermoregulation (at approximately 37-38 °C).

Mouse Catheterizations

The right carotid is exposed and a miniature catheter is then inserted and advanced through the aortic arch and aortic valve, into the LV chamber. While imaging modalities, including portable C-arm X-ray fluoroscopic, and ultrasonic systems may allow catheter visualization and correct placement during this process, they are often associated with prohibitive high-costs and may not be readily available at all research sites. Real-time recordings of the characteristic pressure-conductance volume signals (using dedicated software) from the carotid, aortic arch, and LV can instead allow the user to ascertain correct placement and positioning (Figure 2.3). The correct catheter placement can also be confirmed post-mortem.

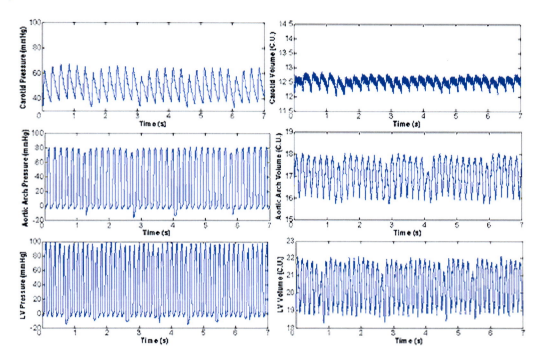

Figure 2.3. Typical real-time (left) pressure and (right) conductance volume recordings using a dedicated Millar mouse micro-catheter from a C57BL/6 mouse from (top) the right carotid, (mid) the aortic arch, and (bottom) the LV chamber. Correct catheter placement can be ensured and ascertained by the userd based on real-time recordings of pressure and volume signals throughout the process, in the absence of available non-invasive imaging modalities.

Once the catheter is in place, and before onset of recordings, an inferior vena cava (IVC) or an aortic maneuver is often attempted (transient occlusion), to ensure capability to record at various loading conditions, accidental catheter contact with intracardiac structures, and that baseline conditions are correctly re-established at reperfusion upon release. LV pressure-volume recordings can span several minutes to an hour and can be concurrently tagged with pharmacological challenges or interventions, using intraperetoneal, or venous (jugular) infusions of inotropic or other agents. To facilitate completion of the protocol for quantification of hemodynamics, catheterization studies are often followed by a hypertonic saline (10-30%) infusion injection into the arterial circulation [femoral artery, aorta] (to allow measurement of the parallel conductance), and exposure of the aorta to allow flow-stroke volume calibrations using invasive, ultrasonic Doppler flowmeters, and dedicated mouse flowprobes, as described below.

Often, in prolonged imaging or bench studies, additional surgeries post-catheterization can prove detrimental to the animal's status and survivability (anesthesia-induced effects, intubation for open chest surgery, and elicited physiologically-induced changes in respiration, oxygen tensions, and electrolytes) and are thus avoided, since they can jeopardize the accuracy of elicited hemodynamic recordings. An alternative approach may involve separate in-vivo catheterizations and flow-stroke volume calibrations in a time-synchronous fashion, as shown in Figure 2.4.

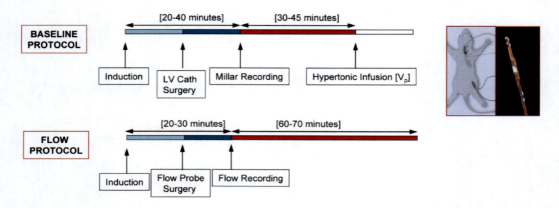

Figure 2.4. Experimental protocol for mouse hemodynamic and flow catheterization studies over a 90-minute period post-anesthesia induction. Estimated approximate time spans for the relevant surgical procedures are indicated.

2.2.2. Conductance to Volume

Recorded catheter conductance volume must be converted to absolute volume units. Such conversion can be achieved either within the analysis software environment or with specialized routines developed easily in house. Conversion is invariably based on the modified Baan's original equation [Baan 1984]:

$$V' = a(V - V_p) \tag{1}$$

where V' is the converted volume, V is the conductance volume, V_p is the parallel conductance, and α is the conversion factor representing the conductance to absolute volume scaling, according to an adopted methodology from the ones listed below.

The displacement volume of the placed catheter (distal part within the LV) is estimated to be approximately 0.245 µl. Quantification of hemodynamic parameters is therefore unaffected by such volume.

I. Phantom Calibrations

An easy and practical approach introduced early on employs the use of constructed plexiglass phantoms (Figure 2.2) with drilled cylindrical holes of specific diameters and known volume content. Filling the phantom with saline or heparinized blood and careful immersion of the effective terminal catheter part (containing the emission and sense electrodes) can yield a conductance-absolute volume calibration curve. Subsequent in-vivo recordings can be referred to such curve for conversion of volume to µl. Despite its practical significance, limited success has been associated with this technique due to overestimated in-vivo volume values [Pacher 2008], primarily due to altered catheter electric field penetration and interaction with the surrounding plastic (in contrast to in-vivo effects).

II. Stroke Volume Calibrations

A more accurate (and widely employed method) uses a Doppler ultrasonic flowmeter and dedicated mouse flow-probes to measure the α-conversion factor in Baan's equation, from the ratio of the beat-to-beat stroke volume $[SV_{flow}]$ of the in-vivo mouse (from the thoracic or ascending aorta) and the catheter's stroke volume $[SV_{cath}]$ (from recorded differences of end-diastolic (EDV) and end-systolic (ESV) volumes in conductance units, according to:

$$a = \left[\frac{SV_{flow}}{SV_{cath}} \right] \quad (2)$$

Such a calibration can often be conducted at the end of recordings and can span a few minutes in duration [Georgakopoulos 1998, Pacher 2008]. It requires, however, surgical expertise, in studies where mice do not undergo strenuous procedures or are exposed to anesthesia for prolonged time periods.

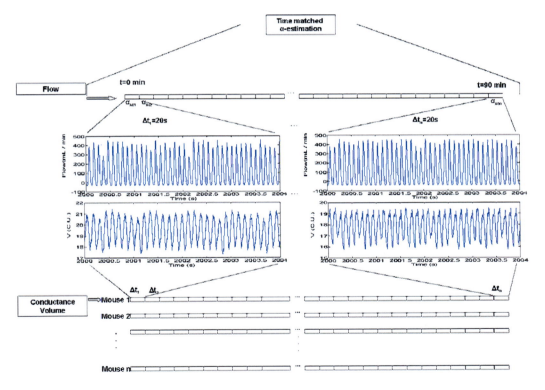

Figure 2.5. Stroke volume flow calibration procedure based on ultrasonic flowmeter recordings in the ascending aorta in studied C57BL/6 mice. Graphical representation showing typical flow- and volume-matched temporal recordings (only 4-2 s of the total time intervals for data acquired at 1 kHz sampling rate) for volume correction factor estimation in normal C57BL/6 mice, according to Baan's equation.

An alternative approach, recommended for prolonged acquisition studies, involves time-matched, but separate flow and catheter measurements, conducted in separate sex-, age-, and weight-matched mice of the same strain. Such an approach assumes stable mouse responses which can be easily achieved if attention is paid in proper animal preparation and anesthesia maintenance protocols [Constantinides2011_ILAR, Constantinides2011_ABME]. To calibrate the relative volume changes (in conductance units) measured by the catheter conductance signal, stroke volumes can be calculated by beat-to-beat integration of the aortic volume-flow signal. The acquired flow data can then be divided in 20-second intervals (sufficiently narrow temporal window to facilitate fast and efficient data post-processing given typical data acquisition rates of 1000 samples/s), and the mean stroke volume can be computed for each interval, for multiple normal control mice of the same strain. Mean stroke volume calculation can be achieved using maximum and minimum flow waveform detection techniques and area waveform calculations [Constantinides 2011_ABME]. The 20-second intervals can then be time-matched (given that the onset of useful recording for both flow and catheterization data was synchronized in time) for all aortic flow mouse studies, to allow the estimation of mean stroke volume at every 20-second interval of recorded flow datasets (Figure 2.5). The stroke volume calculation can be based on the ratio of the total flow area to the number of detected maxima points within the specific 20-second time interval. Independent estimates of the stroke volume can be obtained (in conductance units) from the recorded pressure-volume catheterization data, yielding interval α-correction factors. Typical mean values from male C57BL/6 mice are SV_{flow}=13.5±0.5 μl and α=5.5±0.4.

The series of α-conversion factors of all time intervals can then be used to convert conductance volume V to V' that contains the corrected volume data in absolute volume units, and processed in PVAN (or other dedicated software programs), at 20-second time intervals, for the estimation of the hemodynamic parameters.

III. Other Approaches

Other approaches exist to allow conductance volume to μl conversion, including thermodilution [Georgakopoulos 1998], sonomicrometric [Little 1985], and MRI- or CT-based approaches [Zhang 2008, Wiesmann 2001, Frydrychowicz 2007]. While such approaches are associated with varying degrees of difficulty, complexity, and accuracy, these are beyond the scope of this chapter and the interested reader is referred to relevant published work.

2.2.3. Parallel Conductance Estimation

To calculate V_p, finite amounts (5-10 μl) of 10-30% hypertonic saline are injected in the arterial vasculature and the PV loops recorded. Hypertonic saline injection must occur at a steady and slow rate to ensure maintenance of maximum systolic pressures and physiological homeostasis. The P-V loops that correspond to the time-interval of the hypertonic saline injection can be subsequently carefully selected (exemplary of the characteristic volume shifts, with pressure maintained at constant levels) [Figure 2.6]. These datasets can be further analyzed in PVAN (or exported for analysis in custom-written software) and a regression plot of the V_{es}-V_{ed} relationship plotted. The fitted regression:

$$V_{es} = mV_{ed} + n \tag{3}$$

allows the estimation of the slope *m*, and intercept *n*, and V_p (in conductance units), according to:

$$V_p = \frac{n}{1-m} \qquad (4)$$

assuming that $V_p = V_{ed} = V_{es}$.

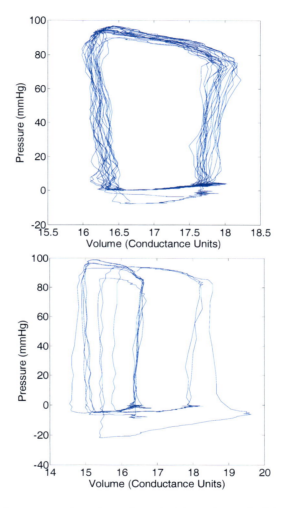

Figure 2.6. (Left) Typical pressure volume loops from the LV cavity, and (right) PV loop shifts upon administration of 10-20 μl hypertonic saline infusion.

Dependency of V_{ed}-V_{es}

While prior and recent work presents evidence and argues for a non-linear dependence of EDV and ESV in-vivo [Szwarc 1995, Wei 2005], nevertheless, recent mouse work [Constantinides2011_ABME] and other prior publications (further to Baan's initial work [Baan 1984]), are based on the linearity assumption of the V_{es}-V_{ed} relationship [Nielsen 2007, Boltwood 1989], for quantification of parallel conductance using the hypertonic saline method (a direct result of the changing blood conductivity and left ventricular volume with injection). This non-linearity argument has also been challenged by Porterfield et al. [Porterfield 2009] indicating that recently proposed correction schemes that account for the proposed non-linear dependency [Wei 2005] lead to minimal benefits in smaller animals, such as mice.

The data distributions in recorded studies in this laboratory suggest the validity of the linearity assumption and yield estimated mean values of $V_{p,control}$=14.8±1.4 µl. Representative V_{es}-V_{ed} plots are depicted in Figure 2.7.

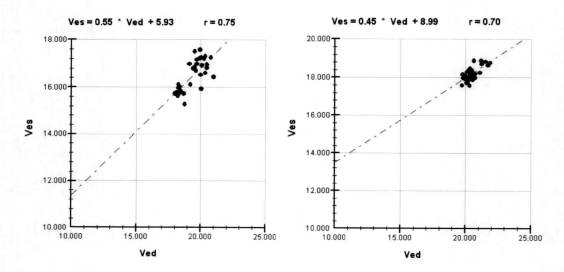

Figure 2.7. Parallel conductance estimation (V_{es} vs. V_{ed} fits) post-hypertonic saline injection in the left ventricular cavity in two control mouse studies (volumes are in conductance units).

2.2.4. Other Approaches – The Concept of Tissue Admittance

Wei et al [Wei 2005, Wei 2007] and Porterfield et al. [Porterfield 2009] have recently proposed the real-time estimation of parallel conductance and gain variability during the cardiac cycle, based on dynamic myocardial admittance (inverse of conductance). This elegant approach, which has recently been translated to a commercial product (ADVantage, Scisence, London, Ontario, Canada), computes contributions in real-time admittance of blood from myocardial sources and compensates for time-varying gains (implicitly dependent on the catheter's electric field interaction within the myocardium and surrounding structures). In this sense, the estimated total signal is less sensitive to the catheter's orientation within the chamber.

3. Quantification of Murine Hemodynamics

The importance and usefulness of in-vivo pressure-volume recordings, exemplified through the intense scientific interest in the areas of molecular physiology, molecular biology (targeted transgenesis), and pharmacology, lies in their direct analogy and correspondence to myocardial material properties, chamber morphology, muscle energetics, and extracellular matrix (ventricular-vascular coupling). Concurrent to prior catheterization work and quantification of hemodynamics in the mouse, have also been recent attempts and strides utilizing imaging methodologies (including, but not limited to, MRI, CT, ultrasound [US], and optical modalities) for isotropic, high-resolution (approximately equal to the size of the cardio-myocyte), image-based phenotyping, studies, during prolonged (> 30 minute) studies with injectable, or inhalational anesthesia exposure. Critical requirement in such efforts has been the achievement and maintenance of stable baseline physiological conditions and hemodynamics [Constantinides_2011_ILAR, Constantinides_2011_ABME], allowing comparative correlations in genetic challenges and translational efforts.

While it would be reasonable to attempt at this stage a detailed description and analysis of important hemodynamic parameters and their physiological significance, nevertheless, such have been summarized in recent, excellent review reports by Suga [Suga 1994], Pacher et al. [Pacher 2008], and Cingolani et al. [Cingolani 2011] from the Kass's group, to which the reader's attention in redirected. Instead, a succinct reference to the most important physiological hemodynamic indices of function is attempted below, for the sake of completeness.

Systolic and Diastolic Function

Myocardial contractile performance can be characterized based upon specific hemodynamic indices of function [Katz 2001, Shioura 2008, Pacher 2008, Cingolani 2011]. Such include the heart rate (HR), stroke volume (SV), cardiac output (CO), arterial elastance (E_a), end-systolic pressure (P_{es}) or aortic impedance [commonly referred to as the afterload], end-diastolic pressure (P_{ed}), end-systolic (ESV) and end-diastolic volumes (EDV) [also known as the preload], and dP/dt_{max}. Commonly used and reliable indices of contractility (inotropy) and relaxation (lusitropy) also include (among others), ejection fraction (EF), stroke work (SW), $[dP/dt_{max}]/EDV$, Power-adjusted maximum power (PAMP), end-systolic elastance (E_{es}), preload-recruitable stroke work (PRSW) the end-systolic pressure-volume relationship (ESPVR), and $[dP/dt_{min}]/EDV$, τ_{weiss}, and τ_{glantz}, and the end-diastolic pressure volume relationship (EDPVR) [Table 3.1].

From such, HR can potentially have a direct effect on cardiac contractility and relaxation and can be a determinant of chronotropic changes (treppe phenomenon) [Shioura 2008, Lorenz 1997] and of myocardial oxygen demand [Reyes 2003]. However, the minimal force-frequency inotropy modulation observed in various mouse strains (FVB, C57BL, Black Swiss) [Janssen 2010, Roof 2011] compared to human (rapid calcium cycling kinetics and sarcoplasmic-reticulum (SR) dominance of Ca^{2+} buffering) [Georgakopoulos 2001], in addition to the limited cardiac reserve in this species, downplay its potential role. PAMP represents the maximum power developed during the cardiac cycle, whereas arterial elastance (E_a), is an index of arterial stiffness [Suga 1994]. Additional LV chamber indices of contractility and relaxation include $[dP/dt_{max}]/EDV$, $[dP/dt_{min}]/EDV$, ESPVR, and EDPVR [Price 1980, Pacher 2008, Shioura 2008, Kass 2000], with the latter (ESPVR) being traditionally used to assess inotropic function (with implicit relevance and correlation to contractile protein function at the sarcomere level), and lusitropic (EDPVR) function relevant to calcium detachment from troponin C (TnC) and actin-myosin decoupling. Of lesser importance, yet critical to cardiac contractility has also been the possible dependence of ESPVR on heart size [Price 1980], a factor that has been accounted for in mouse studies by proper selection of age- and weight-matched mice. Increased usefulness has also been established for $dP/dt_{max}/EDV$, an index proved to be more sensitive to inotropic changes from protein-kinase A (PKA) phosphorylation [Little 1985], compared to ESPVR, an index that reflects overall contractile change [Katz 2001]. Relaxation parameters, such as the dP/dt_{min} are reflective of the onset of diastolic LV filling, whereas the relaxation constants (τ_{glantz}, τ_{weiss}) are the mono-exponential decay constants from EDPVR fits.

Table 3.1. Listing of the most important hemodynamic indices to characterize murine cardiac function

Hemodynamic Indices of Cardiac Function	
Cardiac Mechanical Index	
Heart Rate (HR) [bpm]	
MAP [mmHg]	
End Systolic Pressure (ESP) [mmHg]	
End Diastolic Pressure (EDP) [mmHg]	
End Systolic Volume (ESV) [µl]	
End Diastolic Volume (EDV [µl]	
Stroke Volume (SV) [µl]	
Cardiac Output (CO) [ml/min]	
Arterial Elastance (E_a) [mmHg/µl]	
Systolic Function	**Diastolic Function**
Ejection Fraction (EF) [%]	dP/dt_{min} (mmHg/s)
dP/dt_{max} (mmHg/s)	Weiss Relaxation constant (τ_{weiss}) [ms]
$dP/dt_{max}/EDV$ (mmHg/s/µl)	Glantz Relaxation constant (τ_{glantz}) [ms]
Stroke Work (SW) [mmHg/µl]	EDPVR
PAMP [mW/ml^2]	
PRSW [mmHg]	
E_{es} [mmHg/µl]	
Efficiency [%]	
ESPVR	

4. Catheter Limitations and Pitfalls – New Methodologies and Approaches

Despite the extensive use of catheter-based measurements in animal models for quantification of global cardiac function and hemodynamics, conductance catheter ventricular volume estimates, are however, confounded by the catheter's non-homogeneous emission field and parallel conductance. In practice, in most studies, volume estimates are based on the assumptions that the catheter's electric field is homogeneous and that parallel conductance is constant, despite prior results showing that these assumptions are incorrect [Lankford 1990, White 1996, Kornet 2001]. In accordance to such efforts, new strides, based on imaging technology (microCT and MRI), including the development of accurate computational models of the murine anatomy, have led to new evidence that challenges the accuracy of cardiac hemodynamic estimations, and to the proposition of new, improved catheter designs, to ameliorate prior shortcomings and pitfalls.

4.1. Computational Mouse Morphology and Catheter Models

4.1.1. Computational Mouse Morphology Models

High-resolution (at approximately cardio-myocyte resolution at $110 \times 110 \times 110$ μm^3) MRI cardiac short and long axis imaging throughout the cardiac cycle has recently become available using high-throughput protocol acquisitions with three-dimensional (3D) coverage, in approximately 30-40 minutes [Bucholz 2008, Bucholz 2010]. Standard imaging processing techniques allow subsequent image segmentation, registration, binary mask extraction, and surface model construction [Constantinides 2009, Perperidis 2011]. The surface models and constructed 3D surfaces can be routinely imported in dedicated, powerful software for electric field simulations (Figure 4.1).

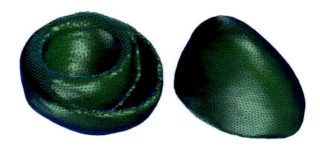

Figure 4.1. Finite element representations of the left and right ventricular myocardium of the C57BL/6 mouse using MRI.

4.1.2. Computational Catheter Models

Accurate models of the catheter have also become available [Constantinides 2011_TBME] recently using commercial computational design software (Autocad Desktop, USA). Such models can be subsequently imported in powerful computational simulation packages, such as XFdtd (Remcom Inc., PA, USA), to emulate in a realistic manner, the catheter, material properties of its constituent parts (polymide sheath, ring-electrodes, inner driving cabling), catheter orientation, electrical material properties (permittivity and conductivity of catheter, mouse blood, tissue structures), driving source characteristics (Figure 4.2), and the simulation environment (murine cardiac anatomy).

Construction of the composite catheter-mouse model involves importing the geometrical myocardial model (at ES or ED, or at any other phase of the cardiac cycle) and the catheter in the simulation environment of XFdtd, as shown in Figures 4.1, 4.2.

If the straight catheter ED model is used to drive the simulation, then the catheter protrudes out of the LV myocardial chamber and extends into the LV atrial cavity (basal myocardium contracts and displaces towards the apex at ES - Figure 4.2). The XFdtd simulation subsequently fails since the protruding catheter part (that extends into the atrium), inaccurately remains in free space.

Given the reduced LV dimensions at ES, the distal part of the catheter-ES model is often adjusted (bent) to accommodate the entire catheter (emission and sense electrodes) in the contracted LV chamber (Figure 4.2). While such an approach is still empirical, more elaborative validation approaches (for accurate ES catheter orientation) can be employed, as described below. The simulation process invariably assumes homogeneous conductivity and permeability blood pool electrical characteristics during both the ED and ES cardiac phases.

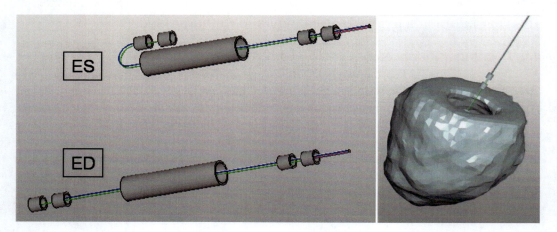

Figure 4.2. (Left) Computer model of the micro-catheter showing the pressure transducer, emission, sense electrodes, and interconnecting cabling at the ES and ED catheter orientations; (right) reconstruction of a typical ES catheter-myocardial model, indicating the protrusion of the straight catheter (ED model) beyond the spatial extent of left ventricular myocardial tissue.

4.2. Emission Electric Field Simulations

The simulation is constructed using a current source for emission, with the electrical characteristics defined previously. The current is defined to flow to the outermost emission ring electrode, while the inner emission electrode is grounded. The simulation grid is often constructed with 20-50 μm^3 cells, with defined materials comprised of free space, perfect electric conductors (catheter electrodes), and the catheter sheath made of polymide, defined as a non-dispersive material, electrically isotropic, with a relative permeability of 3, conductance of 1.17x10^{-13} S/m, with a density ρ = 1430 kg/m^3.

Blood is set as an electrically isotropic material with a relative permittivity ε_r=1000.34, a conductance σ=0.93 S/m, and density ρ=1060 kg/m^3, as defined previously [Burger 1961, Wei 2007]. Myocardium is also assigned electrical isotropic material properties with σ=0.17 S/m, and ρ=1050 kg/m^3 [Wei 2007, Raghavan 2009], and a relative permittivity of ε_r=11844, 33615, and 98800, in accordance to results reported by Porterfield et al. [Porterfield 2009] at a frequency of 20 kHz, Raghavan et al. [Raghavan 2009] at 30 kHz, and Gabriel et al. at 20 kHz [Gabriel 1996_I, Gabriel 1996_II], in CD-1, C57BLKS, and C57BL/6 mouse strains, respectively.

Figure 4.3 shows indicative, overlaid electric-field simulations on a mean myocardial model of the C57BL/6 mouse (constructed from five age-, sex-, and weight-matched mouse datasets from the same cohort), at the ED cardiac phase. Also shown are corresponding results for the geometric model (ED frame), that includes the LV blood cavity and myocardium (separately and additively). From such results and axial electric-field profiles (sensing electrode level), the electric-field falls to 10% of its peak value (ε_r=11844, 33615, 98800) within 1.1-2.0 mm of the centerline electrode (catheter surface) location. Within 5 mm of the electrode centerline position, the field drops to 0.4-2% of its peak value. An asymmetry in the electric-field profiles is also observed in such results, the end-result of the field interactions with the endocardium and the ventricular and atrial blood cavities. Additional simulations at ED yield a power leakage < 1% of the total input power into surrounding tissue structures and blood-cavities and vessels, for two values of tissue permittivity (ε_r=33615 and 11844). More than 99% of the input electrical power is deposited in myocardial tissue and LV blood, in a relatively uniform fashion.

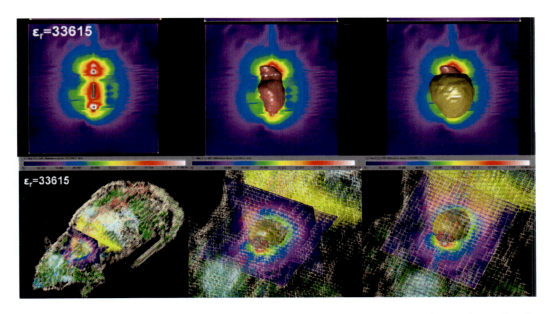

Figure 4.3. (Top, left to right) End-Diastolic (ED) depiction of the heterogenous micro-catheter electric field excitation pattern, based on realistic simulations using the composite computational model of LV blood, myocardium, and catheter; (Bottom, left to right) Simulated electric field overlaid on the mouse computational model (available in XFdtd) showing penetration within the LV cavity and surrounding structures at ED [Image is a partial reproduction from Constantinides et al. IEEE-TBME 58(11):3260-3268, 2011 – Copyright IEEE].

Overall, the total catheter conductance signal can be expressed as the weighted sum ($w_{E\text{-}i}$) of conducting (temporally varying) emanating electric field signals, of inherent conductivity (G_i), from structures and blood-filled vessels and cavities, according to:

$$G_{total}(t) = w_{E-S}(t) \cdot G_{surrounding structure}(t) + w_{E-LVblood}(t) \cdot G_{LVblood}(t) + w_{E-LVmyo}(t) \cdot G_{LVmyo}(t)$$
$$+ w_{E-bloodtimevarying}(t) \cdot G_{blood\_flow}(t) \quad (5)$$

where $w_{E\text{-}S}$, $w_{E\text{-}LVblood}$, $w_{E\text{-}LVmyo}$, $w_{E\text{-}blood}$, represent the time varying weight factors for the fixed surrounding structures, LV blood, myocardium, and time varying blood flow in major vessels, respectively. The most important contributory term ($w_{LVblood}$) to the total recorded signal refers to LV blood conductance. Another term (which accounts primarily for the temporal variations of V_p throughout the cardiac cycle) refers to the conductance contributory term from surrounding structures (primarily blood vessels), as a result of the time-varying component of the blood flowing through them, during the cardiac cycle ($w_{blood,\ time\ varying}$). There are two additional terms, namely, the left ventricular myocardial contribution (w_{LVmyo}), and the contribution from stationary, external (to the heart) conducting tissue structures ($w_{E\text{-}S}$). In terms of their relative contribution and relevance, the following inequality holds:

$$w_{LVblood} > w_{blood,\ time\ varying} > w_{LVmyo} > w_{E-S} \qquad (6)$$

However, the temporal dependence of all such terms and their changing relative contribution to the total conductance (throughout the cardiac cycle), including the additional difficulty to verify accurately the catheter's exact orientation throughout the cardiac cycle and during the study, preclude easy and practical determination of their quantitative values.

4.3. Parallel Conductance and Imaging Studies – Computational Validation

While parallel conductance can be estimated using methodologies described previously, prior work in large mammals [Gopakumaran 2000, Staal 2003], and recent work [Porterfield 2009], also refer to its temporal variation during the cardiac cycle. Staal et al. [Staal 2003] proposes percentage relative changes in V_p throughout the entire cardiac cycle, with a noted 10% maximum excursion from the mean parallel conductance value. Also observed are higher than mean values during systole and lesser than mean values during diastole. The potential explanation proposed refers to systolic-V_p increases as a result of the increase of the contributory conductance from in-flowing blood from surrounding structures [$w_{E-blood\ time\ varying}(t)$] (due to atria being filled with blood, and the pulmonary circulation increasing in blood volume), and decreases during diastole as a result of the decrease of contributory conductance from blood emptying in the left and right ventricular chambers (due to the pulmonary circulation and atria emptying into the heart and its ventricles).

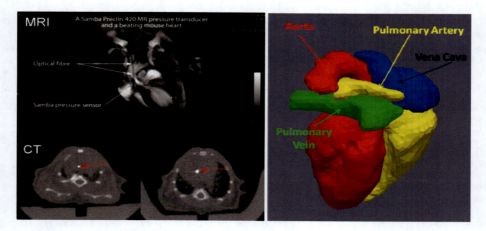

Figure 4.4. (Left) MRI (using a commercial Samba Preclin MR-compatible transducer – www.sambasensors.com), and CT (using the Millar mouse microcatheter) of the in-vivo mouse heart, showing catheter orientation during the cardiac cycle. (Right) Composite, 3D model of the murine heart (ventricular blood chambers) and large vessels constructed from segmentation and classification of major tissue structures. [MRI image: courtesy of Drs. Michael Horn and Anna Wickman, Centre for Physiology and Bio-Imaging, The Sahlgrenska Academy, University of Gothenburg, Sweden – www.cf.gu.se/CPI].

The contribution of parallel conductance to the measured total conductance signal and its variation has been quantified previously using dilution methods and invasive conductance measurements [Staal 1993]. Arguably, given the complexity of such experimental efforts, newly emerging computational efforts ought to be able to easily quantify V_p values and cardiac-cycle variation. Nevertheless, important issues exist that preclude easy and direct quantification, including the:

i. Possible physiological effects, due to non-optimized or adverse anesthesia effects during prolonged cardiac studies
ii. Difficulty to accurately simulate the electric field excitation at ES (as a result of the altered and unknown catheter orientation) within the ventricular chamber
iii. Contributing dynamic effects of inflowing blood in various neighboring compartments and the inability to computationally model flow (at present) in a dynamic fashion, throughout the cycle, in the mouse

Despite such difficulties, recent research efforts have identified and minimized anesthesia-induced effects [Constantinides2011_ILAR] in the mouse, and have employed state-of-the-art imaging modalities [Constantinides2011_TBME], to accurately predict catheter orientation in the ventricular chamber (Figure 4.4). Accurate, computational modeling of blood flow in the mouse heart is, nevertheless, challenging. To some level of adequate approximation, and given accurate construction of 4D MR image-based models of cardiac anatomy (Figure 4.4), flow modeling can be attempted, in synergy with Phase Contrast imaging methods [Janiczek 2011].

Even still, computational driven quantification of physiological-relevant parameters (such as V_p) is limited by the lack of intuitive understanding of the conductance-volume relationship, shortcomings of phantom experiments to emulate in-vivo catheter field response, and the inability to emulate physiologically-elicited changes in the estimation of such parameters (e.g. hypertonic saline infusions and transient LV SV volume changes) without effects on the total blood volume (which is approximately 2.5 ml in the mouse). Nevertheless, attempts are promising, in search of a robust and automated methodology to convert conductance to absolute volume and quantify parallel conductance in a dynamic fashion.

Conclusion

An overview of the most recent engineering advances in the field of murine cardiac catheterization, calibration and quantification methodologies, and new computational efforts (in association to imaging) has been presented.

It is hoped that the interested reader will treat this chapter as a reference guide for new and exciting applications of microcatheters in murine molecular cardiovascular physiology.

Acknowledgments

Particular thanks are deserved to Professor G. A. Johnson, Professor L. Hedlund, Dr. E. Bucholz, Dr. C. Badea, and Mrs. Y. Qi at the Center for In Vivo Microscopy at Duke Medical Center for the provision of the MRI data and support with CT catheter studies.

I am grateful for the hard work and dedication of my students and research fellows Mr. S. Angeli, Mr. P. Ktorides, Mr. R. Mean, for the design, modeling, simulations, and physiological in-vivo mouse recordings and processing.

Special thanks and appreciation is deserved for Mrs. L. Smith, Mrs. S. Lucas, Mr. J. Stack, Mr. Tarun, Mr. J. Rokita at Remcom Inc. for their tremendous help and support with the XFdtd simulations, and to Mr. M. Davis, and Mrs. P. Croft at ADI Instruments Inc. for their continuous technical support with the PVAN and ADI recording environment and the Millar equipment.

Grants

The work was partly funded by the Hellenic Bank grant "HEART" and by the Research Promotion Foundation grants on International collaboration STOXOS/0308/02 and TECH-NOLOGY/MHXAN/0609(BE)/05.

References

Auerbach SS; Thomas R; Shah R; Xu H; Vallant MK; Nyska A; Dunnick JK. Comparative assessment of cardiac pathology, physiology, and expression in C3H/HeJ, C57BL/6J, and B6C3F1/J mice, *Toxicol Pathol* 2010 38(6), 923-942.

Baan, J; van der velde, ET; de Bruin, HG; Smeenk, GJ; Koops, J; van Duk, AD; Temmerman, D; Senden, J; Buts, B. Continuous measurement of left ventricular volume in animals and humans by conductance catheter, *Circulation* 1984 70(5),812-823.

Barbee, RW; Perry, BD; Re, RN; Murgo, JP; Field, LJ. Hemodynamics in Transgenic Mice with Overexpression of Atrial Natriuretic Factor, *Circ. Res.* 1994 74,747-751.

Boltwood, CM; Appleyard, RF; Glantz, SA. Left ventricular measurement by conductance catheter in intact dogs, *Circulation* 1989 80, 1360-1377.

Bucholz, E; Ghaghada, K; Qi, Y, Mukundan, S; Johnson, GA. Four-dimensional MR microscopy of the mouse heart using radial acquisition and liposomal gadolinium contrast agent, *Magnetic Resonance in Medicine* 2008 60, 111-118.

Bucholz, E; Ghaghada, K; Qi, Y; Mukundan, S; Rockman, HA; Johnson, GA. Cardiovascular phenotyping of the mouse heart using a 4D radial acquisition and liposomal Gd-DTPA-BMA, Magnetic *Resonance in Medicine* 2010 63, 979-987.

Burger, HC; van Dongen, R. Specific electrical resistance of body tissues, *Phys Med Biol* 1961 5, 431-437.

Cingolani, OH; Kass, DA. Pressure-Volume relation analysis of mouse ventricular function, *American Journal of Physiology* 2011 301(6), H2198-206, doi:10.1152/ajpheart. 00781. 2011.

Constantinides, C; Aristocleous, A; Johnson, A; Perperidis, D. Static and Dynamic Cardiac modeling: initial strides and results towards a quantitatively accurate mechanical heart model, *Proceedings of the IEEE Society on Biomedical Imaging (SBI), Rotterdam,* February 2009.

Constantinides, C; Mean, R; Janssen, BJA. *Effects of isoflurane anesthesia on the murine cardiac function of the C56BL/6 mouse,* ILAR 2011 52, e21-e31.

Constantinides, C; Angeli, S; Mean, R. Murine cardiac hemodynamics following manganese administration under isoflurane anesthesia, *Annals of Biomedical Engineering* 2011 39(11), 2706-2720. doi: 10.1007/s10439-011-0367-5, 2011.

Constantinides, C; Angeli, A; Mean, R. Murine cardiac catheterizations and hemodynamics: On the issue of parallel conductance, *IEEE Transactions of Biomedical Engineering* 58(11), 3260-3268, 2011.

Epstein, FH, Yang, Z, Gilson, WD, Berr, SS, Kramer, CM, French, BA. MR tagging early after myocardial infarction in mice demonstrates contractile dysfunction in adjacent and remote regions. *Magnetic Resonance in Medicine* 2002 48(2), 399-403.

Feldman, MD; Mao, Y; Valvano, JW; Pearce, JA; Freeman, GL. Development of a multifrequency conductance catheter-based system to determine LV function in mice, *Am J Physiol Heart Circ Physiol* 2000 279, H1411-H1420.

Frank, O. Die Grundform des Arteriellen Pulses, Ztschr f Biol 1899 37, 483. Translated version by Sagawa, K, Lie, RK, Schaefer, J, *J. Mol Cell Cardiol* 1990 22, 253-277.

Frydrychowicz, A; Spindler, M; Rommel, E; Ertl, G; Haase, A; Neubauer, S; Wiesmann F. Functional assessment of isolated right heart failure by high resolution in-vivo cardiovascular magnetic resonance in mice, *Journal of Cardiovascular Magnetic Resonance* 2007 9, 623-627.

Gabriel, S; Lau, RW; Gabriel, C. The dielectric properties of biological tissues: II. Measurements in the frequency range 10 Hz to 20 GHz, *Phys. Med. Biol.* 1996 41(11), 2251-2269.

Gabriel, S; Lau, RW; Gabriel, S. The dielectric properties of biological tissues: III. Parametric models for the dielectric spectrum of tissues, *Phys. Med. Biol.* 1996 41(11), 2271-2293.

Georgakopoulos, D; Mitzner, W; Chen, CH; Byrne, BJ; Millar, HD; Hare, JM; Kass, DA. In vivo murine left ventricular pressure-volume relations by miniaturized conductance micromanometry, *Am J Physiol Heart Circ Physiol* 1998 274(43), H1416-H1422.

Georgakopoulos, D; Kass DA. Estimation of parallel conductance by dual-frequency conductance catheter in mice, *Am J Physiol Heart Circ Physiol* 2000 279, H443-H450.

Georgakopoulos, D; Kass DA. Minimal force-frequency modulation of inotropy and relaxation of in situ murine hearts, *Journal of Physiology* 2001 534(2), 535-545.

Gehrmann, J; Hammer, PE; Maguire, CT; Wakimoto, H; Triedman. JK; Berul, CI. Phenotypic screening for heart rate variability in the mouse, *Am. J. Physiol. Heart Circ Physiol* 2000 279(2), H733-H740.

Gopakumaran, B; Petre, JH; Sturm, B; White, RD; Murray, PA. Estimate of current leakage in left and right ventricular conductance volumetry using a dynamic finite element model, *IEEE Trans. Biomed. Eng.* 2000 47(11), 1476-1486.

Hoit, BD; Ball, N; Walsh, RA. Invasive hemodynamics and force-frequency relationships in open- versus closed-chest mice, *Am J Physiol Heart Circ Physiol* 1997 42, H2528-H2533.

Hoit, BD. New Aapproaches to Pphenotypic Aanalysis in Aadult Mmice, *J. Mol. Cell Cardiol.* 2001 33, 27-35.

Janiczek, RL; Blackman, BR; Roy, J; Meyer, CH; Acton, ST; Epstein, FH. Three-dimensional phase contrast angiography of the mouse aortic arch using spiral MRI, *Magnetic Resonance in Medicine* 2011 66(5), 1382-1390. doi.:10.1002/mrm.22937.Epub 2011 Jun 7.

Janssen, PM. Kinetic of cardiac muscle contraction and relaxation are linked and determined by properties of the cardiac sarcomere, *Am J Physiol Heart Circ Physiol* 2010 299(4), H1092-9.

Joho, S; Ishizaka, D; Sievers, R; Foster, R; Simpson, PC; Grossman, W. Left ventricular pressure-volume relationship in conscious mice, *Am J Physiol Heart Circ Physiol* 2006 292, H369-H377.

Kass, DA; Midei, M; Brinker, J; Maughan, WL. Influence of coronary occlusion during PTCA on end-systolic and end-diastolic pressure-volume relations in humans, *Circulation* 1990 81, 447-460.

Kass, DA; Chen, CH; Curry, C; Talbot, M; Berger, R; Fetics, B; Nevo, E. Improved left ventricular mechanics from acute VDD pacing in patients with dilated cardiomyopathy and ventricular conduction delay, *Circulation* 1999 99, 1567-1573, 1999.

Kass, DA. Assessment of diastolic dysfunction. Invasive modalities, Cardiol Clin 2000 18, 571-586.

Katz, A.M. *Physiology of the Heart. Philadelphia*: Lippincott Williams and Wilkins; 2001.

Kornet, L; Schreuder, JJ; van der Velde, ET; Jansen, JRC. The volume-dependency of parallel conductance throughout the cardiac cycle and its consequence for volume estimate of the left ventricle in patients, *Cardiovascular Research* 2001 51, 729-735.

Lankford, EB; Kass, DA; Maughan, WL; Shoukas, AA. Does volume catheter parallel conductance vary during a cardiac cycle? *Am J Physiol* 1990 258 (6 Pt 2), H1933-H1942.

Leatherbury, L; Yu, Q; Lo, CW. Noninvasive phenotypic analysis of cardiovascular structure and function in mice using ultrasound. *Birth Defects Res C Embryo Today* 2003 69(1), 83-91.

Little, WC. The left ventricular dP/dtmax-end-diastolic volume relation in closed-chest dogs, *Circulation Research* 1985 56, 808-815.

Litwin, SE; Katz, SE; Litwin, CM; Morgan, JP; Douglas, PS. Gender differences in postinfarction left ventricular remodeling, *Cardiology* 1999 91(3), 173-183.

McGowan, GA; Du, C; Cowan, DB; Stamm, C; McGowan, FX; Solaro, RJ; Koretsky, AP; DelNido, PJ. Ischemic dysfunction in transgenic mice expressing troponin I lacking protein kinase C phosphorylation sites, Am. J. Physiol. Heart Circ. Physiol. 2001 280, H835-H843.

Mercure, C; Yogi, A; Callera, GE; Aranha, AB; Bader, M; Ferreira, AJ; Santos, RA; Walther, T; Touyz, RM; Reudelhuber, TL. Angiotensin(1-7) blunts hypertensive cardiac remodeling by a direct effect on the heart, *Circ Res* 2008 103(11), 1319-26.

Milano, CA; Allen, LF; Rockman, HA; Dolber, PC; McMinn, TR; Chien, TR; Johnson, TD; Bond, RA; Lefkowitz, RJ. Enhanced myocardial function in transgenic mice overexpressing the beta-adrenergic receptor, *Science* 1994 264, 5158:582-586.

Nielsen, JM; Kristiansen, SB; Ringgaard, S; Nielsen, TT; Flyvbjerg, A; Redington, AN; Botker, HE. Left ventricular volume measurement in mice by conductance catheter: evaluation and optimization of calibration, *Am. J. Physiol. Heart Circ. Physiol.* 2007 293, H534-H540.

Oosterlinck, W; Vanderper, A; Flameng, W; Herijgers, P. Glucose tolerance and left and ventricular pressure-volume relationships in frequently used mouse strains, *Journal of Biomedicine and Biotechnology* 2011 2011, 1-7.

Pacher, Pal; Nagayama, T; Mukhopadhyay, P; Batkal, S; Kass, DA. Measurement of cardiac function using pressure-volume conductance catheter technique in mice and rats. *Nat Protocols* 2008 3(9), 1422-1434.

Pallares, P; Gonzalez-Bulnes, A. Non-invasive ultrasonographic characterization of phenotypic changes during embryo development in non-anesthetized mice of different genotypes. *Theriogenology* 2008 70(1), 44-52.

Perperidis, D; Bucholz, E; Johnson, GA, Constantinides, C. Morphological studies of the murine heart based on probabilistic and statistical atlases, *Computerized Medical Imaging and Graphics*, doi:10.1016/j.compmedimag.2011.07.001.

Porterfield, JE; Kottam, ATG; Raghavan, K; Escobedo, D; Jenkins, JT; Larson, ER; Trevino, RJ; Valvano, JW; Pearce, JA; Feldman, MD. Dynamic correction for parallel conductance, G_p, and gain factor, α, in invasive murine left ventricular volume measurements, *J Appl Physiol* 2009 107, 1693-1703.

Raghavan, K; Porterfield, JE; Kottam, ATG; Feldman, MD; Escobedo, D; Valvano, JW; Pearce, JA. Electrical conductivity and permittivity of murine myocardium, *IEEE Trans. Biomed. Eng.* 2009 56(8), 2044-2053.

Reyes, M; Freeman, GL; Escobedo, D; Lee, S; Steinhelper, ME; Feldman, MD. Enhancement of contractility with sustained afterload in the intact murine heart, *Circulation* 2003 107, 2962-2968.

Reyes, M; Steinhelper, M; Alvarez, J; Escobedo, D; Pearce, JA; Valvano, JW; Pollock, B; Wei, CL; Kottam, ATG; Altman, D; Lee, S; Bailey, S; Thomsen, SL; Freeman, G; Feldman, MD. Impact of physiologic variables and genetic background on myocardial frequency-resistivity relations in the intact beating murine heart, *Am J Physiol Heart Circ Physiol* 2006 291(4), H1659-H1669.

Roof, SR; Shannon, TR; Janssen, PM; Ziolo, MT. Effects of increased systolic Ca^{2+} and phospholamban phosphorylation during adrenergic stimulation on Ca^{2+} transient kinetics in cardiac myocytes, *Am J Physiol Heart Circ Physiol* 2011 301(4), H1570-8.

Ross, AJ; Yang, Z; Berr, SS; Gilson, WD; Peterssen, WC; Oshinski, JN; French, BA. Serial MRI evaluation of cardiac structure and function in mice after reperfused myocardial infarction, *Magnetic Reson. Med.* 2002 47(6), 1158-68.

Ruff, J; Wiesmann, F; Hiller, KH; Voll, S; von Kienlin, M; Bauer, WR; Rommel, E; Neubauer, S; Haase, A. Magnetic resonance microimaging for noninvasive quantification of myocardial function and mass in the mouse, *Magn. Reson. Med.* 1998 40, 43-48.

Sagawa, K, Maughan, W.L., Suga, H, Sunagawa K. *Cardiac Contraction and the Pressure-Volume Relationship*. New York: Oxford University Press, 1988.

Sampath, H; Batra, AK; Vartanian, V; Carmical, JR; Prusak, D; King, IB; Lowell, B; Early, LF; Wood, TG; Marks, D; McCullogh, AK; Stephen RL. Variable penetrance of metabolic phenotypes and development of high-fat diet induced adiposity in NEIL-1 deficient mice, *Am J Physiol Endocrinol Metab* 2011 300(4), E724-34.

Schwartz, LA; Zuurbier, CJ ; Ince, C. Mechanical ventilation of mice. *Basic Research in Cardiology* 2000 95, 510-520.

Segers, P; Georgakopoulos, D; Afanasyeva, M; Champion, HC; Judge, DP; Millar, HD; Verdonck, P; Kass, DA; Stergiopoulos, N; Westerhof, N. Conductance catheter-based assessment of arterial input impedance, arterial function, and ventricular-vascular interaction in mice, *Am J Physiol Heart Circ Physiol* 2005 288, H1157-H1164.

Shioura, K; Geenen, DL; Goldspink, PH. Assessment of cardiac function with the pressure-volume conductance system following myocardial infarction in mice, *Am J Physiol Heart Circ Physiol* 2007 293, H2870-H2877.

Shioura, K; Geenen, DL; Goldspink, PH. Sex-related changes in cardiac function following myocardial infarction in mice, *Am J Physiol Regul Integr Comp Physiol* 2008 295, R528-R534.

Staal, EM; Steendijk, P; Baan J. The trans-cardiac conductance method for on-line measurement of left ventricular volume: assessment of parallel conductance offset volume, *IEEE Trans. Biomed. Eng.* 2003 50(2), 234-240.

Starling, EH: *Linacre Lecture on the Law of the Heart.* Longmans, Green and Co, London, 1918.

Suga, H. Analysis of left ventricular pumping by its pressure-volume coefficient (in Japanese with English abstract), *Japanese Journal Med Electr Biol Eng* 1969 7, 406.

Suga, H. Paul Dudley White International Lecture: Cardiac Performance as Viewed Through the Pressure-Volume Window (Special Article), *Japanese Heart Journal* 1994 35, 263-280.

Szwarc, RS; Laurent, D; Allegrini, PR; Ball, HA. Conductance catheter measurement of left ventricular volume: evidence for nonlinearity within cardiac cycle, *Am. J. Phys.* 1995 268 (4 Pt 2) 37, H1490-H1498.

Tankersley, CG; Fitzgerald, RS; Kleeberger, SR. Differential control of ventilation among inbred strain of mice, *American Journal Physiology* 1994 267(36), R1371-1377.

Thomas, AC; Potts, EN; Chen, BT; Slipetz, DM; Foster, WM; Driehuys, B. A robust protocol for regional evaluation of methacholine challenge in mouse models of allergic asthma using hyperpolarized ^{3}He MRI, *NMR Biomed* 2009 22(5), 502-15.

Wei, C; Valvano, JW; Feldman, MD; Pearce, JA. Nonlinear conductance-volume relationship for murine conductance catheter measurement system, *IEEE Trans Biomed Eng* 2005 52(10), 1654-1661.

Wei, C; Valvano, JW; Feldman, MD; Nahrendorf, M; Peshock, R; Pearce, JA. Volume catheter parallel conductance varies between end-systole and end-diastole, *IEEE Trans Biomed Eng* 2007 54(8), 1480-1489.

White, PA; Chaturvedi, RR; Bishop, AJ; Brookes, CIO; Oldershaw, PJ; Redington AN. Does parallel conductance vary during systole in the human right ventricle? *Cardiovascular Research* 1996 32, 901-908.

Wiesmann, F; Ruff, J; Engelhardt, S; Hein, L; Dienesch, C; Leupold, A; Illinger, R; Frydrychowicz, A; Hiller, KH; Rommel, E; Haase, A; Lohse, MJ; Neubauer, S. Dobutamine-Stress Magnetic Resonance Microimaging in mice: acute changes of cardiac geometry and function in normal and failing murine hearts, *Circulation Research* 2001 88(6), 550-551.

Yang, B; Larson, DF; Watson, R. Age-related left ventricular function in the mouse: analysis based on in vivo pressure-volume relationships, *Am J Physiol Heart Circ Physiol 1999* 277(5), H1906-H1913.

Yang Q; Osinska H; Klevitsky R; Robbins J. Phenotypic deficits in mice expressing a myosin binding protein C lacking titin and myosin binding domains, *J Mol Cell Cardiol* 2001 33(9), 1649-58.

Zhang, W; ten Hove, M; Schneider, JE; Stuckey, DJ; Sebag-Montefiore, L; Bia, BL; Radda, GK; Davies, KE; Neubauer, S; Clarke K. Abnormal cardiac morphology, function and energy metabolism in the dystrophic mdx mouse: An MRI and MRS study, *Journal of Molecular and Cellular Cardiology* 2008 45(6), 754-760.

In: Hemodynamics: Monitoring, Theory and Applications
Editor: Hideaki Senzaki

ISBN: 978-1-62257-361-5
© 2013 Nova Science Publishers, Inc.

Chapter 4

Analysis of Arterial Waveform: Noninvasive Estimation of Ventricular Contractility Using Arterial Pressure Waveform

Hidenori Kawasaki and Hideaki Senzaki
Department of Pediatric Cardiology, Saitama Medical University, Saitama, Japan

Introduction

Comprehensive information about the vascular system can be best obtained by impedance analysis. However, useful information about vascular and even ventricular properties can be much more easily obtained by a detailed assessment of the arterial waveform with a precise understanding of the background physiology of the vascular system. Aortic waveform analysis also has the potential for noninvasive assessment of the ventricular-vascular pathophysiology.

In this chapter, the basic theory involved in the arterial waveform will be discussed first, and the clinical application of arterial waveform analysis in pediatric cardiovascular disease will be presented in the second part.

1. Aortic Pressure

The pressure and blood flow of the ascending aorta (AAo) are determined by a complex interaction between the left ventricle (LV) and arterial system. The driving force for the movement of blood from the LV into the AAo is dependent on LV contractility, LV morphology, and heart rate (HR). This driving force is opposed by arterial impedance, which is determined by peripheral vascular resistance (including blood viscosity), inertia, and compliance related to arterial distensibility [1]. Arterial wave reflections also contribute to forming arterial impedance. Therefore, all of such information is included in the aortic pressure waveform, and thus, can be deduced by a detailed assessment of the aortic pressure waveform.

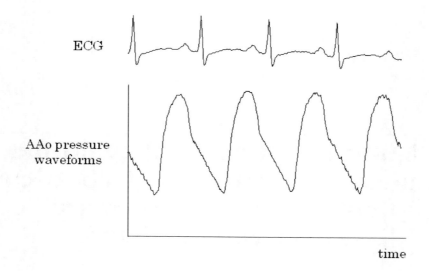

Figure 1.

A typical record of the AAo pressure wave is shown in figure 1. AAo pressure rises rapidly in early systole, which is often termed as anacrotic limb. It is known that the anacrotic limb consists of 2 parts, that is, sharp upstroke in the early phase and slow rise to peak pressure; thus, the maximum rate of AAo pressure rise occurs slightly earlier than the peak pressure [2]. After its peak, AAo pressure declines with an incisura, which is caused by closure of the aortic valve.

The pressure pulse of the proximal portion of the aorta is transmitted along the arterial tree with various changes in shape (figure 2). The velocities of pressure pulse transmission, which are inversely proportional to the compliance of each vascular segment, change from 3 to 5 m/s in the aortas, 7 to 10 m/s in large arterial branches, and 15 to 35 m/s in small arteries [3]. Furthermore, because of resistance to blood movement in the vessels and compliance of the vessels, the pressure pulse diminishes progressively along the arterial tree in the smaller arteries, arterioles, and, especially, capillaries [3]. This phenomenon is called damping of the pressure pulses. The differences in mean and diastolic pressure between the aorta and peripheral arteries are small, but the differences in systolic pressure and pressure waveform are large [4].

For a given blood flow ejected into the arterial system, the ascending rim of the aortic pressure trajectory is determined by the mechanical properties of the arterial bed, including characteristic impedance (Z_c), peripheral resistance (R_t), and total arterial compliance (C). An increase in Z_c causes a rise in peak aortic pressure without a change in minimum (diastolic) pressure, whereas an increase in R_t results in increases in both peak and minimum pressure. On the other hand, an increase in C increases the maximum pressure but decreases the minimum pressure without a change in the mean pressure. Since the ventricular contractility is a key to determine the blood flow ejected into the arterial system, one may be able to estimate ventricular contractility from the aortic pressure waveform using the relationships between arterial properties and aortic pressure as mentioned above. This possibility is discussed in the following section.

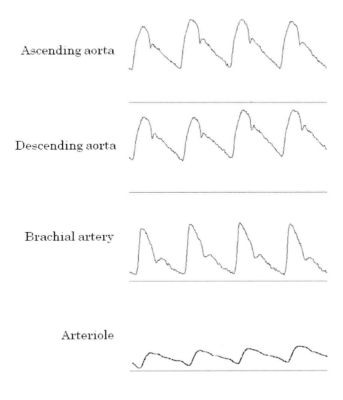

Figure 2.

2. Estimation of LV Contractility by Aortic Pressure

There have been some studies as to whether an index of AAo pressure may become a marker of LV contractility, focusing on the maximum rate of pressure rise (dp/dt_{max}). LV dp/dt_{max} is an index of LV contractility [5, 6], with apparent dependence on preload [7], and without dependence on afterload as well as LV morphology or structural abnormalities [8]. Although invasive monitoring of the intraventricular pressure by cardiac catheterization is required to measure LV dp/dt_{max}, LV dp/dt_{max} reflects the change in LV contractility in both acute and chronic conditions [9, 10]. Various methods for noninvasive estimation of LV dp/dt_{max} have been proposed, mainly depending on Doppler echocardiography of mitral regurgitation [11-13].

There have been previous studies showing considerable variation in the relationship between AAo dp/dt_{max} and LV dp/dt_{max} under conditions in which the vascular properties were markedly altered [14, 15]. However, by investigating 30 healthy children (controls) and 45 children with congenital heart disease (without aortic valvular disease or LV outflow obstruction), we identified a constant relationship between LV dp/dt_{max} and AAo dp/dt_{max}^2:

AAo dp/dt_{max}/LV dp/dt_{max} = 0.641 + 1.445*10^{-4}*Zc − 3.73*10^{-3}*MAP
(Zc, characteristic impedance; MAP, mean AAo pressure; $P < 0.0001$; $r = 0.87$).

In theory, vascular properties should affect the Ao dp/dt_{max}-LV dp/dt_{max} relationship by changing Ao dp/dt_{max}, even when LV contractility (LV dp/dt_{max}) is unchanged. In addition, changes in HR alone without changes in cardiac output or vascular properties also change pulse pressure and, thereby, potentially affect the Ao dp/dt_{max}-LV dp/dt_{max} relationship. However, in human heart, changes in each property affect the ventricular ejection; thus, increases in Zc and Rt and a decrease in C significantly reduce the ventricular ejection. Using an isolated canine heart model which enables the evaluation of independent and quantitative effects of changes in vascular properties on ventricular ejection, Sunagawa et al. demonstrated that Rt is a major determinant of stroke volume, while Zc and C had a significant but only minimal effect on ejection. Therefore, increases in Rt should reduce the stroke volume and, thereby, counteract the effect of Rt change on the rise in Ao dp/dt_{max}. MAP represents the result of such interaction between Rt and stroke volume, including the HR effects, which may explain why MAP, but not Rt or HR per se, is an important determinant of the Ao-LV dp/dt_{max} relationship. The reason why Zc but not C significantly affects the Ao-LV dp/dt_{max} relationship may also be related to the balance between their effects on aortic pressure trajectory and those on ventricular ejection (changes in Ao dp/dt_{max} outweigh the changes in ventricular ejection when Zc changes, whereas changes in Ao dp/dt_{max} are counterbalanced by changes in ejection when C changes).

The constant Ao dp/dt_{max}-LV dp/dt_{max} relationship implies that LV contractility can be estimated noninvasively from aortic pressure measurements. However, since computing Zc requires a complex calculation, we further tested whether AAo dp/dt_{max}/LV dp/dt_{max} can be estimated using MAP only[2]. We found that AAo dp/dt_{max}/LV dp/dt_{max} can be estimated by MAP as follows:

AAo dp/dt_{max}/LV dp/dt_{max} = 0.694 − 4.00 * 10^{-3} * MAP

Furthermore, we discovered that a linear regression exists between AAo dp/dt_{max} and the descending aorta (DAo) dp/dt_{max} (our unpublished data) as well as between AAo dp/dt_{max} and the peripheral artery (BrA, brachial artery; RaA, radial artery) dp/dt_{max} among children with congenital heart disease [16].

AAo dp/dt_{max} = 0.738 * DAo dp/dt_{max} + 134.4 ($n = 27$, $P < 0.0001$, $r = 0.92$)

AAo dp/dt_{max} = 0.299 * BrA dp/dt_{max} + 210.6 ($n = 17$, $P = 0.0002$, $r = 0.78$)

AAo dp/dt_{max} = 1.442 * RaA dp/dt_{max} + 165.9 ($n = 14$, $P = 0.0001$, $r = 0.87$)

In our study population, these findings were adopted irrespective of ventricular morphological abnormalities and existence of various aortopulmonary connections such as patent ductus arteriosus and major aortopulmonary collateral arteries. Although there are problems in that the coefficients differ largely between the monitoring points, these findings may lead to noninvasive continuous bedside monitoring of LV contractility, using umbilical artery lines or peripheral artery lines.

References

[1] Alexander RW, Schlant RC, Fuster V, O'Rourke RA, Roberts R, Sonnenblick EH. *Hurst's the Heart: Arteries and Veins.* 9th ed; 1998.

[2] Masutani S, Iwamoto Y, Ishido H, Senzaki H. Relationship of Maximum Rate of Pressure Rise Between Aorta and Left Ventricle in Pediatric Patients. *Circ J* 2009.

[3] Guyton AC, Hall JE. Textbook of Medical Physiology. 10th ed; 2000.

[4] Westerhof BE, Guelen I, Stok WJ, Lasance HA, Ascoop CA, Wesseling KH, et al. Individualization of transfer function in estimation of central aortic pressure from the peripheral pulse is not required in patients at rest. *J Appl Physiol* 2008;105(6):1858-63.

[5] Quinones MA, Gaasch WH, Alexander JK. Influence of acute changes in preload, afterload, contractile state and heart rate on ejection and isovolumic indices of myocardial contractility in man. *Circulation* 1976;53(2):293-302.

[6] Furnival CM, Linden RJ, Snow HM. Inotropic changes in the left ventricle: the effect of changes in heart rate, aortic pressure and end-diastolic pressure. *J Physiol* 1970;211(2):359-87.

[7] Little WC. The left ventricular dP/dtmax-end-diastolic volume relation in closed-chest dogs. *Circ Res* 1985;56(6):808-15.

[8] Rhodes J, Udelson JE, Marx GR, Schmid CH, Konstam MA, Hijazi ZM, et al. A new noninvasive method for the estimation of peak dP/dt. *Circulation* 1993;88(6):2693-9.

[9] Senzaki H, Isoda T, Paolocci N, Ekelund U, Hare JM, Kass DA. Improved mechanoenergetics and cardiac rest and reserve function of in vivo failing heart by calcium sensitizer EMD-57033. *Circulation* 2000;101(9):1040-8.

[10] Senzaki H, Paolocci N, Gluzband YA, Lindsey ML, Janicki JS, Crow MT, et al. beta-blockade prevents sustained metalloproteinase activation and diastolic stiffening induced by angiotensin II combined with evolving cardiac dysfunction. *Circ Res* 2000;86(7):807-15.

[11] Bargiggia GS, Bertucci C, Recusani F, Raisaro A, de Servi S, Valdes-Cruz LM, et al. A new method for estimating left ventricular dP/dt by continuous wave Doppler-echocardiography. Validation studies at cardiac catheterization. *Circulation* 1989;80(5):1287-92.

[12] Chen C, Rodriguez L, Guerrero JL, Marshall S, Levine RA, Weyman AE, et al. Noninvasive estimation of the instantaneous first derivative of left ventricular pressure using continuous-wave Doppler echocardiography. *Circulation* 1991;83(6):2101-10.

[13] Chung N, Nishimura RA, Holmes DR, Jr., Tajik AJ. Measurement of left ventricular dp/dt by simultaneous Doppler echocardiography and cardiac catheterization. *J Am Soc Echocardiogr* 1992;5(2):147-52.

[14] Taylor SH, Snow HM, Linden RJ. Relationship between left ventricular and aortic dP-dt (max). *Proc R Soc Med* 1972;65(6):550-2.

[15] Sharman JE, Qasem AM, Hanekom L, Gill DS, Lim R, Marwick TH. Radial pressure waveform dP/dt max is a poor indicator of left ventricular systolic function. *Eur J Clin Invest* 2007;37(4):276-81.

[16] Kawasaki H, Seki M, Saiki H, Masutani S, Senzaki H. Noninvasive assessment of left ventricular contractility in pediatric patients using the maximum rate of pressure rise in peripheral arteries. *Heart Vessels* 2011.

In: Hemodynamics: Monitoring, Theory and Applications
Editor: Hideaki Senzaki
ISBN: 978-1-62257-361-5
© 2013 Nova Science Publishers, Inc.

Chapter 5

Assessment of Arterial Stiffness in Children

Ryo Nakagawa, Akiko Tamai and Hideaki Senzaki
Department of Pediatric Cardiology,
Saitama International Medical Center, Saitama, Japan

Introduction

Arterial stiffness directly influences left ventricular afterload and coronary perfusion, and it also appears to approximately parallel the extent of atherosclerosis in adults. Arterial stiffening may be sufficient on its own to cause endothelial dysfunction. In addition, in recent longitudinal studies of several diseases and conditions, arterial stiffness has been shown to be an independent predictor of cardiovascular morbidity and mortality, including strokes, abdominal aortic aneurysm, peripheral artery disease, heart failure and coronary heart disease. In contrast, arterial stiffness and its effects on overall hemodynamics are not well understood in children. Pulse wave velocity (PWV) is a useful and widely accepted measure of arterial stiffness, and is derived by noninvasive techniques.

In this chapter, methodological and theoretical issues regarding measuring arterial stiffness by PWV will be discussed to begin with, and then pathophysiological changes in atrial stiffness (PWV) will be presented.

1. Basics of PWV

1.) What is PWV?

The heart intermittently ejects blood by pumping it at regular intervals. However, the actual blood flow in the blood vessels is not intermittent but continuous. Because energy stored during the systolic phase in elastic vessels, mainly consisting of the proximal aorta, is released during the diastolic phase, pulsatile flow is converted to steady flow. This can be explained by the Windkessel model (Figure 1).

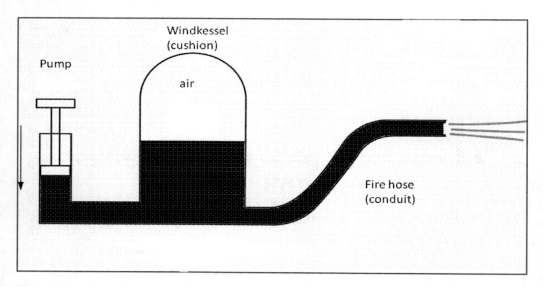

Figure 1.

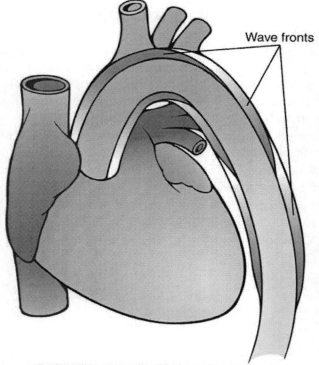

Figure 2.

Even though blood is pumped out from the heart into the blood vessels during the systolic phase, it does not immediately flow to the periphery due to inertia. First, the proximal aorta distends, and the pressure in the center gradually increases. When the pressure reaches a cutoff level, waves of extension spread to the periphery along the aorta (Figure 2), representing transmission of the pulse wave to the peripheral arteries. In other words, the pulse wave itself represents transmission of pressure, but does not indicate advance of blood flow. PWV is a measure of the velocity of the transmission.

In 1878, Moens and Korteweg defined PWV using the following equation:

$PWV^2 = (E \times h)/(2r \times \rho)$
E: Young's modulus
h: arterial wall thickness
r: diameter of the blood vessel
ρ: blood viscosity

The above equation indicates that the PWV decreases as the caliber of the blood vessel increases. This has already been shown by several studies reporting measurement of the PWV in arterial segments.

Moreover, Young's modulus indicates the stiffness inherent to elastic bodies and is associated with resilience against pressure. The modulus is defined by the following equation:

$E = \Delta P/h \times \Delta D$

ΔP and ΔD are the changes in blood pressure and the caliber of the blood vessel, respectively. The greater the stiffness of the vessel wall, the larger the value of Young's modulus and the greater the PWV. The modulus can be considered to indicate the association between PWV and arterial stiffening.

In 1922, Bramwell and Hill derived the following equation:

$$PWV^2 = (\Delta P \times \rho)(V/\Delta V) \qquad [1]$$

ΔP: Ps-Pd
ρ: blood density
V: volume of blood vessel
ΔV: change of V

They applied this equation to clinical practice for the first time. However, due to the high cost of the measuring instruments and cumbersome procedures, only few studies were conducted until Mackay et al. reported, in the 1960's, the use of applanation tonometry (Figure 3) for the measurement. In Japan, an instrument which measures the PWV by using volume pulse waves recorded by an oscillometry-based blood pressure measuring cuff (Form PWV/ABI [ankle-brachial pressure index], Nihon Koden) was developed in 2000. This instrument has made the measurement of PWV short and simple, and also allows simultaneous measurement of the ABI, resulting in an explosive proliferation of studies involving measurement of the PWV.

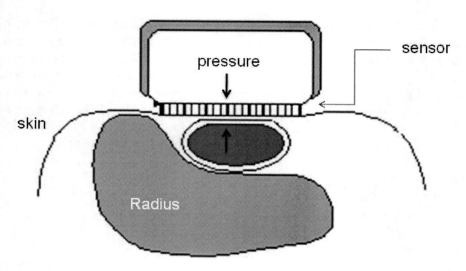

Figure 3.

2.) Types of PWV

Although the arteries have a 3-layer structure, consisting of the intima, media and adventitia, the detailed properties of the blood vessels differ markedly depending on their segments. The central arteries, represented by the aorta, have a media containing abundant elastin and collagen, called elastic vessels. Meanwhile, the medium- and small-sized arteries, such as the brachial and femoral arteries, have a media containing much smooth muscle, and are called muscular arteries. PWV is also measured by various methods in various segments of the arterial tree. Because PWV values differ among different blood vessels, attention should be paid to this point while interpreting the results. At present, mainly heart-ankle PWV (haPWV), carotid-femoral PWV (cfPWV), heart-femoral PWV (hfPWV), and brachial-ankle PWV (baPWV) are used in clinical practice. Figure 4 shows the blood vessels included in the measurement range for each type of PWV. Factors for ideal PWV measurement would include a measurement range including many central arteries, a simple procedure, reproducibility, and abundant epidemiologic data. Mainly in Europe and the United States, cfPWV has been regarded as the so-called gold standard. In fact, large-scale clinical studies on antihypertensive therapy using cfPWV have been conducted, and the usefulness of cfPWV measurement has been demonstrated. [2, 3] However, the problems with cfPWV measurement are that the measurement requires exposure of the groin and some special techniques to record pulse waves. In Japan, baPWV has been previously regarded as the standard, because its measurement is easier and the method used allows simultaneous measurement of the ABI. In regard to the problems related to baPWV measurement, it is of concern that the baPWV might be insufficient for assessment of the central arteries, because the measurement range includes mostly muscular arteries. However, a subsequent comparative study between the cfPWV and baPWV revealed a good correlation between the two (r = 0.76). [4] Although baPWV may not be perfect, it is considered to be sufficiently reliable for the assessment of central arterial stiffness. In contrast, comparison of each type of PWV may be helpful for determining the sites of vessel stiffness.

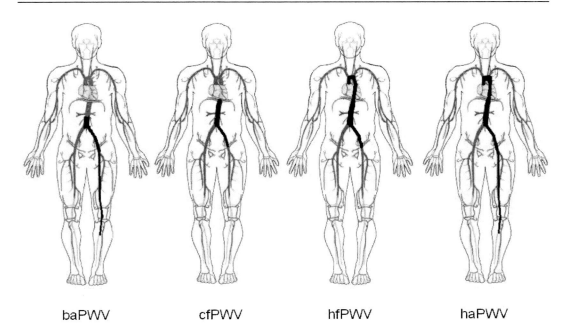

Figure 4.

3.) Factors Influencing PWV

Age and Gender

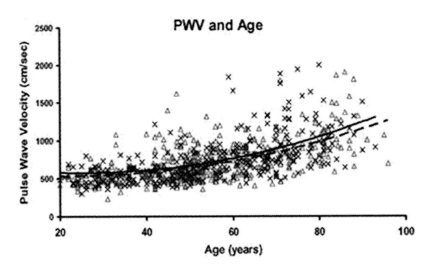

Figure 5.

PWV is known to increase with age (Figure 5), [5-7] which may be mainly attributable to arterial stiffness. As shown by the Moens-Korteweg equation, increase in the arterial stiffness is directly associated with increase of the PWV. In regard to increase of the arterial stiffness due to aging, the intima-media thickness (IMT) increases by approximately twice between ages of 20 and 90 years. [8] Moreover, a significant correlation between IMT and cfPWV was demonstrated in a study of healthy volunteers. [9] In regard to the influence of gender on the PWV, the PWV is significantly lower in women than in men. However, it is known to rapidly increase after menopause, and the gender difference is no longer seen in people aged 60 years or older. [10] In women, the increase of the PWV after menopause may reflect the rapidly developing estrogen deficiency observed after menopause.

Blood Pressure

The influence of blood pressure on the PWV has been reported in several studies, most of which report a significant correlation between the systolic blood pressure and the PWV. In other words, the PWV in the same blood vessel may vary drastically with varying blood pressure levels. This is attributable to the fact that increased blood pressure increases vascular tension, which causes stiffening of the blood vessels. The influence of blood pressure is determined by Laplace's law (tension [T] = internal pressure [P] × radius [R]). Asmar et al., who conducted a study in 418 men and women ranging in age from 18 to 77 years, reported that the cfPWV is proportionally associated with the systolic blood pressure and age in both normotensive and hypertensive groups. [11] Similarly, the study on baPWV in 10,000 Japanese persons conducted by Yamashina et al. showed that systolic blood pressure is an independent factor influencing the baPWV, in addition to the age and gender. [12]

Heart Rate

Lantelme et al. have reported the changes in the blood pressure and PWV associated with changes in the heart rate (HR) in elderly people with an implanted pacemaker. The PWV increased steadily with the HR. The PWV values (mean ± SD) were 13.7 ± 3.1, 13.7 ± 2.6, 14.2 ± 3.6, 14.6 ± 3.7, and 15.1 ± 4.3 m/s for heart rates of 60, 70, 80, 90, and 100 b/min, respectively. [13] A leading hypothesis for this association is that the viscous components of the blood vessel change depending on the HR, resulting in decreased distensibility of the arteries with increasing HR. This hypothesis, however, remains to be confirmed.

4.) Cardio-Ankle Vascular Index

Recently, the cardio-ankle vascular index (CAVI), which was developed as a new arterial stiffness index independent of the blood pressure, has been drawing attention in Japan. [14] The theoretical basis of CAVI is the stiffness parameter β theory, [15] which is defined as follows:

$$\beta = \ln(P_s/P_d)/\{\Delta D/D\} \tag{1}$$

Ps: systolic blood pressure
Pd: diastolic blood pressure
D: diameter of the blood vessel
ΔD: change of D

This means that the stiffness parameter β is a ratio of the logarithm of the systolic/diastolic blood pressure and the relative change of the blood vessel diameter.

Next, this equation is converted in scale according to the following procedure in order to determine the CAVI.

Bramwell-Hill equation

$$PWV^2 = (\Delta P/\rho) \times (V/\Delta V) \tag{2}$$

Then, the relation equation between volume displacement and change of the blood vessel diameter is used.

$$V/\Delta V \cong (D/\Delta D)/2 \tag{3}$$

By substituting equation (3) into equation (2), the following equation is obtained:

$$D/\Delta D = (2\rho/\Delta P) \times PWV^2 \tag{4}$$

By substituting equation (4) into equation (1), the following equation is obtained:

$$CAVI_0 = \{(2\rho/\Delta P) \times \ln(Ps/Pd)PWV^2\}$$
(Figure 6)

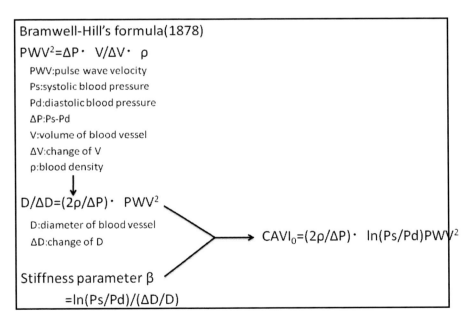

Figure 6.

Currently, the actual CAVI is determined by the following procedure based on the haPWV:

haPWV is determined by dividing the vascular length (L) from the aortic valve to the ankle, as calculated from the body height by the propagation time (T) of pulse wave. This propagation time (T) is determined by adding the time differences between the 2nd heart sound and the initial rise of the brachial arterial pulse wave (tb) and between the initial rise of the brachial arterial pulse wave and that of the pulse wave at the ankle (tba). Thus, haPWV is determined by the following equation: haPWV = L/(tb + tba) = L/T. CAVI is calculated by simultaneously plugging the measured blood pressure into the following equation (Figure 7).

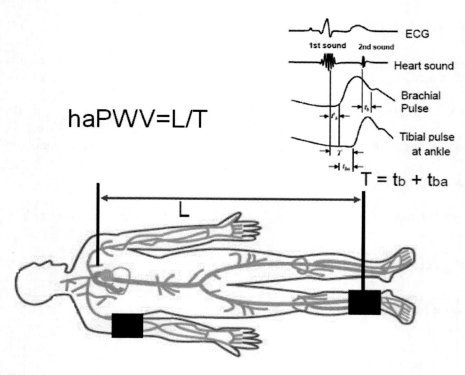

Figure 7.

CAVI = a{($2\rho/\Delta P$) × ln(Ps/Pd)haPWV^2} + b
Ps: systolic blood pressure
Pd: diastolic blood pressure
ΔP: Ps-Pd
PWV: pulse wave velocity,
ρ: blood density
a and b: constants

CAVI is ultimately approximated to the hfPWV by constants a and b, so that it can be compared with conventional PWV.

The CAVI is reportedly little influenced by the blood pressure, and the measurement range is from the orifice of a cardiac valve to the ankle artery. In other words, stiffness parameter β for the central arteries is calculated. In addition, the measurement procedure itself is the same as that of the baPWV and the simplest among those currently used in tests. Of course, the CAVI is influenced by various factors in common with the PWV. The CAVI is also reported to show a weak proportional relationship to the systolic blood pressure (r = 0.423). [16] However, overall, the CAVI may be the most ideal index of arterial stiffening at present, and there have been many clinical reports endorsing this notion. [16-18] Moreover, CAVI has been shown to be useful to assess interaction with the cardiac function. A significant correlation has been reported of the CAVI with the left atrial dimension (r = 0.2, *P* = 0.03) and the ratio of the peak early diastolic velocity to peak atrial diastolic velocity in the left ventricular blood flow patterns (r = −0.47, *P* < 0.001) determined by echocardiography. [19] Studies not only in Japan, but also on a global scale are expected in the future.

5.) Ankle-Brachial Pressure Index

The ankle-brachial pressure index (ABI) is a measure for examining stenosis and occlusion of the arteries from the iliac artery downstream. ABI is briefly mentioned here because it is often simultaneously measured with the baPWV.

Although ABI was originally developed for the diagnosis of arteriosclerosis obliterans, subsequent reports have shown that ABI can be a predictor of onset of various atherosclerotic diseases. While ABI is useful by itself, it is also helpful for interpreting the baPWV values. With occlusion of the blood vessels and decrease in blood pressure in the lower limbs, the baPWV appears to decrease, that is, when the bilateral ABI is less than 0.9, measured values of the baPWV become less reliable.

2. Pathophysiological Changes in Arterial Stiffness Indicated by the PWV and ABI

1.) Neural Factors

Arterial stiffness is controlled by not only the structure of the arterial wall, but also by the vascular smooth muscle tone. Kingwell et al. compared the PWV across the aorta and the artery of the lower limb before and after a 30-minute bicycle exercise in healthy young volunteers. They reported a significant decrease of the PWV at 30 minutes after the end of the exercise, with the values returning to those recorded before the exercise by 60 minutes after the end of the exercise. [20] Sugawara et al., who conducted a study in which healthy young volunteers performed bicycle exercise using only one lower limb for 5 minutes, reported that the PWV decreased in only the exercised limbs. Short-term changes in the PWV are speculated to be attributable to involvement of the vascular sympathetic nerves and vasoactive substances derived from the vascular endothelium. These findings show that the PWV may easily change depending on the measurement conditions. [21]

2.) Renal Function

Many studies have revealed that the PWV in dialysis patients with renal failure is high, irrespective of the arterial segment measured. [22, 23] Moreover, the PWV has been known to be associated with the degree of renal function impairment, even from the early stage of renal dysfunction. The urinary albumin excretion has been reported to be positively correlated with the baPWV in healthy volunteers, and with the aortic PWV (AoPWV) in patients with mild hypertension. [24] Decrease of the glomerular filtration rate has also been reported to be correlated with the AoPWV, [25] and the degree of change of the AoPWV has been shown to be larger in patients with higher serum levels of creatinine. [26] Furthermore, it is of great interest that according to one study, while the PWV in the central arteries (carotid artery and the aorta) was higher in patients with a higher stage of diabetic nephropathy, no significant change was observed in the PWV of the peripheral arteries (upper and lower limb arteries). [27]

3.) Hypertension

The essential objective of antihypertensive therapy is to prevent various target organ diseases associated with hypertension rather than to reduce the blood pressure *per se*. Even blood pressure reduction may not reduce the risk of cerebro- and cardiovascular diseases without amelioration of arteriall stiffening. In fact, a comparative study on the effects of calcium channel antagonists, angiotensin-converting enzyme inhibitors (ACE-Is), and angiotensin receptor blockers (ARBs) on the PWV, plasma aldosterone level, and blood pressure showed that while the hypotensive effects of the 3 drugs were equivalent, only the ACE-Is reduced the PWV and plasma aldosterone levels. [28] In regard to ARBs, it has been reported that their administration in combination with ACE-Is may additively improve the PWV. [29] Furthermore, administration of renin-angiotensin-aldosterone inhibitors at low doses has been reported to improve the PWV while having no effect on the blood pressure. [30]

4.) Children, Coronary Heart Disease, and Kawasaki Disease

Niboshi et al. published a report on the values of the baPWV in 970 healthy Japanese children. While the values were higher in boys than in girls, the influences of age, systolic blood pressure and heart rate on the baPWV were the same in the children as those in adults. [31]

There have been several reports of the PWV values in children with congenital heart diseases. We have reported a significant increase of the AoPWV in children after operation for tetralogy of Fallot. [32, 33] This may be attributable to the concomitant increase in the diameter of the aorta. Moreover, we have reported that arterial stiffness, as measured by the effective arterial elastance, increased in children after repair of coarctation of aorta. [33] Furthermore, an increase of the AoPWV in children after repair of coarctation of the aorta has recently been reported by Kenny et al. [34] They suggested that this increase was associated with a decrease of the baroreceptor reflex sensitivity.

Kawasaki disease, which was first discovered by Dr. Tomisaku Kawasaki in 1967, is a disease characterized by vasculitis involving the medium- and small-sized arteries in the entire body. [35] In particular, coronary arterial lesions may progress from dilational lesions to coronary artery aneurysms and cause ischemic heart disease via inducing stenotic lesions. Thus, Kawasaki disease is clinically very important. It has often been pointed out that a history of Kawasaki disease may be a risk factor for arterial stiffening. [36, 37] We have also reported increases in the wall stiffness of the proximal and distal aorta and of the peripheral pulmonary vascular bed in Kawasaki disease, based on the data on cardiac catheterization performed in children with coronary arterial lesions. [38]

Although children without coronary arterial lesions or with only transient coronary artery dilatation constitute the vast majority of those undergoing cardiac catheterization, the long-term prognosis still remains unknown. Of course, occurrence of qualitative changes in the vascular bed is highly likely in children with Kawasaki disease without coronary arterial lesions or with only transient mild coronary artery dilatation.

Thus, we conducted a comparative study of the baPWV and CAVI in 194 children with Kawasaki disease without coronary arterial lesions or with only transient mild coronary artery dilatation and 199 normal control subjects. The results revealed baPWV values of 915 ± 122 cm/s in the Kawasaki (mucocutaneous lymph-node syndrome [MCLS]) group and of 887 ± 144 cm/s in the normal control group ($P < 0.05$), being significantly higher in the MCLS group. There was no significant difference in the CAVI between the two groups. We consider that a significant difference was observed only in baPWV, the measurement range of which includes medium- and small-sized arteries, as Kawasaki disease is characterized by lesions of the medium- and small-sized arteries.

Conclusion

PWV and CAVI derived from the PWV are indices of vessel stiffness that can be easily determined. They are helpful in the assessment of many pathological conditions. In the future, these indices are expected to be applied to a wide range of clinical populations, from children to adult, to elucidate the pathophysiological mechanism of more disease conditions.

References

[1] M.A. JCB, M.A. AVH. Velocity of transmission of the pulse-wave: And elasticity of arteries. *Lancet*. 1922;1:891-892

[2] Asmar R, Topouchian J, Pannier B, Benetos A, Safar M. Pulse wave velocity as endpoint in large-scale intervention trial. The complior study. Scientific, quality control, coordination and investigation committees of the complior study. *Journal of hypertension*. 2001;19:813-818

[3] Asmar RG, London GM, O'Rourke ME, Safar ME. Improvement in blood pressure, arterial stiffness and wave reflections with a very-low-dose perindopril/indapamide combination in hypertensive patient: A comparison with atenolol. *Hypertension*. 2001;38:922-926

[4] Sugawara J, Hayashi K, Yokoi T, Cortez-Cooper MY, DeVan AE, Anton MA, Tanaka H. Brachial-ankle pulse wave velocity: An index of central arterial stiffness? *Journal of human hypertension*. 2005;19:401-406

[5] Vaitkevicius PV, Fleg JL, Engel JH, O'Connor FC, Wright JG, Lakatta LE, Yin FC, Lakatta EG. Effects of age and aerobic capacity on arterial stiffness in healthy adults. *Circulation*. 1993;88:1456-1462

[6] Tomiyama H, Yamashina A, Arai T, Hirose K, Koji Y, Chikamori T, Hori S, Yamamoto Y, Doba N, Hinohara S. Influences of age and gender on results of noninvasive brachial-ankle pulse wave velocity measurement--a survey of 12517 subjects. *Atherosclerosis*. 2003;166:303-309

[7] Najjar SS, Scuteri A, Lakatta EG. Arterial aging: Is it an immutable cardiovascular risk factor? *Hypertension*. 2005;46:454-462

[8] Nagai Y, Metter EJ, Earley CJ, Kemper MK, Becker LC, Lakatta EG, Fleg JL. Increased carotid artery intimal-medial thickness in asymptomatic older subjects with exercise-induced myocardial ischemia. *Circulation*. 1998;98:1504-1509

[9] Taniwaki H, Kawagishi T, Emoto M, Shoji T, Kanda H, Maekawa K, Nishizawa Y, Morii H. Correlation between the intima-media thickness of the carotid artery and aortic pulse-wave velocity in patients with type 2 diabetes. Vessel wall properties in type 2 diabetes. *Diabetes care*. 1999;22:1851-1857

[10] Tomiyama H, Kushiro T, Okazaki R, Yoshida H, Doba N, Yamashina A. Influences of increased oxidative stress on endothelial function, platelets function, and fibrinolysis in hypertension associated with glucose intolerance. *Hypertension research : official journal of the Japanese Society of Hypertension*. 2003;26:295-300

[11] Asmar R, Benetos A, Topouchian J, Laurent P, Pannier B, Brisac AM, Target R, Levy BI. Assessment of arterial distensibility by automatic pulse wave velocity measurement. Validation and clinical application studies. *Hypertension*. 1995;26:485-490

[12] Yamashina A, Tomiyama H, Arai T, Koji Y, Yambe M, Motobe H, Glunizia Z, Yamamoto Y, Hori S. Nomogram of the relation of brachial-ankle pulse wave velocity with blood pressure. *Hypertension research : official journal of the Japanese Society of Hypertension*. 2003;26:801-806

[13] Lantelme P, Mestre C, Lievre M, Gressard A, Milon H. Heart rate: An important confounder of pulse wave velocity assessment. *Hypertension*. 2002;39:1083-1087

[14] Shirai K, Utino J, Otsuka K, Takata M. A novel blood pressure-independent arterial wall stiffness parameter; cardio-ankle vascular index (cavi). *Journal of atherosclerosis and thrombosis*. 2006;13:101-107

[15] Kawasaki T, Sasayama S, Yagi S, Asakawa T, Hirai T. Non-invasive assessment of the age related changes in stiffness of major branches of the human arteries. *Cardiovascular research*. 1987;21:678-687

[16] Okura T, Watanabe S, Kurata M, Manabe S, Koresawa M, Irita J, Enomoto D, Miyoshi K, Fukuoka T, Higaki J. Relationship between cardio-ankle vascular index (cavi) and carotid atherosclerosis in patients with essential hypertension. *Hypertension research : official journal of the Japanese Society of Hypertension*. 2007;30:335-340

[17] Kubozono T, Miyata M, Ueyama K, Nagaki A, Otsuji Y, Kusano K, Kubozono O, Tei C. Clinical significance and reproducibility of new arterial distensibility index. *Circulation journal : official journal of the Japanese Circulation Society*. 2007;71:89-94

[18] Shirai K, Hiruta N, Song M, Kurosu T, Suzuki J, Tomaru T, Miyashita Y, Saiki A, Takahashi M, Suzuki K, Takata M. Cardio-ankle vascular index (cavi) as a novel indicator of arterial stiffness: Theory, evidence and perspectives. *Journal of atherosclerosis and thrombosis*. 2011;18:924-938

[19] Sakane K, Miyoshi T, Doi M, Hirohata S, Kaji Y, Kamikawa S, Ogawa H, Hatanaka K, Kitawaki T, Kusachi S, Yamamoto K. Association of new arterial stiffness parameter,

the cardio-ankle vascular index, with left ventricular diastolic function. *Journal of atherosclerosis and thrombosis.* 2008;15:261-268

[20] Kingwell BA, Berry KL, Cameron JD, Jennings GL, Dart AM. Arterial compliance increases after moderate-intensity cycling. *The American journal of physiology.* 1997;273:H2186-2191

[21] Sugawara J, Maeda S, Otsuki T, Tanabe T, Ajisaka R, Matsuda M. Effects of nitric oxide synthase inhibitor on decrease in peripheral arterial stiffness with acute low-intensity aerobic exercise. *American journal of physiology. Heart and circulatory physiology.* 2004;287:H2666-2669

[22] Shoji T, Nishizawa Y, Kawagishi T, Kawasaki K, Taniwaki H, Tabata T, Inoue T, Morii H. Intermediate-density lipoprotein as an independent risk factor for aortic atherosclerosis in hemodialysis patients. *Journal of the American Society of Nephrology : JASN.* 1998;9:1277-1284

[23] London G, Guerin A, Pannier B, Marchais S, Benetos A, Safar M. Increased systolic pressure in chronic uremia. Role of arterial wave reflections. *Hypertension.* 1992;20:10-19

[24] Mule G, Cottone S, Vadala A, Volpe V, Mezzatesta G, Mongiovi R, Piazza G, Nardi E, Andronico G, Cerasola G. Relationship between albumin excretion rate and aortic stiffness in untreated essential hypertensive patients. *Journal of internal medicine.* 2004;256:22-29

[25] Mourad JJ, Pannier B, Blacher J, Rudnichi A, Benetos A, London GM, Safar ME. Creatinine clearance, pulse wave velocity, carotid compliance and essential hypertension. *Kidney international.* 2001;59:1834-1841

[26] Benetos A, Adamopoulos C, Bureau JM, Temmar M, Labat C, Bean K, Thomas F, Pannier B, Asmar R, Zureik M, Safar M, Guize L. Determinants of accelerated progression of arterial stiffness in normotensive subjects and in treated hypertensive subjects over a 6-year period. *Circulation.* 2002;105:1202-1207

[27] Kimoto E, Shoji T, Shinohara K, Hatsuda S, Mori K, Fukumoto S, Koyama H, Emoto M, Okuno Y, Nishizawa Y. Regional arterial stiffness in patients with type 2 diabetes and chronic kidney disease. *Journal of the American Society of Nephrology : JASN.* 2006;17:2245-2252

[28] Rajzer M, Klocek M, Kawecka-Jaszcz K. Effect of amlodipine, quinapril, and losartan on pulse wave velocity and plasma collagen markers in patients with mild-to-moderate arterial hypertension. *American journal of hypertension.* 2003;16:439-444

[29] Mahmud A, Feely J. Reduction in arterial stiffness with angiotensin ii antagonist is comparable with and additive to ace inhibition. *American journal of hypertension.* 2002;15:321-325

[30] Ichihara A, Hayashi M, Kaneshiro Y, Takemitsu T, Homma K, Kanno Y, Yoshizawa M, Furukawa T, Takenaka T, Saruta T. Low doses of losartan and trandolapril improve arterial stiffness in hemodialysis patients. *American journal of kidney diseases : the official journal of the National Kidney Foundation.* 2005;45:866-874

[31] Niboshi A, Hamaoka K, Sakata K, Inoue F. Characteristics of brachial-ankle pulse wave velocity in japanese children. *European journal of pediatrics.* 2006;165:625-629

[32] Seki M, Kurishima C, Kawasaki H, Masutani S, Senzaki H. Aortic stiffness and aortic dilation in infants and children with tetralogy of fallot before corrective surgery: Evidence for intrinsically abnormal aortic mechanical property. *European journal of*

cardio-thoracic surgery : official journal of the European Association for Cardio-thoracic Surgery. 2011

[33] Senzaki H, Iwamoto Y, Ishido H, Matsunaga T, Taketazu M, Kobayashi T, Asano H, Katogi T, Kyo S. Arterial haemodynamics in patients after repair of tetralogy of fallot: Influence on left ventricular after load and aortic dilatation. *Heart*. 2008;94:70-74

[34] Kenny D, Polson JW, Martin RP, Caputo M, Wilson DG, Cockcroft JR, Paton JF, Wolf AR. Relationship of aortic pulse wave velocity and baroreceptor reflex sensitivity to blood pressure control in patients with repaired coarctation of the aorta. *American heart journal*. 2011;162:398-404

[35] Kawasaki T. [acute febrile mucocutaneous syndrome with lymphoid involvement with specific desquamation of the fingers and toes in children]. *Arerugi = [Allergy]*. 1967;16:178-222

[36] Dhillon R, Clarkson P, Donald AE, Powe AJ, Nash M, Novelli V, Dillon MJ, Deanfield JE. Endothelial dysfunction late after kawasaki disease. *Circulation*. 1996;94:2103-2106

[37] Niboshi A, Hamaoka K, Sakata K, Yamaguchi N. Endothelial dysfunction in adult patients with a history of kawasaki disease. *European journal of pediatrics*. 2008;167:189-196

[38] Senzaki H, Chen CH, Ishido H, Masutani S, Matsunaga T, Taketazu M, Kobayashi T, Sasaki N, Kyo S, Yokote Y. Arterial hemodynamics in patients after kawasaki disease. *Circulation*. 2005;111:2119-2125

In: Hemodynamics: Monitoring, Theory and Applications
Editor: Hideaki Senzaki

ISBN: 978-1-62257-361-5
© 2013 Nova Science Publishers, Inc.

Chapter 6

Wave Intensity Analysis

Mitsuru Seki[1,2] *and Hideaki Senzaki*[1]
[1] Saitama Medical University, Saitama, Japan
[2] Gunma Children's Medical Center, Gunma, Japan

Introduction

Aortic pressure and aortic flow waveforms result from complex interactions between the dynamics of the left ventricular contraction and the mechanical properties of the arteries. The wave intensity (WI) is a new hemodynamic index that can be defined at any site in the circulatory system and that provides information about the dynamic behavior of the heart, the vascular system, and their interaction. In 1972, Westerhof et al. introduced a linear method based on impedance analysis for separating the measured pressure and velocity into their forward and backward waveforms. [1] Then, in 1988, Parker et al. also introduced a linear method based on the method of characteristics for the separation of pressure and velocity waves. [2] At first, the WI had a dimension of rate of energy flux per unit area, defined as the product of ΔP and ΔU. This original WI depends on the sampling time interval. It is difficult to compare WI measured at different sampling rate. Therefore, Ramsey and Sugawara et al. proposed a new WI as the product of the derivatives of P and U, dP/dt and dU/dt. [3] This definition indicates that WI has meanings of not only the positive and negative waves but the magnitude of the wave since WI is normalized by time.

Waveforms have four distinct types: the forward, backward, compression, and expansion types. [2] Arterial waveforms can be made by forward wave fronts (from the heart to the periphery) and backward wave fronts (from the periphery to the heart). The terms "compression" and "expansion" are used as standard terms in compressible gas dynamics: an increase in pressure compresses a gas, and a fall in pressure causes a gas to expand. At the arterial caliber, if a wave front carries a positive rate of pressure change, it is of compression type and tends to steepen as it travels. Conversely, if the rate of pressure change is negative, then it is of expansion type and broadens as it travels.

Theory

The arterial waveform is considered to be composed of the summation of sequential infinitesimal wave fronts, where a wave front is the temporal change in pressure or velocity over one sampling interval (dP and dU).

The theoretical basis of wave intensity analysis is the solution of the classical one-dimensional equations for the conservation of mass and momentum, and the following equations were derived by Parker and Jones.[4] The net WI, dI, is

$$dI = dPdU, \tag{1}$$

where dP and dU are the pressure and velocity differences over one sampling period, respectively. Briefly, the water hammer equation for the forward (+) and backward (−) waves is

$$dP_\pm = \pm\rho c\, dU_\pm \tag{2}$$

where ρ is the density of the blood and c is the wave speed. Eq. (2) can be used for determining the wave speed only if the waves are all passing by the measurement site in one direction.

The pressure and velocity differences across the measured wave fronts are assumed to be the sums of the differences between the forward and backward wave fronts; $dP = dP_+ + dP_-$ and $dU = dU_+ + dU_-$. This assumption enables us to write the pressure and velocity differences across the forward and backward wave fronts as

$$dP_\pm = 1/2\,(dP \pm \rho c\, dU), \tag{3}$$

$$dU_\pm = 1/2\,(dU \pm dP/\rho c). \tag{4}$$

The intensities of the forward and backward waves can then be written as

$$dI_\pm = \pm 1/4\rho c\,(dP \pm \rho c\, dU)^2. \tag{5}$$

Note that the WI is always positive for forward waves and negative for backward waves.

This original WI defined by Parker and Jones depends on the sampling interval, dt, which makes it difficult to compare data taken at different sampling rates. The rates of change in pressure and velocity at a fixed point in an artery caused by a forward and a backward wave are again related according to the water hammer equation, which is now

$$dP_f/dt = \rho c\, dU_f/dt \text{ for a forward wave, and} \tag{6}$$

$$dP_b/dt = -\rho c\, dU_b/dt \text{ for a backward wave.} \tag{7}$$

Here, dP_f/dt and dU_f/dt are the rates of change in pressure and velocity, respectively, caused by a forward wave, and dP_b/dt and dU_b/dt are those caused by a backward wave. The subscript "f" refers to the forward direction, and the subscript "b," to the backward direction.

The measured rates of change in pressure and velocity, dP/dt and dU/dt, are the sum of the rates of change caused by forward and backward waves:

$$dP/dt = dP_f/dt + dP_b/dt \tag{8}$$

and

$$dU/dt = dU_f/dt + dU_b/dt . \tag{9}$$

Using the above four equations (6)–(9), WI can be written as

$$WI = (dP/dt)(dU/dt)$$

$$= [(dP_f/dt)^2 - (dP_b/dt)^2]/\rho c \tag{10}$$

$$= \rho c[(dU/dt)^2 - (dU/dt)^2] \tag{11}$$

From Eqs. (10) and (11), we can see that if WI > 0, the rates of change caused by the forward wave, dP_f/dt and dU_f/dt, are greater than those caused by the backward wave, dP_b/dt and dU_b/dt. On the other hand, if WI < 0, the rates of change caused by the backward wave are greater than those caused by the forward wave.

WI as a Physical Property

As described above, physical property WI contains some important information about blood circulation. Figure 1 shows simultaneously recorded pressures and flow velocities and the WI calculated using these parameters at the ascending aorta of a normal pediatric subject. WI has the following three phases in the cardiac systolic cycle:

a) a first positive peak in the early ejection period (W1),
b) a flat wave in the midsystolic period, when WI is almost zero or negative, and
c) a second positive peak in the late ejection period (W2).

The first positive peak (W1) coincides with rising pressure and acceleration and is therefore a compression wave composed of compression-type wave fronts. This wave corresponds to the acceleration period of the aortic flow. During midsystole, between the positive peaks of WI, the wave is either zero or negative. This means that blood flows mainly under the influence of inertia during this period. In addition, a negative wave appears just after the first positive peak, and this negative wave is considered to be the reflection wave from the periphery. This area of wave (negative area) is considered to represent the magnitude of reflection wave from the periphery. [5] The second positive peak coincides with falling pressure and deceleration and is therefore an expansion wave composed of expansion-type wave fronts. Although WI is positive during this second wave period, both pressure and flow are decreasing. Therefore, the wave that decreases the aortic pressure and flow, that is, the expansion wave, propagates from the ventricle to the periphery. It is suggested that the heart itself stops the flow of blood from the ventricle to the periphery during late ejection. [2]

It is believed that there are two mechanisms causing the expansion wave during late systole. One is the decay in left ventricle pressure caused by the rapid isovolumic myocardial relaxation. Another is that the ventricle stops pumping out blood to the periphery a short time before the isovolumic relaxation phase begins. After the ventricle stops its ejection, the blood, once set into motion, will remain in motion because of its inertia. Therefore, the rapid decay of the left ventricular pressure occurs even before myocardial relaxation. [6,7]

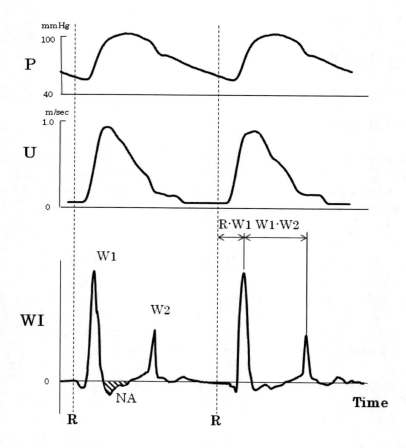

Figure 1. Representative recordings of aortic pressure (*P*), flow velocity (*U*), and wave intensity (WI) in the ascending aorta of a healthy pediatric subject. The area highlighted in mid-systole shows negative area (NA). The vertical dotted lines indicated the average R wave on the electrocardiogram. R-W1 shows the time interval between peak of R wave and W1 (nearly equal to pre-ejection period). W1-W2 shows the time interval between W1 and W2 (nearly equal to ejection time).

In addition, WI is useful for time phase analysis. The time interval between R wave of electrocardiogram and peak of W1 is nearly equal to pre-ejection period. The time interval between W1 and W2 is nearly equal to ejection time.

Hemodynamic Characteristics of WI

The physical meaning of WI is simple. If WI is positive at a particular instant, the effects of the waves travel from the ventricles to the periphery. On the other hand, if WI is negative, the effects of the reflected waves from the periphery dominate. WI is applicable to any part of the circulation and can be derived easily at any site through simultaneous measurements of pressure and velocity. [3] Although its physical meaning is simple, WI also has important physiological meanings, since it changes as changes in the working condition of the heart interact with the arterial system.

Theoretically, W1 and W2 can be described with the following formulas: [3,8]

$$W1 \propto (\max dP/dt)^2/\rho c \qquad (12)$$

$$W2 \propto \rho c (\max dU/dt)^2 \qquad (13)$$

Here, max dP/dt is the maximum rate of left ventricular pressure increase, max dU/dt is the maximum aortic deceleration toward the end of ejection period, ρ is the density of blood, and c is the wave speed. Eq. (12) shows that the height of W1 reflects the change due to ventricle contraction or, in other words, the maximum rate of left ventricular pressure increase during the early systolic phase. On the other hand, the height of W2 is considered to reflect the ventricular relaxation, since W2 increases with increasing maximum aortic deceleration, max dU/dt, as shown in Eq. (13).

Figure 2 shows the change in WI measured in the ascending aorta of an anesthetized dog both under control conditions and after administration of dobutamine, which is primarily a β_1-adrenergic receptor agonist, or propranolol, a nonselective β-adrenergic receptor antagonist. [9] After dobutamine infusion, W1, the peak compression WI during early systole, is greatly increased; however, W2, the peak expansion WI, is unchanged. After propranolol infusion, the height of W1 is markedly decreased, although the height of W2 has no statistically significant change. These changes are predicted by Eqs. (12) and (13).

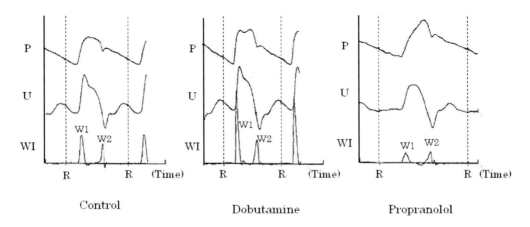

Figure 2. Recordings of pressure (P), velocity (U), and wave intensity (WI) in the ascending aorta of a dog, calculated under control conditions and after administration of dobutamine and propranolol, plotted against time.

Figure 3 shows the change in WI measured in the ascending aorta of an anesthetized dog after administration of nitroglycerin, a vasodilating agent, and methoxamine, an α_1-adrenergic receptor agonist. [9] After nitroglycerin infusion, W1 is consistently reduced, and W2 is also reduced. Although the values are not high, the midsystolic wave intensity becomes positive; that is, the forward waves predominate. Nitroglycerin influenced the travel of forward compression and expansion waves. The most likely explanation for the reduced compression wave (W1) amplitude is reduced venous left ventricular filling, or preload. In addition, nitroglycerin selectively influences expansion wave travel. Forward expansion wave fronts ($dP/dt < 0$) appear relatively early in midsystole and reach a relatively low late systolic peak (W2). Nitroglycerin might be expected to reduce the pulse wave speed c and cause W2 to decrease according to Eq. (13).

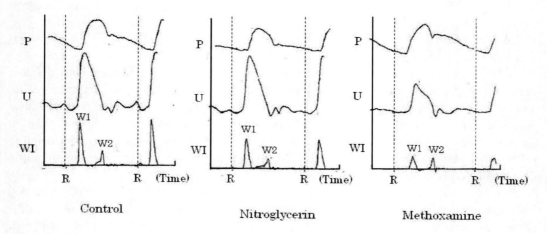

Figure 3. Recordings of pressure (P), velocity (U), and wave intensity (WI) in the ascending aorta of a dog, calculated under control conditions and after administration of nitroglycerin and methoxamine, plotted against time.

After methoxamine infusion, W1 is reduced; however, W2 is unchanged. WI takes relatively large negative values after the descent from W1, and the midsystolic wave intensity remains negative until near the rapid ascent toward W2; that is, the reflecting waves predominate. The aortic pressure was increased considerably by methoxamine, indicating that the external load markedly increased. A direct negative inotropic effect of high-dose methoxamine has also been suggested previously by open-chest studies performed on a dog. [] Therefore, the fall in W1 may be caused by the increase in pressure, which causes an increase in c, and the decrease in max dP/dt.

Relationship between WI and Systolic or Diastolic Performance

Figure 4 shows the relationship between W1 and the maximum rate of left ventricular pressure increase (max dP/dt). [11] The magnitude of W1 is significantly correlated with max dP/dt. Figure 5 shows the relationship between W2 and the time constant of left ventricular relaxation (τ) [11]. The amplitude of W2 is significantly correlated with τ. In addition, the amplitude of W2 is greater in patients with an inertia force of late their systolic aortic flow than in those without an inertia force. Therefore, these findings indicate that W2 reflects the left ventricular diastolic performance during the period from late systole to isovolumic relaxation.

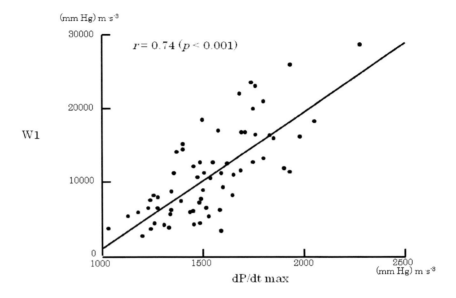

Figure 4. Relation between peak compression wave intensity (W1) and maximum rate of increase in left ventricular pressure (max dP/dt).

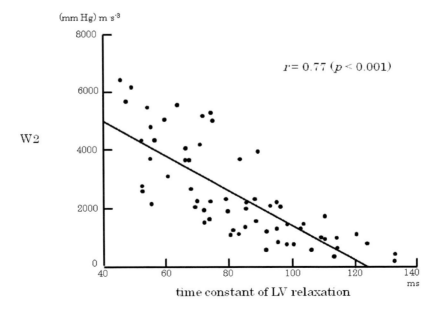

Figure 5. Relation between peak expansion wave intensity (W2) and the time constant of left ventricular relaxation (τ).

However, attention is required to use WI as a systolic and diastolic parameter clinically. As is the case for several other parameters, WI is affected hemodynamic factors: afterload, preload, and the density of the blood. An increase in aortic stiffness causes an increase in the reflection wave from the periphery, which then affects the heights of both the compression and expansion waves. Since WI is affected by max dP/dt, a preload-dependent contractile parameter, and the aortic flow velocity according to Eqs. (12) and (13), the height of WI is affected by changes in the preload. Preload-adjusted WIs are more correlated with cardiac contractile and relaxation indices than nonadjusted WIs. [12]

Conclusion

WI may be a useful tool for defining and investigating the hemodynamics of ventriculoarterial interaction, since WI is sensitive to the ventricular inotropic change and several external loads and is related to diastolic performance.

References

[1] Westerhof, N., Sipkema, P., van den Bos, G.C. & Elzinga, G. Forward and backward waves in the arterial system. *Cardiovasc Res* 6, 648-56 (1972).
[2] Parker, K.H., Jones, C.J., Dawson, J.R. & Gibson, D.G. What stops the flow of blood from the heart? *Heart Vessels* 4, 241-5 (1988).
[3] Ramsey, M.W. & Sugawara, M. Arterial wave intensity and ventriculoarterial interaction. *Heart Vessels* Suppl 12, 128-34 (1997).
[4] Parker, K.H. & Jones, C.J. Forward and backward running waves in the arteries: analysis using the method of characteristics. *J Biomech Eng* 112, 322-6 (1990).
[5] Bleasdale, R.A. et al. Wave intensity analysis from the common carotid artery: a new noninvasive index of cerebral vasomotor tone. *Heart Vessels* 18, 202-6 (2003).
[6] Jones, C.J. & Sugawara, M. "Wavefronts" in the aorta--implications for the mechanisms of left ventricular ejection and aortic valve closure. *Cardiovasc Res* 27, 1902-5 (1993).
[7] Sugawara, M. et al. Aortic blood momentum--the more the better for the ejecting heart in vivo? *Cardiovasc Res* 33, 433-46 (1997).
[8] Niki, K. et al. A noninvasive method of measuring wave intensity, a new hemodynamic index: application to the carotid artery in patients with mitral regurgitation before and after surgery. *Heart Vessels* 14, 263-71 (1999).
[9] Jones, C.J., Sugawara, M., Kondoh, Y., Uchida, K. & Parker, K.H. Compression and expansion wavefront travel in canine ascending aortic flow: wave intensity analysis. *Heart Vessels* 16, 91-8 (2002).
[10] Stanfield, C.A. & Yu, P.N. Hemodynamic effects of methoxamine in mitral valve disease. *Circ Res* 8, 859-64 (1960).
[11] Ohte, N. et al. Clinical usefulness of carotid arterial wave intensity in assessing left ventricular systolic and early diastolic performance. *Heart Vessels* 18, 107-11 (2003).
[12] Nakayama, M. et al. Preload-adjusted 2 wave-intensity peaks reflect simultaneous assessment of left ventricular contractility and relaxation. *Circ J* 69, 683-7 (2005).

Chapter 7

Hemodynamic Assessment by Echocardiographic Tissue Imaging

Hirofumi Saiki and Hideaki Senzaki
Department of Pediatric Cardiology, Saitama Medical University,
Saitama, Japan

Introduction

There is no doubt that echocardiography is one of the most powerful tools in evaluating children's hearts. This modality provides anatomical information, which is essential for surgical repair of congenital heart defects, and also visualizes the ventricular motion that directly represents the cardiac output. The fundamental evaluation obtained by echocardiography provides the "insight" evidence of physical examinations such as auscultation, palpation, and visual examination. The technological advance of Doppler echocardiography enables us to detect small shunt flow or regurgitation of the valve, which provides information to understand the complex hemodynamic status of the patients. For example, the waveform of the mitral regurgitation represents information about the left ventricular (LV) systolic pressure profile, and the aortic velocity time integral represents the function of the stroke volume. The inflow pattern of the atrioventricular valve and pulmonary venous return waveform suggest the status of ventricular relaxation and stiffness [1] (Figure 1).

Recent advances of echo devices enable us to confirm not only blood flow, but also tissue mechanical motion, which contributes profoundly to the understanding of the physiology of the heart. Doppler signals derived from tissues, eg, myocardium or valve, were conventionally considered to be artifacts that make it difficult to detect blood flow signals. However, when we try to evaluate the status of the myocardium, signals from the myocardial tissue will provide us with much valuable information. These Doppler signals derived from myocardial tissue enable us to obtain information relatively independent from the load status, eg, preload, afterload, and heart rate, compared to the conventional assessment. For example, the myocardial acceleration and deceleration during isovolumic constriction and relaxation is considered to exclude the preload influence and represent the characteristics of the myocardium itself, providing much valuable information on hemodynamics.

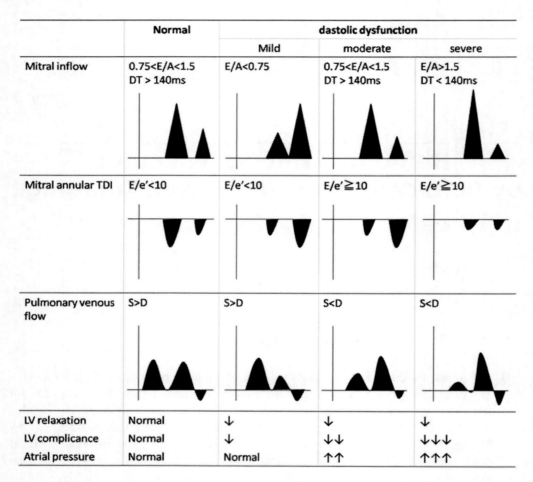

Figure 1. Doppler criteria for classification of diastolic function. Normal to severe diastolic dysfunction is classified by Doppler echocardiography. The mitral annular velocity is useful in differentiating between normal and mild dysfunction and between mild and moderate dysfunction. E: peak early filling velocity, A: velocity at atrial contraction, DT: mitral E wave deceleration time, Adur: A duration, ARdur: AR duration, S: systolic forward flow, D: diastolic forward flow, AR: pulmonary venous atrial reverse flow, e': velocity of mitral annulus early diastolic motion, a': velocity of mitral annulus motion with atrial systole

Furthermore, recent advances also enable us to obtain detailed information about localized myocardial movements. During constriction and relaxation, the local myocardium exhibits a complex movement of shortening, thickening, and rotation, resulting in a twisting movement, which is derived from the characteristic structure consisting of 3 muscular sheet layers, ie, transverse, longitudinal, and oblique layers. In particular, though the rotational movement could be evaluated only with magnetic resonance imaging (MRI) in the past, the development of speckle tracking imaging in echocardiography makes it possible to evaluate such complex movements with the significant advances in spatial and temporal resolution.

These technologies are applied in routine evaluations of patients with heart disease and are expected to elucidate the pathophysiologic mechanisms in congenital heart disease.

In addition, cardiac resynchronization therapy (CRT) improved the outcomes of chronic heart failure in recent years. Simultaneous multisite evaluations of the tissue Doppler imaging (TDI) or speckle tracking method have shown that they are also promising methods to select the pacing site or to decide the indication of CRT because these methods enable us to compare the movements of each part of the myocardium.

The following discussion highlights the basic and clinical applications of tissue imaging, including TDI and speckle tracking, by echocardiography with the latest findings of clinical research.

1. Tissue Doppler Imaging

The Basic Concepts of TDI

The principle of TDI is the same as that of color Doppler imaging and color Doppler velocity measurement, which are calculated by using the autocorrelation method. When the ultrasonic pulse wave is reflected from the range of interest (ROI), it includes blood flow signals as well as tissue signals, eg, from the myocardium and valvular tissue. We can easily detect tissue signals in the velocity spectrum of pulse wave Doppler images without observing blood flow signals only by filtering low echo levels and higher velocity signals, [2] since the echo levels derived from tissues are about 100 times higher than those of the blood stream and since the velocity from the tissue is much lower than that from the blood stream (Figure 2). During sampling, the sending and receiving frequencies need to be reduced because sufficient time is required to observe the slow velocity ranges.

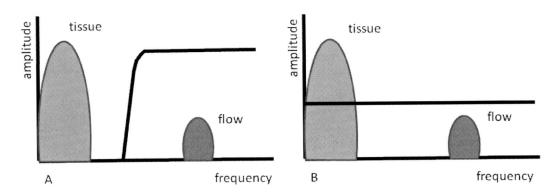

Figure 2. Schema of setting differences between color Doppler and tissue Doppler echocardiography. Signals of low frequency with high amplitude indicate tissue-derived signals, whereas signals of high frequency with low amplitude indicate blood flow signals. The solid line in the graph indicates the filter setting. A: Color flow Doppler. B: Tissue Doppler.

After the first report of pulse TDI by Isaaz, [2] TDI has been applied to color and M-mode TDI, which are visualized with colors representing velocity information. Because both pulse Doppler method and color Doppler method are based on the same Doppler principle, angle dependency (Figure 3) is an important point of weakness, and the measuring point may be outside the ROI due to tissue motion corresponding to the cardiac cycle or respiration, if the echo device does not have a tracking function. In addition, tissue imaging by TDI is affected to a significant extent by surrounding tissues. Because the ROI is usually surrounded by myocardium in every direction, tissue imaging has always the potential to be affected by tethering. Upon data analysis, we have to note which method has been applied in each study, because color TDI represents average velocity within the specific lesions and pulse TDI represents peak velocity. In this session, we will highlight pulse TDI, because this method is suitable and adjustable to the small heart with higher heart rates.

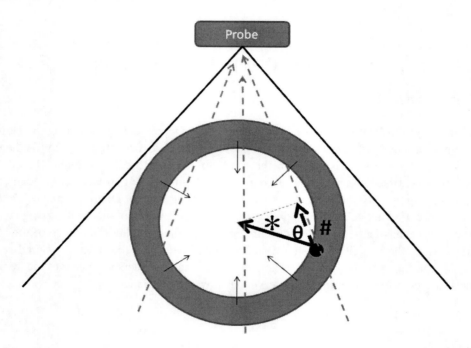

Figure 3. Angle dependency of the assessment based on the Doppler method. The left ventricular short axis view is shown. The solid line indicates tissue velocity directed to the center of the constriction. The velocity signals from the myocardium, which are received by the probe, are only the opposite components directed to the probe (dotted line). If the angle made between solid and dotted lines is relatively small, angle correction would be applied, whereas if the angle is larger than 30 degrees, the reliability of angle correction decreases. Solid line: real tissue velocity of the myocardium in the region of interest (ROI). Dotted line: tissue velocity component directed to the probe.

Cardiac Function and Hemodynamic Assessment by TDI

The myocardial velocity parameters that can be obtained by TDI generally consist of 3 kinds of waves: E' and A' waves in diastole and S wave in systole (Figure 4). For the small heart with high heart rates, it is sometimes difficult to visualize each wave clearly, and each wave is affected by the loading status. In principle, assessment by the waveform of the TDI, which represents velocity of the local myocardium, is useful for a limited range of the heart because of its angle-dependent properties. However, by selecting the ROI appropriately, the status of the heart can be estimated. For example, mitral and tricuspid annular velocities from the apical 4-chamber view represent the myocardial function between each sampling volume on the annulus and the cardiac apex just below the probe, while the velocity in the LV posterior wall in the short axis view only represents local partial velocity. We will describe typical measurements and their characteristics in TDI utilized in daily practice.

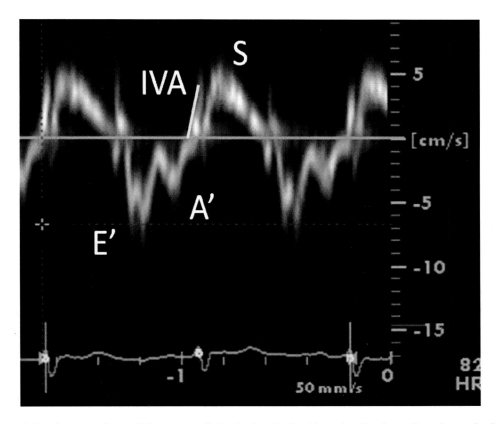

Figure 4. Typical waveform of the myocardial velocity obtained by using the tissue Doppler method. S wave: The systolic positive wave consists of 2 components. The first component is acceleration during isovolumic constriction, of which amplitude and slope (isovolumic ventricular acceleration: IVA) represent the ventricular systolic property relatively independent from loading status. The second component is also representing the ventricular systolic function, which is reported to be associated with the ventricular systolic index, eg, ejection fraction. E' wave: Early diastolic negative wave begins before atrioventricular valve opening, thus representing the relative preload independent of the diastolic property of the ventricle. A' wave: The latter diastolic negative wave appears at the constriction of the atrium. In combination with the E' wave, the diastolic ventricular property is indicated.

1.) Mitral Annular Velocity

The Meaning of Velocity

The mitral annular velocity is easily visualized in the apical 4-chamber view, which is considered to be representative of the myocardial function between sampling volume and apex.

The S wave is seen in systole and representative of the systolic ventricular movement (Figure 4). The early diastolic peak wave, E', and the later diastolic peak wave, A', represent the diastolic properties of the heart. In an adult study, Yip et al. reported that the systolic S wave and diastolic E' wave were reduced in heart failure patients despite preserved ejection fraction. [3] This report emphasized the usefulness of tissue imaging in unmasking heart failure with preserved ejection fraction. A similar observation was also reported by Vinereanu et al. [4] for aortic regurgitation; reduction in the longitudinal mean velocity gradient was sensitive to subclinical LV dysfunction in asymptomatic patients.

The amplitude of E', which represents the diastolic velocity in the longitudinal direction, was also reported to correlate with the time constant of the LV diastolic pressure decline (τ), which is representative of diastolic relaxation. [5] According to this report, an early peak diastolic mitral annular velocity (E') of <8.5 cm/s is useful to differentiate pseudonormalization of the mitral inflow pattern, independent of the preload status. Because the E' wave in TDI arises earlier than the E wave of the mitral inflow, and because the timing when the E' wave arises is close to the timing of ventricular active relaxation, the E' wave is considered to be more independent from the effect of preload and more precise to detect diastolic dysfunction than the E wave. However, we have to keep in mind that E' in TDI is also affected by preload, because E' represents the velocity, and the diastolic τ is not completely independent from the loading status.

The mitral annular velocity in adult patients is equivalent to the annular excursion if the patient's heart rate is assumed to be similar. When the mitral annular velocity is applied to pediatric patients, it is also essential to have information about the normal value of its velocity, which is dependent on age, body size, and heart rate. [6,7] In fact, Robertson [8] reported the importance of normalization in evaluating the cardiac function in children. They found a good correlation between global LV ejection fraction and longitudinal TDI in the mitral annulus velocity S wave standardized by the distance between mitral annulus and LV apex.

On the other hand, Border [9] reported the diastolic function in children with congenital heart disease without standardizing heart size and rate. They compared TDI parameters with invasively obtained pressure data and found that the early peak diastolic mitral annular velocity significantly correlated to the diastolic τ. They recommended to measure mitral annular velocity in the septal annulus because of the relative independence of myocardial rotation and translation. Nonetheless, we always have to consider the effect of heart rate, body size, and age when applying TDI for children, though these effects might be negligible in a specific situation. In our experience, the mitral annular velocity seems to be a good indicator of cardiac function for following up the same patient, but it may not be adequate for comparing the heart function among different patients.

The Velocity-Derived Index of Systolic Myocardial Performance: IVA

As discussed in the former paragraph, tissue velocity is affected by body size and loading status. Recently, acceleration during isovolumic contraction has been proposed as an independent index of load and body size, termed myocardial acceleration during isovolumic contraction (IVA). [10] This parameter is mainly developed in the pediatric ward, and reports for adult cardiac disease are rare. In an animal model, IVA in the mitral annulus correlated well with a load-independent index of contractility (end-systolic elastance [Ees]) [11]. Similarly, IVA in RV free wall immediately below the insertion of the tricuspid valve leaflet had a good correlation with Ees and preload recruitable stroke work, which is also load independent [12]. Furthermore, both of these correlations were also validated during pacing.

The same group [13] also reported the clinical usefulness of IVA in the evaluation of cardiac function in postoperative congenital heart disease. However, in our clinical experience, it is sometimes difficult to delineate the waveform of acceleration, which seems to be dependent on the way of assessment.

The Velocity-Derived Index of Diastolic Myocardial Performance: E/E'

The ratio of early to late peak of mitral inflow velocity by echocardiography conventionally serves as an index of the ventricular diastolic status. The ratio of E wave to A wave of mitral inflow in normal adults is more than 0.75 and less than 1.5, and relaxation abnormalities cause a decrease in E/A to less than 0.75. However, this ratio returns to normal range, which is called pseudonormalization, when the diastolic dysfunction worsens due to the compensatory increase in preload and atrial pressure. [1] Pseudonormalization occurs because the E wave depends on the preload status. As mentioned before, because the preload affects the early peak velocity of the mitral annulus (E') to a lesser extent, E/E' is reported to be able to estimate the preload condition of the ventricle. To be precise, an increase in E/E' is suggestive of an increase in preload. Ommen et al. [14] reported that the ratio of mitral velocity to early diastolic velocity of the mitral annulus (E/E') showed a better correlation with the mean LV diastolic pressure than other Doppler variables. According to their report, an E/E' of <8 is accurately suggestive of a normal mean LV diastolic pressure, and an E/E' of >15 predicts an increased mean LV filling pressure in adult patients. The usefulness of E/E' in estimating LV filling pressure was also reported in healthy volunteers [15] and in post-transplant patients. [16] However, there is also a debate about the accuracy of predicting the LV pressure by using this method. Mullens et al. [17] reported that the E/E' may not be very reliable for predicting increased LV filling pressure in patients with an ejection fraction of less than 30%. They concluded in their report that a large LV volume, severely impaired cardiac output, and presence of CRT might result in discordance between E/E' and LV filling pressure. Therefore, as shown in Figure 1, a multimodality approach would be recommended to evaluate heart failure, especially in patients with severely impaired cardiac function. [1]

We rarely encounter extremely increased end diastolic pressure in the pediatric population because of the high heart rate with relatively short diastolic filling time. Because the wide range of different diastolic functions and different loading statuses can show the same LV filling pressure, it seems to be challenging to predict the LV filling pressure in children [9] by using a single index, eg, E/E'.

2.) Tricuspid Annular Velocity

Anatomically, the tricuspid valve belongs to the right ventricle. Therefore, the annular velocity should reflect the right ventricular (RV) function. So far, catheter-based RV angiography and pressure measurements were the gold standard in evaluating RV function. The development of Doppler echocardiography allows the noninvasive assessment of RV function and enables us to estimate the RV pressure by evaluating the tricuspid regurgitation flow.

By comparing TDI and MRI, Pavlicek et al. [18] reported that a systolic peak of the tricuspid annular velocity (S wave) of <11 cm/s represents a mildly decreased RV ejection fraction of <50%. In addition, a myocardial performance index of >0.50 is suggestive of a decreased ejection fraction of <30% in adults.

Similar observations in children were reported by Kutty et al. [19], ie, the tricuspid peak systolic velocity (S) had a good correlation with the ejection fraction evaluated by MRI, and S > 8.4 cm/s and IVA > 95 cm/s^2 predicted an RV ejection fraction of >45%. Thus, the tricuspid annular velocity could be a surrogate of the RV function in case of normal RV morphology. The evaluation of RV adaptation against increased preload and/or afterload by morphological anomaly is often important to estimate the cardiac reserve function when patients undergo surgical repair for congenital heart defects.

Because the same approach can be applied for the LV assessment in children with congenital heart disease, the tricuspid annular velocity may have meritorious roles in noninvasive assessments of the RV systolic and diastolic function in this population.

3.) Application of TDI to Single Ventricular Circulation

Fontan surgery was developed for patients with single-ventricle circulation. The successful establishment of this circulation is supported by a good pulmonary condition as well as excellent ventricular diastolic properties, which are comprehensively estimated by the end-diastolic pressure (EDP). Menon et al. [20] found that the E/E' of the atrioventricular annulus in a single-ventricle heart is loosely correlated to EDP, and an E/E' of <8 is predictive of an EDP of <12 mmHg.

Although this report is innovative in noninvasively evaluating the diastolic property in single-ventricle circulation, where to sample the annular velocity remains to be solved. Therefore, *additional efforts should be directed towards developing approaches that* provide a more precise prediction of the cardiac function, which is only possible by using invasive methods in cases of single-ventricle circulation.

4.) Analysis of Myocardial Deformations

TDI could be applied to kinematic analyses of the myocardium (Figure 5). In addition to tissue velocity, strain, strain rate, and displacement are used to qualitatively assess myocardial movements and are reported to be highly sensitive to detect an ischemic myocardium. [21-24] Because of the angle dependency, these parameters measured by TDI are inferior to those obtained by speckle tracking imaging but still have an irreplaceable value in deformation analysis. For example, Bansal et al. [25] reported that deformation analysis using TDI was more sensitive in predicting myocardial viability by dobutamine challenge than the analysis using speckle tracking echocardiography.

This is thought to be associated with the high temporal resolution and high reproducibility of TDI. TDI is also suitable for evaluating longitudinal properties. As Jones et al. [26] reported, because longitudinal fibers begin to contract before radial fibers do, the longitudinal function is initially affected by myocardial ischemia and is, therefore, possibly suitable for ischemic monitoring.

The postsystolic strain index [24] measured by TDI was also reported to be sensitive in defining transmurality of chronic myocardial infarction. [27] In addition, Palka et al. [28] reported that the assessment of strain rate could accurately discriminate hypertrophic cardiomyopathy from hypertrophy in athletes.

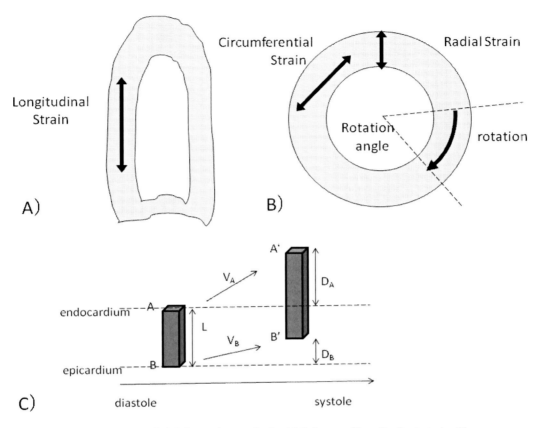

Figure 5. Schema of myocardial deformation analysis. A) Schema of longitudinal strain. The longitudinal strain, which is mostly used by tissue Doppler imaging (TDI), is the ventricular deformity of the basal-apical direction. The disposition of myocardium makes the longitudinal constriction occur earlier than the other directional constrictions and thus, shows high sensitivity to ventricular ischemia and dysfunction. B) Schema of radial and circumferential strain and rotation. The radial strain, which can be assessed by both TDI and speckle tracking, represents the thickening of the ventricular wall. When the myocardium is subjected to ischemia, the thickness of its inner part is reduced during constriction. In addition, employing radial strain enables physicians to describe postsystolic thickening, the index of the ischemic change. The meaning of circumferential strain remains still unclear. However, rotation and circumferential strain are indices representing disposition along the myocardium and are expected to help elucidating the physiology of heart failure. C) Schema of myocardial strain. A: epicardium at diastole, A': epicardium at systole. B: endocardium at diastole, B': endocardium at systole. L: initial length of the myocardium. DA: displacement of point A, DB: displacement of point B. VA: myocardial velocity of point A, VB: myocardial velocity of point B. Strain is defined as the change in length divided by the original length. Strain = $\Delta L/L$ = $(DA - DB)/L$. Strain rate is the first derivative of strain with respect to time, represented by the velocity difference of both sides of the objective myocardium divided by the initial myocardial length. Strain rate = $\Delta strain/\Delta T$ = $(\Delta DA/\Delta T - \Delta DB/\Delta T)/L$ = $(VA - VB)/L$.

As shown above, deformation analysis derived from TDI has significantly contributed to elucidate the pathophysiology of heart diseases, particularly in adult patients. In addition, the high temporal resolution of TDI seems to provide an important advantage in evaluating heart diseases in pediatric patients who have higher heart rates than adults.

Dyssynchrony	Direction		Index	Method	normal	cutoff
Intra-ventricular	longitudinal	Time to peak	Opposing wall delay, 2sites	Color TDI Peak velocity	<50 ms	≧65 ms
			Maximum wall delay, 12sites	Color TDI Peak velocity	<90 ms	≧100 ms
			Yu index	Color TDI 12-segment SD	<30 ms	≧33 ms
		Delayed contraction	Delay in onset of systolic velocity	Pulse TDI	<80 ms	≧100 ms
	radial		Septal to posterior wall delay	M-mode	<50ms	≧130ms
			Septal to posterior wall delay	Radial strain	<40ms	≧130ms
Inter-ventricular			Interventricular mechanical delay	Pulse Doppler	<20 ms	≧40ms
			Left ventricular pre-ejection period	Pulse Doppler		≧140ms

Figure 6 Algorism for evaluating ventricular synchronicity by echocardiography. The principal dyssynchrony indices are shown. Most of the reported methods consisted of tissue Doppler-derived methods in adult patients. For pediatric patients, there are some case reports concerning the indication and effect of cardiac resynchronization therapy (CRT). Further investigation is warranted.

5.) Analysis of Tissue Synchronicity

Pulse TDI has the advantage to be suitable for evaluating the systolic and diastolic synchronicity of myocardial movements. Comparing the myocardial velocity among different parts enables us to assess the systolic and diastolic synchronicity. Many methods for synchronicity assessment [29] have been reported (Figure 6). Although synchronicity analysis by using TDI has the advantage of temporal resolution and little dependency on the angle, the possibility of misunderstanding the synchronicity could not be necessarily avoided in patients with severe heart failure with shuffling motion because of adjacent segmental movements, including tethering, translocation, and rotation. In addition, the accuracy in evaluating concentric motion from the vertical direction is problematic because of the angle dependency, even if the angle effect might be small.

Some modifications in the assessment of ventricular synchronicity (Figure 6) are reported in the clinical settings. Yu et al. [30] had also reported an asynchrony index in patients with CRT, measuring the electromechanical delay in 12 segments of the LV. Bax et al. [31] reported the Ts-4w method to quantify dyssynchrony, which is defined as the delay between the onset of the QRS complex of the surface electrocardiogram and peak systolic velocity of the LV wall derived by TDI. They reported that Ts-4w > 65 ms provides a good distinction between responders and nonresponders to CRT. These methods have been applied to pediatric heart failure in normally structured hearts, for example, as reported by Verma. [32] They reported the possible usefulness of the Ts-4w method derived by TDI in determining the optimal pacing site. Although easy and rapid acquisition is an important advantage of TDI, synchronicity assessment derived from the speckle tracking method is also advantageous in visualizing myocardial (dys)synchronicity.

2. Speckle Tracking Echocardiography

The term "speckle pattern" in echocardiography refers to the granular structure, which looks like maculation, generated by irregular echoreflection. Because this pattern is preserved and moves following the myocardial movement in a relatively short time interval, the ROI containing multiple speckle patterns can be pursued if these speckle patterns were recognized in the former frame. The speckle patterns are tracked frame by frame, and thus, the direction and distance of the speckle movement can be calculated. This technique of echocardiography is called speckle tracking, and the method to calculate varieties of parameters based on speckle pattern displacement by two-dimensional (2D) echocardiography is called 2D speckle tracking.

Application of the 2D Speckle Tracking Method in Pediatric Patients

Most of the parameters obtained by 2D speckle tracking provide information regarding localized myocardial deformities, including myocardial velocity, strain, strain rate, translation, rotation, and rotation angle. Strain and myocardial velocity are also obtained by the pulse TDI method as discussed earlier. While the most important disadvantage of the TDI method is its angle dependency, the speckle tracking method, which is based on the displacement by B-mode echocardiography, is angle independent or at least much less dependent than TDI. [33] Conversely, tracking itself might sometimes be impossible, eg, if the speckle pattern is difficult to be recognized because of poor imaging of the myocardium and/or interference of the lung. In addition, when the frame rate cannot be adjusted to match the velocity of myocardial movement, the speckle patterns of the ROI will be out of the range of the traceable area in the next frame. Therefore, using the speckle tracking method might be very difficult in some patients, especially in small children whose hearts are beating very fast with an extremely small range of movement. Although a frame rate of 50/s to 80/s is in general used for the assessment of the pediatric heart, appropriate instrumental adjustment is needed according to the patient's age, heart size, and heart rate. If tracking seems to be inappropriate, it would be better to perform an evaluation by using the TDI method, which has frame rates of more than 150/s with commercially available devices. A frame rate of >500/s can be achieved with a high tracking device.

Assessment and Clinical Application of the Speckle Tracking Method

The heart with normal structure and function is beating with complex movements, including shortening, thickening, and twisting during contraction. In diastole, a converse movement is observed in each part of the myocardium. These complex movements are originated from the myocardial-specific sheet structure (Figure 7). The speckle tracking method enables precise evaluation of these local myocardial deformities, even in small children. This feature is in sharp contrast to MRI tagging, which is applicable only to adult patients. With the speckle tracking method, we can construct excellent images of the myocardial movement, even in children, with higher temporal and spatial resolution than MRI.

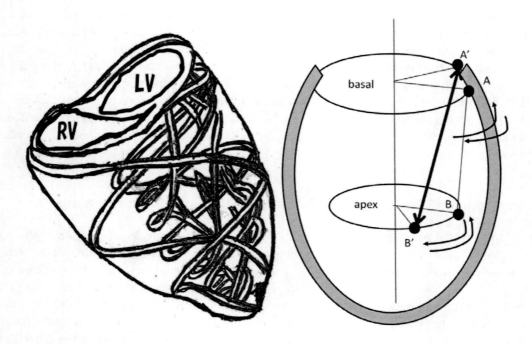

Figure 7. Schema of the myocardial layer structure and basic concepts of myocardial torsion. Left: The picture shows the schema of disposition in the myocardium in both ventricles. The myocardial deformation is mainly distributed to the left ventricle, forming spiral dispositions. Right: The schema shows the torsion and rotation of the left ventricle. As shown in the figure, point A in basal and point B in apex are in correspondence. The left ventricular (LV) apex usually rotates counter clockwise (B→B′), when viewed from the apex, while the basal myocardium rotates clockwise (A→A′). These myocardial displacements along to circumferential direction are called rotation, and its angle is called rotation angle. The angle that is made between the basal part of the myocardium and its corresponding part in the apex (angle between A′ and B′) is called torsion angle.

1.) Assessment of Myocardial Deformity by the Speckle Tracking Strain Method

Myocardial contractions in both ventricles are anisotropic in the normal heart; the LV lateral wall predominantly contracts in the circumferential direction, whereas the free wall of the RV contracts predominantly in the longitudinal direction. In addition, anisotropic contraction is also observed within the same ventricle. Such anisotropic movements between both ventricles and within each ventricle are called myocardial deformity, which changes in accordance with the loading status of the heart.

The parameters of myocardial deformity consist of strain, strain rate, and displacement. Strain is an index of myocardial contractile deformity without dimension, ie, the change in myocardial length divided by the original length of the specific myocardium (Figure 5). The shortening movement, eg, longitudinal contraction, is expressed as change of a minus value, and the thickening movement, eg, radial contraction, as change of a plus value. Strain rate is the first derivative of strain with respect to time, represented by the velocity difference of both sides of the objective myocardium divided by the initial myocardial length (Figures 5,

8). Strain rate is less preload dependent than strain. Displacement is the index of the displaced distance, calculated as the integral of velocity by time. Employing these indices to quantify the local myocardial deformity, we are able to evaluate and classify the contractile and diastolic properties. The accuracy of these myocardial deformity indices derived from the speckle tracking 2D strain method has been validated by using animal models and in adult patients. [34,35] While these parameters of myocardial deformity can be assessed by using TDI, the assessment by TDI is mostly limited to longitudinal strain because of its angle dependency. On the other hand, circumferential and radial strain can be evaluated by using the speckle tracking method.

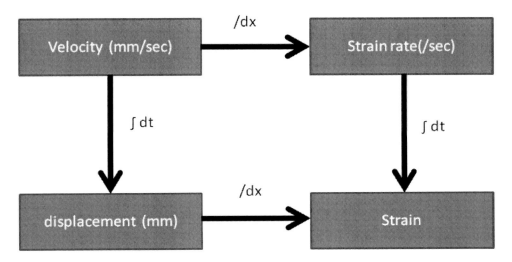

Figure 8. Transformation relationship between each myocardial deformation index. The relationship between each deformity index is shown. Transformation is performed by integration or differentiation with respect to time or distance.

Myocardial Deformity Analysis for Insights of the Physiology

With the progression of heart failure, reductions in radial and circumferential strain become prominent, while the reduction in strain is only limited to the longitudinal strain in the early stage of heart failure. [36] The advent of speckle tracking echocardiography enables us to evaluate the angle-independent radial strain and renowned parameters, eg. circumferential strain and twisting, which have never been assessed by using TDI (Figure 7).

Radial strain, which is a parameter used to visualize systolic wall thickening, is best applied to evaluate ischemic heart disease and to assess myocardial damage. The systolic thickening of the LV is not uniform across all layers. In the normal myocardium, the radial strain of the inner layer is 1.4 to 11 times larger than that of the outer layer, [37, 38] and the peak of the myocardial velocity gradient is in the subendocardial layer, whereas it shifts to the subepicardial layer in the ischemic myocardium. These characteristics of the ischemic heart were demonstrated in experimental and clinical studies. [39, 40]

Circumferential strain is attracting attention in nonresponders of CRT. Knabel et al. reported that there is a remarkable difference in circumferential strain between responders and nonresponders after CRT. [41] The fact that the dyssynchrony of circumferential strain is associated with the frequency of premature ventricular contraction from the RV outflow tract is one of the findings showing the importance of circumferential strain.

Myocardial Deformation Analysis in Pediatric Patients

There are several issues that have to be overcome to successfully apply speckle tracking methods to pediatric patients. In addition to the technical issues already mentioned, controlling their age and body size in the assessment of strain is really challenging because of the nonlinear change in strain. [42, 43] Marcus et al. [42] found a strong second-order polynomial relation between global peak systolic strain and age, with the peak systolic strain observed in the young adult group.

Another important limitation is that the reference values are not necessarily equivalent among different echocardiographs. Koopman et al. reported that in children, longitudinal and circumferential strains are comparable, whereas radial strain is significantly different between iE33 (Phillips) and Vivid7 (General Electric). [44] Therefore, we have to keep in mind which vendor is used. In addition, we should be familiar with the principle and setting of echocardiography.

Despite these limitations, varieties of important findings have been reported in pediatric patients. Cheung et al. [45] found that RV dilatation reduces LV circumferential strain in postoperative tetralogy of Fallot (TOF). Van der Holst et al. also analyzed this LV-RV interaction by comparing RV and LV strain and concluded that the LV dysfunction was affected by RV through adverse ventricular-ventricular interactions. [46]

There are many other trials using local myocardial deformity analysis to clarify the mechanical properties and hemodynamics of single-ventricle circulation. In the analysis concerning systemic RV strain of each surgical stage in patients with hypoplastic left heart syndrome (HLHS), the longitudinal strain in the free wall decreased after Norwood [47] and Glenn [48] procedures. Khoo et al. [49] also reported in the analysis of HLHS after Norwood procedure that RV deformation changed in a LV-like style and that the suspected subclinical ischemic change represented by postsystolic shortening was observed. These are clinically based novel research works that might affect the treatment strategy of these functional single ventricles in the future. On the other hand, there are some reports about limitations of the functional assessment by using the 2D strain method. Singh et al. [50] had questioned the accuracy of 2D strain in evaluating local deformations of single-ventricle circulation because of its specific anatomical feature.

Thus, the assessment of myocardial deformities in pediatric patients, especially in single-ventricle hearts, is often difficult. Nonetheless, the speckle tracking method is expected to serve as a key to elucidate the myocardial properties in congenital heart defects in combination with other imaging modalities. [51] Future instrumental development, in particular, combination with 3D echocardiography, which will possibly enable us to evaluate deformities along the myocardial layer, is strongly expected.

2.) Analysis of Torsion — Twisting and Untwisting

Cardiac torsion is a fundamental motion that originates from the disposition of the myocardial sheet structure. The evaluations of twisting and untwisting were experimentally and based on invasively performed methods using radiopaque markers or sonomicrometry in the myocardium. The properties of cardiac torsion [52-54] are as follows: when viewed from the apex, the apex rotates counter clockwise against the basal myocardium in systole. The twisting angle in the inner and near apex myocardium is larger than that of the outer and basal myocardium. These findings of twisting can also be evaluated by using the speckle tracking method [55] and validated with data from the MRI tissue tagging method.

Changes in twisting and untwisting are age-dependent. Notomi et al. [56] reported the trends of torsion property in detail. Although LV twisting and untwisting rates increase with aging, the underlying mechanisms are different. The increase in LV twisting during childhood is caused by the increase in basal rotation, whereas that in adult is caused by the increase in apical rotation. These differences might indicate the process of the developing heart and adaptation to stiffened arteries due to aging.

Untwisting of the ventricular torsion begins just before the end-systole; 40% of untwisting occurs during the isovolumic relaxation period, before opening of the mitral valve. [53] The velocity of untwisting during isovolumic relaxation, which is called recoil rate, [57] was shown to correlate with the relaxation (τ) by using the MRI tissue tagging method. The same authors also reported that the recoil rate is independent of the left atrial and aortic pressure. In the older age group, the rate of untwisting was significantly prolonged in early diastole, representing a relaxation disorder in the left ventricle. [53] The remaining 60% of untwisting during diastole is believed to cause an intraventricular pressure gradient (IVPG), which causes sucking from the atrium to the ventricle. On the basis of these findings, untwisting could be a renowned index of relaxation.

The Ventricular Torsion in Sick Heart

There are some reports of ventricular torsion in myocardial disease. In patients with LV hypertrophy due to valvular stenosis, [58] torsion is known to be increased compared to that of normal patients. This phenomenon is interpreted as thickened ventricular wall, which causes a distance between the endocardium and epicardium, increases the torque in the outer layer of the myocardium, and results in increased torsion. Interestingly, torsion assessed by MRI in hypertrophic cardiomyopathy [59] is also reported to be increased, despite of myocardial disarray. However, Palka et al. [28] reported a significant difference in the myocardial velocity gradient between hypertrophic cardiomyopathy and ventricular hypertrophy. Similarly, untwisting in both LV hypertrophy [60] and hypertrophic cardiomyopathy [61] were reported to be reduced. Popescu et al. [62] investigated patients with dilated cardiomyopathy (DCM) and found that torsion in DCM is reduced and that the apex rotates adversely.

In patients with ischemic heart disease, the status of torsion and rotation are reported to be different, depending on the region and degree of ischemia. [63,64] According to these reports, LV torsion, which is, in general, mostly affected by apical myocardial motion, is significantly associated with the systolic function.

As indicated in this section, torsion seems to have a significant interaction with cardiac systolic and diastolic function. This renowned index is promising in further elucidating the hidden pathophysiology and mechanisms of heart failure.

3.) Synchronicity Analysis of the Myocardium: Application to CRT

Despite the disadvantage of temporal resolution in the speckle tracking method over TDI, the 2D speckle tracking strain method is often used in adult heart failure patients to evaluate synchronicity [62,65] and to select responders as a part of the trial of CRT. [66,67] Though CRT often drastically improves the decompensating heart, [68,69] it is difficult to differentiate responders and nonresponders to the CRT. Therefore, not all improvements in dyssynchrony can be directly linked to the clinical improvement of the patient's life. [70]

In pediatric patients, Hui et al. [71] studied the feasibility of measuring RV synchronicity and reported that 2D speckle tracking and TDI were suitable to analyze RV synchronicity in 63% and 95% of patients, respectively. However, as mentioned before, because of the advantages of angle independence and reduced adjunctive tissue influence, the speckle tracking method is appropriate in patients with congenital heart disease. Usually, dyskinesis and dyssynchrony occur between the atrium and the ventricle (interventricle and intraventricle). Especially in congenital heart disease with large ventricular septal defect (VSD) or single ventricle, inter- and intraventricular dyssynchrony makes some part of the myocardium act as a damping chamber. In such situation, the total cardiac output will be reduced, thereby inducing heart failure symptoms, even if contraction of the myocardium *per se* is preserved. In order to solve these physiological issues, we can apply CRT. [72,73] Although reports regarding the effects of CRT on treating heart failure are increasing, [74-77] as already shown in adult patients during the Predictors of Response to Cardiac Resynchronization Therapy (PROSPECT) [67] study, identifying responders to CRT [74,78] among pediatric patients is very challenging. However, selecting the pacing site by using speckle tracking methods [72,79-81] and performing synchronicity assessment by using 3D speckle tracking methods [82,83] are increasingly reported. Further accumulation of information about CRT in pediatric patients is warranted to improve the prognosis of children with severe heart failure.

Conclusion

The renowned tissue imaging by echocardiography occupies one of the most important parts of the noninvasive hemodynamic assessment. Knowledge of adequate evaluation based on the latest modality and the ability to command it should be acquired by cardiologists to treat patients, including frail children. Remarkable advances in medical engineering and technology enable us to recognize the detailed properties of the heart and vessels and serve to enhance the therapeutic standards for the benefit of the patient's outcome.

References

[1] Redfield MM, Jacobsen SJ, Burnett JC, Jr., Mahoney DW, Bailey KR, Rodeheffer RJ. Burden of systolic and diastolic ventricular dysfunction in the community: appreciating the scope of the heart failure epidemic. *JAMA* 2003;289:194-202.

[2] Isaaz K, Thompson A, Ethevenot G, Cloez JL, Brembilla B, Pernot C. Doppler echocardiographic measurement of low velocity motion of the left ventricular posterior wall. *Am J Cardiol* 1989;64:66-75.

[3] Yip G, Wang M, Zhang Y, Fung JW, Ho PY, Sanderson JE. Left ventricular long axis function in diastolic heart failure is reduced in both diastole and systole: time for a redefinition? *Heart* 2002;87:121-5.

[4] Vinereanu D, Ionescu AA, Fraser AG. Assessment of left ventricular long axis contraction can detect early myocardial dysfunction in asymptomatic patients with severe aortic regurgitation. *Heart* 2001;85:30-6.

[5] Sohn DW, Chai IH, Lee DJ, Kim HC, Kim HS, Oh BH, Lee MM, Park YB, Choi YS, Seo JD, Lee YW. Assessment of mitral annulus velocity by Doppler tissue imaging in the evaluation of left ventricular diastolic function. *J Am Coll Cardiol* 1997;30:474-80.

[6] Eidem BW, McMahon CJ, Cohen RR, Wu J, Finkelshteyn I, Kovalchin JP, Ayres NA, Bezold LI, O'Brian Smith E, Pignatelli RH. Impact of cardiac growth on Doppler tissue imaging velocities: a study in healthy children. *J Am Soc Echocardiogr* 2004;17:212-21.

[7] Roberson DA, Cui W, Chen Z, Madronero LF, Cuneo BF. Annular and septal Doppler tissue imaging in children: normal z-score tables and effects of age, heart rate, and body surface area. *J Am Soc Echocardiogr* 2007;20:1276-84.

[8] Roberson DA, Cui W. Tissue Doppler imaging measurement of left ventricular systolic function in children: mitral annular displacement index is superior to peak velocity. *J Am Soc Echocardiogr* 2009;22:376-82.

[9] Border WL, Michelfelder EC, Glascock BJ, Witt SA, Spicer RL, Beekman RH, 3rd, Kimball TR. Color M-mode and Doppler tissue evaluation of diastolic function in children: simultaneous correlation with invasive indices. *J Am Soc Echocardiogr* 2003;16:988-94.

[10] Dalsgaard M, Snyder EM, Kjaergaard J, Johnson BD, Hassager C, Oh JK. Isovolumic acceleration measured by tissue Doppler echocardiography is preload independent in healthy subjects. *Echocardiography* 2007;24:572-9.

[11] Vogel M, Cheung MM, Li J, Kristiansen SB, Schmidt MR, White PA, Sorensen K, Redington AN. Noninvasive assessment of left ventricular force-frequency relationships using tissue Doppler-derived isovolumic acceleration: validation in an animal model. *Circulation* 2003;107:1647-52.

[12] Vogel M, Schmidt MR, Kristiansen SB, Cheung M, White PA, Sorensen K, Redington AN. Validation of myocardial acceleration during isovolumic contraction as a novel noninvasive index of right ventricular contractility: comparison with ventricular pressure-volume relations in an animal model. *Circulation* 2002;105:1693-9.

[13] Cheung MM, Smallhorn JF, Vogel M, Van Arsdell G, Redington AN. Disruption of the ventricular myocardial force-frequency relationship after cardiac surgery in children: noninvasive assessment by means of tissue Doppler imaging. *J Thorac Cardiovasc Surg* 2006;131:625-31.

[14] Ommen SR, Nishimura RA, Appleton CP, Miller FA, Oh JK, Redfield MM, Tajik AJ. Clinical utility of Doppler echocardiography and tissue Doppler imaging in the estimation of left ventricular filling pressures: A comparative simultaneous Doppler-catheterization study. *Circulation* 2000;102:1788-94.

[15] Firstenberg MS, Levine BD, Garcia MJ, Greenberg NL, Cardon L, Morehead AJ, Zuckerman J, Thomas JD. Relationship of echocardiographic indices to pulmonary capillary wedge pressures in healthy volunteers. *J Am Coll Cardiol* 2000;36:1664-9.

[16] Sundereswaran L, Nagueh SF, Vardan S, Middleton KJ, Zoghbi WA, Quinones MA, Torre-Amione G. Estimation of left and right ventricular filling pressures after heart transplantation by tissue Doppler imaging. *Am J Cardiol* 1998;82:352-7.

[17] Mullens W, Borowski AG, Curtin RJ, Thomas JD, Tang WH. Tissue Doppler imaging in the estimation of intracardiac filling pressure in decompensated patients with advanced systolic heart failure. *Circulation* 2009;119:62-70.

[18] Pavlicek M, Wahl A, Rutz T, de Marchi SF, Hille R, Wustmann K, Steck H, Eigenmann C, Schwerzmann M, Seiler C. Right ventricular systolic function assessment: rank of echocardiographic methods vs. cardiac magnetic resonance imaging. *Eur J Echocardiogr*;12:871-80.

[19] Kutty S, Zhou J, Gauvreau K, Trincado C, Powell AJ, Geva T. Regional dysfunction of the right ventricular outflow tract reduces the accuracy of Doppler tissue imaging assessment of global right ventricular systolic function in patients with repaired tetralogy of Fallot. *J Am Soc Echocardiogr*;24:637-43.

[20] Menon SC, Gray R, Tani LY. Evaluation of ventricular filling pressures and ventricular function by Doppler echocardiography in patients with functional single ventricle: correlation with simultaneous cardiac catheterization. *J Am Soc Echocardiogr*;24:1220-5.

[21] Edvardsen T, Gerber BL, Garot J, Bluemke DA, Lima JA, Smiseth OA. Quantitative assessment of intrinsic regional myocardial deformation by Doppler strain rate echocardiography in humans: validation against three-dimensional tagged magnetic resonance imaging. *Circulation* 2002;106:50-6.

[22] Kukulski T, Jamal F, Herbots L, D'Hooge J, Bijnens B, Hatle L, De Scheerder I, Sutherland GR. Identification of acutely ischemic myocardium using ultrasonic strain measurements. A clinical study in patients undergoing coronary angioplasty. *J Am Coll Cardiol* 2003;41:810-9.

[23] Skulstad H, Edvardsen T, Urheim S, Rabben SI, Stugaard M, Lyseggen E, Ihlen H, Smiseth OA. Postsystolic shortening in ischemic myocardium: active contraction or passive recoil? *Circulation* 2002;106:718-24.

[24] Weidemann F, Dommke C, Bijnens B, Claus P, D'Hooge J, Mertens P, Verbeken E, Maes A, Van de Werf F, De Scheerder I, Sutherland GR. Defining the transmurality of a chronic myocardial infarction by ultrasonic strain-rate imaging: implications for identifying intramural viability: an experimental study. *Circulation* 2003;107:883-8.

[25] Bansal M, Jeffriess L, Leano R, Mundy J, Marwick TH. Assessment of myocardial viability at dobutamine echocardiography by deformation analysis using tissue velocity and speckle-tracking. *JACC Cardiovasc Imaging*;3:121-31.

[26] Jones CJ, Raposo L, Gibson DG. Functional importance of the long axis dynamics of the human left ventricle. *Br Heart J* 1990;63:215-20.

[27] Hanekom L, Jenkins C, Jeffries L, Case C, Mundy J, Hawley C, Marwick TH. Incremental value of strain rate analysis as an adjunct to wall-motion scoring for assessment of myocardial viability by dobutamine echocardiography: a follow-up study after revascularization. *Circulation* 2005;112:3892-900.

[28] Palka P, Lange A, Fleming AD, Donnelly JE, Dutka DP, Starkey IR, Shaw TR, Sutherland GR, Fox KA. Differences in myocardial velocity gradient measured throughout the cardiac cycle in patients with hypertrophic cardiomyopathy, athletes and

patients with left ventricular hypertrophy due to hypertension. *J Am Coll Cardiol* 1997;30:760-8.

[29] Gorcsan J, 3rd, Abraham T, Agler DA, Bax JJ, Derumeaux G, Grimm RA, Martin R, Steinberg JS, Sutton MS, Yu CM. Echocardiography for cardiac resynchronization therapy: recommendations for performance and reporting--a report from the American Society of Echocardiography Dyssynchrony Writing Group endorsed by the Heart Rhythm Society. *J Am Soc Echocardiogr* 2008;21:191-213.

[30] Yu CM, Fung WH, Lin H, Zhang Q, Sanderson JE, Lau CP. Predictors of left ventricular reverse remodeling after cardiac resynchronization therapy for heart failure secondary to idiopathic dilated or ischemic cardiomyopathy. *Am J Cardiol* 2003;91:684-8.

[31] Bax JJ, Bleeker GB, Marwick TH, Molhoek SG, Boersma E, Steendijk P, van der Wall EE, Schalij MJ. Left ventricular dyssynchrony predicts response and prognosis after cardiac resynchronization therapy. *J Am Coll Cardiol* 2004;44:1834-40.

[32] Verma AJ, Lemler MS, Zeltser IJ, Scott WA. Relation of right ventricular pacing site to left ventricular mechanical synchrony. *Am J Cardiol*;106:806-9.

[33] Mertens LL, Friedberg MK. Imaging the right ventricle--current state of the art. *Nat Rev Cardiol*;7:551-63.

[34] Amundsen BH, Helle-Valle T, Edvardsen T, Torp H, Crosby J, Lyseggen E, Stoylen A, Ihlen H, Lima JA, Smiseth OA, Slordahl SA. Noninvasive myocardial strain measurement by speckle tracking echocardiography: validation against sonomicrometry and tagged magnetic resonance imaging. *J Am Coll Cardiol* 2006;47:789-93.

[35] Korinek J, Wang J, Sengupta PP, Miyazaki C, Kjaergaard J, McMahon E, Abraham TP, Belohlavek M. Two-dimensional strain--a Doppler-independent ultrasound method for quantitation of regional deformation: validation in vitro and in vivo. *J Am Soc Echocardiogr* 2005;18:1247-53.

[36] Greenbaum RA, Ho SY, Gibson DG, Becker AE, Anderson RH. Left ventricular fibre architecture in man. *Br Heart J* 1981;45:248-63.

[37] Cheng A, Nguyen TC, Malinowski M, Daughters GT, Miller DC, Ingels NB, Jr. Heterogeneity of left ventricular wall thickening mechanisms. *Circulation* 2008;118:713-21.

[38] Cheng A, Langer F, Rodriguez F, Criscione JC, Daughters GT, Miller DC, Ingels NB, Jr. Transmural cardiac strains in the lateral wall of the ovine left ventricle. *Am J Physiol Heart Circ Physiol* 2005;288:H1546-56.

[39] Ishizu T, Seo Y, Baba M, Machino T, Higuchi H, Shiotsuka J, Noguchi Y, Aonuma K. Impaired subendocardial wall thickening and post-systolic shortening are signs of critical myocardial ischemia in patients with flow-limiting coronary stenosis. *Circ J*;75:1934-41.

[40] Ishizu T, Seo Y, Enomoto Y, Sugimori H, Yamamoto M, Machino T, Kawamura R, Aonuma K. Experimental validation of left ventricular transmural strain gradient with echocardiographic two-dimensional speckle tracking imaging. *Eur J Echocardiogr*;11:377-85.

[41] Knebel F, Schattke S, Bondke H, Eddicks S, Grohmann A, Baumann G, Borges AC. Circumferential 2D-strain imaging for the prediction of long term response to cardiac resynchronization therapy. *Cardiovasc Ultrasound* 2008;6:28.

[42] Marcus KA, Mavinkurve-Groothuis AM, Barends M, van Dijk A, Feuth T, de Korte C, Kapusta L. Reference values for myocardial two-dimensional strain echocardiography in a healthy pediatric and young adult cohort. *J Am Soc Echocardiogr*;24:625-36.

[43] Lorch SM, Ludomirsky A, Singh GK. Maturational and growth-related changes in left ventricular longitudinal strain and strain rate measured by two-dimensional speckle tracking echocardiography in healthy pediatric population. *J Am Soc Echocardiogr* 2008;21:1207-15.

[44] Koopman LP, Slorach C, Hui W, Manlhiot C, McCrindle BW, Friedberg MK, Jaeggi ET, Mertens L. Comparison between different speckle tracking and color tissue Doppler techniques to measure global and regional myocardial deformation in children. *J Am Soc Echocardiogr*;23:919-28.

[45] Cheung EW, Liang XC, Lam WW, Cheung YF. Impact of right ventricular dilation on left ventricular myocardial deformation in patients after surgical repair of tetralogy of fallot. *Am J Cardiol* 2009;104:1264-70.

[46] van der Hulst AE, Delgado V, Holman ER, Kroft LJ, de Roos A, Hazekamp MG, Blom NA, Bax JJ, Roest AA. Relation of left ventricular twist and global strain with right ventricular dysfunction in patients after operative "correction" of tetralogy of fallot. *Am J Cardiol*;106:723-9.

[47] Petko C, Uebing A, Furck A, Rickers C, Scheewe J, Kramer HH. Changes of right ventricular function and longitudinal deformation in children with hypoplastic left heart syndrome before and after the Norwood operation. *J Am Soc Echocardiogr*;24:1226-32.

[48] Petko C, Hoffmann U, Moller P, Scheewe J, Kramer HH, Uebing A. Assessment of ventricular function and dyssynchrony before and after stage 2 palliation of hypoplastic left heart syndrome using two-dimensional speckle tracking. *Pediatr Cardiol*;31:1037-42.

[49] Khoo NS, Smallhorn JF, Kaneko S, Myers K, Kutty S, Tham EB. Novel insights into RV adaptation and function in hypoplastic left heart syndrome between the first 2 stages of surgical palliation. *JACC Cardiovasc Imaging*;4:128-37.

[50] Singh GK, Cupps B, Pasque M, Woodard PK, Holland MR, Ludomirsky A. Accuracy and reproducibility of strain by speckle tracking in pediatric subjects with normal heart and single ventricular physiology: a two-dimensional speckle-tracking echocardiography and magnetic resonance imaging correlative study. *J Am Soc Echocardiogr*;23:1143-52.

[51] Hayabuchi Y, Sakata M, Ohnishi T, Kagami S. A novel bilayer approach to ventricular septal deformation analysis by speckle tracking imaging in children with right ventricular overload. *J Am Soc Echocardiogr*;24:1205-12.

[52] Buchalter MB, Weiss JL, Rogers WJ, Zerhouni EA, Weisfeldt ML, Beyar R, Shapiro EP. Noninvasive quantification of left ventricular rotational deformation in normal humans using magnetic resonance imaging myocardial tagging. *Circulation* 1990;81:1236-44.

[53] Rademakers FE, Buchalter MB, Rogers WJ, Zerhouni EA, Weisfeldt ML, Weiss JL, Shapiro EP. Dissociation between left ventricular untwisting and filling. Accentuation by catecholamines. *Circulation* 1992;85:1572-81.

[54] Sandstede JJ, Johnson T, Harre K, Beer M, Hofmann S, Pabst T, Kenn W, Voelker W, Neubauer S, Hahn D. Cardiac systolic rotation and contraction before and after valve

replacement for aortic stenosis: a myocardial tagging study using MR imaging. *AJR Am J Roentgenol* 2002;178:953-8.

[55] Notomi Y, Lysyansky P, Setser RM, Shiota T, Popovic ZB, Martin-Miklovic MG, Weaver JA, Oryszak SJ, Greenberg NL, White RD, Thomas JD. Measurement of ventricular torsion by two-dimensional ultrasound speckle tracking imaging. *J Am Coll Cardiol* 2005;45:2034-41.

[56] Notomi Y, Srinath G, Shiota T, Martin-Miklovic MG, Beachler L, Howell K, Oryszak SJ, Deserranno DG, Freed AD, Greenberg NL, Younoszai A, Thomas JD. Maturational and adaptive modulation of left ventricular torsional biomechanics: Doppler tissue imaging observation from infancy to adulthood. *Circulation* 2006;113:2534-41.

[57] Dong SJ, Hees PS, Siu CO, Weiss JL, Shapiro EP. MRI assessment of LV relaxation by untwisting rate: a new isovolumic phase measure of tau. *Am J Physiol Heart Circ Physiol* 2001;281:H2002-9.

[58] Stuber M, Scheidegger MB, Fischer SE, Nagel E, Steinemann F, Hess OM, Boesiger P. Alterations in the local myocardial motion pattern in patients suffering from pressure overload due to aortic stenosis. *Circulation* 1999;100:361-8.

[59] Young AA, Kramer CM, Ferrari VA, Axel L, Reichek N. Three-dimensional left ventricular deformation in hypertrophic cardiomyopathy. *Circulation* 1994;90:854-67.

[60] Takeuchi M, Borden WB, Nakai H, Nishikage T, Kokumai M, Nagakura T, Otani S, Lang RM. Reduced and delayed untwisting of the left ventricle in patients with hypertension and left ventricular hypertrophy: a study using two-dimensional speckle tracking imaging. *Eur Heart J* 2007;28:2756-62.

[61] Maier SE, Fischer SE, McKinnon GC, Hess OM, Krayenbuehl HP, Boesiger P. Evaluation of left ventricular segmental wall motion in hypertrophic cardiomyopathy with myocardial tagging. *Circulation* 1992;86:1919-28.

[62] Popescu BA, Beladan CC, Calin A, Muraru D, Deleanu D, Rosca M, Ginghina C. Left ventricular remodelling and torsional dynamics in dilated cardiomyopathy: reversed apical rotation as a marker of disease severity. *Eur J Heart Fail* 2009;11:945-51.

[63] Nagel E, Stuber M, Lakatos M, Scheidegger MB, Boesiger P, Hess OM. Cardiac rotation and relaxation after anterolateral myocardial infarction. *Coron Artery Dis* 2000;11:261-7.

[64] Takeuchi M, Nishikage T, Nakai H, Kokumai M, Otani S, Lang RM. The assessment of left ventricular twist in anterior wall myocardial infarction using two-dimensional speckle tracking imaging. *J Am Soc Echocardiogr* 2007;20:36-44.

[65] Tanaka H, Tanabe M, Simon MA, Starling RC, Markham D, Thohan V, Mather P, McNamara DM, Gorcsan J, 3rd. Left ventricular mechanical dyssynchrony in acute onset cardiomyopathy: association of its resolution with improvements in ventricular function. *JACC Cardiovasc Imaging*;4:445-56.

[66] Bank AJ, Kaufman CL, Kelly AS, Burns KV, Adler SW, Rector TS, Goldsmith SR, Olivari MT, Tang C, Nelson L, Metzig A. Results of the Prospective Minnesota Study of ECHO/TDI in Cardiac Resynchronization Therapy (PROMISE-CRT) study. *J Card Fail* 2009;15:401-9.

[67] Chung ES, Leon AR, Tavazzi L, Sun JP, Nihoyannopoulos P, Merlino J, Abraham WT, Ghio S, Leclercq C, Bax JJ, Yu CM, Gorcsan J, 3rd, St John Sutton M, De Sutter J, Murillo J. Results of the Predictors of Response to CRT (PROSPECT) trial. *Circulation* 2008;117:2608-16.

[68] St John Sutton MG, Plappert T, Abraham WT, Smith AL, DeLurgio DB, Leon AR, Loh E, Kocovic DZ, Fisher WG, Ellestad M, Messenger J, Kruger K, Hilpisch KE, Hill MR. Effect of cardiac resynchronization therapy on left ventricular size and function in chronic heart failure. *Circulation* 2003;107:1985-90.

[69] Young JB, Abraham WT, Smith AL, Leon AR, Lieberman R, Wilkoff B, Canby RC, Schroeder JS, Liem LB, Hall S, Wheelan K. Combined cardiac resynchronization and implantable cardioversion defibrillation in advanced chronic heart failure: the MIRACLE ICD Trial. *JAMA* 2003;289:2685-94.

[70] Pouleur AC, Knappe D, Shah AM, Uno H, Bourgoun M, Foster E, McNitt S, Hall WJ, Zareba W, Goldenberg I, Moss AJ, Pfeffer MA, Solomon SD. Relationship between improvement in left ventricular dyssynchrony and contractile function and clinical outcome with cardiac resynchronization therapy: the MADIT-CRT trial. *Eur Heart J*;32:1720-9.

[71] Hui W, Slorach C, Bradley TJ, Jaeggi ET, Mertens L, Friedberg MK. Measurement of right ventricular mechanical synchrony in children using tissue Doppler velocity and two-dimensional strain imaging. *J Am Soc Echocardiogr*;23:1289-96.

[72] Gonzalez MB, Schweigel J, Kostelka M, Janousek J. Cardiac resynchronization in a child with dilated cardiomyopathy and borderline QRS duration: speckle tracking guided lead placement. *Pacing Clin Electrophysiol* 2009;32:683-7.

[73] Cazeau S, Ritter P, Bakdach S, Lazarus A, Limousin M, Henao L, Mundler O, Daubert JC, Mugica J. Four chamber pacing in dilated cardiomyopathy. *Pacing Clin Electrophysiol* 1994;17:1974-9.

[74] Dubin AM, Feinstein JA, Reddy VM, Hanley FL, Van Hare GF, Rosenthal DN. Electrical resynchronization: a novel therapy for the failing right ventricle. *Circulation* 2003;107:2287-9.

[75] Janousek J, Gebauer RA, Abdul-Khaliq H, Turner M, Kornyei L, Grollmuss O, Rosenthal E, Villain E, Fruh A, Paul T, Blom NA, Happonen JM, Bauersfeld U, Jacobsen JR, van den Heuvel F, Delhaas T, Papagiannis J, Trigo C. Cardiac resynchronisation therapy in paediatric and congenital heart disease: differential effects in various anatomical and functional substrates. *Heart* 2009;95:1165-71.

[76] Janousek J, Tomek V, Chaloupecky VA, Reich O, Gebauer RA, Kautzner J, Hucin B. Cardiac resynchronization therapy: a novel adjunct to the treatment and prevention of systemic right ventricular failure. *J Am Coll Cardiol* 2004;44:1927-31.

[77] Senzaki H, Kyo S, Matsumoto K, Asano H, Masutani S, Ishido H, Matunaga T, Taketatu M, Kobayashi T, Sasaki N, Yokote Y. Cardiac resynchronization therapy in a patient with single ventricle and intracardiac conduction delay. *J Thorac Cardiovasc Surg* 2004;127:287-8.

[78] Misra N, Webber SA, DeGroff CG. Adult definitions for dyssynchrony are inappropriate for pediatric patients. *Echocardiography*;28:468-74.

[79] Cua CL, Phillips A, Ackley T, Ro PS, Kertesz N. Optimization of biventricular pacing via strain dyssynchrony measurements in a paediatric patient. *Acta Cardiol*;66:527-30.

[80] Madriago E, Sahn DJ, Balaji S. Optimization of myocardial strain imaging and speckle tracking for resynchronization after congenital heart surgery in children. *Europace*;12:1341-3.

[81] Saito K, Ibuki K, Yoshimura N, Hirono K, Watanabe S, Watanabe K, Uese K, Yasukouchi S, Ichida F, Miyawaki T. Successful cardiac resynchronization therapy in a

3-year-old girl with isolated left ventricular non-compaction and narrow QRS complex: a case report. *Circ J* 2009;73:2173-7.

[82] Tanaka H, Hara H, Saba S, Gorcsan J, 3rd. Usefulness of three-dimensional speckle tracking strain to quantify dyssynchrony and the site of latest mechanical activation. *Am J Cardiol*;105:235-42.

[83] Thebault C, Donal E, Bernard A, Moreau O, Schnell F, Mabo P, Leclercq C. Real-time three-dimensional speckle tracking echocardiography: a novel technique to quantify global left ventricular mechanical dyssynchrony. *Eur J Echocardiogr*;12:26-32.

Chapter 8

Atrial Function

Clara Kurishima and Hideaki Senzaki
Department of Pediatric Cardiology, Saitama Medical University,
Saitama, Japan

Introduction

The ventricle, a pump sending blood to the body and the pulmonary circulation, is unquestionably a primary determinant of cardiac function. Many studies have been conducted on ventricular function and its effects on the circulatory system and pathophysiology. The atrium, in contrast, has received rather little attention because its contraction does not markedly affect the circulatory system in the way or to the extent that ventricular contraction does. However, it is clear that normal atrioventricular coordination is essential for maintenance of proper blood circulation. Inefficient circulation during atrial fibrillation or complete atrioventricular block provides a better understanding of the circulatory disadvantages associated with loss of atrial contraction[1]. Conversely, not only ventricular but also atrial functions are reportedly changed in disease states of the heart such as hypertension, heart failure, myocardial infarction and chronic atrial fibrillation, which strongly suggest that both atrial and ventricular functions are involved in the pathological development of the heart[2-4].

This chapter presents atrial functions, assessment methods, and changes in pathological states, and aims to deepen understanding of the atrial role in circulatory dynamics.

1. Atrial Function

Atrial function consists of three general phases: booster pump, reservoir, and conduit (5-9).

1.) Booster Pump Function

The atrium actively contracts in end-diastole, and contributes 15% to 30% of left ventricular stroke volume in the normal heart and more in cases with reduced left ventricular diastolic performance [10, 11].

Pump function is determined by the contractility of the left atrial muscle itself and left atrial volume in early systole of the left atrium (left atrial preload). This function varies depending on the compliance or end-diastolic pressure of the left ventricle, which correspond to afterload for atrial contraction.

2.) Reservoir Function

The atrium actively expands during systole, due to blood flow into the atria from the pulmonary vein after mitral valve closure. This is associated with left ventricular contraction and pulling of the mitral valve ring downward toward the cardiac apex via this contraction and isovolumic relaxation.

Reservoir function varies depending on the contractility of the left ventricle, right ventricular systolic pressure affecting pulmonary circulation, and characteristics of the left atrium (compliance, relaxation etc.). The left atrial appendage has high compliance and plays an important role in reservoir function under loaded conditions via left atrial pressure and volume [12].

3.) Conduit Function

Diastolic left ventricular pressure falls below left atrial pressure during left ventricular relaxation, and pulmonary venous blood then flows passively into the left ventricle after the mitral valve opens. This conduit function varies depending on characteristics of the left ventricular diastolic period (left ventricular relaxation, early diastolic pressure).

4.) Others

Natriuretic peptide (NP) is a hormone produced by cardiac atrial myocytes. Atrial NP (ANP) is produced by atrial muscle.

Brain NP is produced by both atrial and ventricular muscles, and the central nervous system also makes a contribution to its production. NP exerts the following actions: i) increased secretion of water and electrolytes by acting on the kidney, ii) antagonistic action on renin-aldosterone system, iii) anti-vasoconstriction action, iv) movement of water from blood into interstitial spaces via increased *capillary* permeability[13, 14].

Atrial muscle distension induced by volume-overload is the major determinant of ANP release [15, 16]. Hence, the ANP concentration can serve as a marker of atrial overload.

2. Assessment of Atrial Function

The left atrium is located between four pulmonary veins and the left ventricle. The left atrium opens to the left atrial appendage, and the right atrium opens into the superior vena cava, inferior vena cava, and right atrial appendage. The boundary between the two atria is unclear. Due to this un-closed cavity, the shape of the atria cannot be assumed to be spherical as is that of the ventricles. There are certain challenges in assessing left atrial function due to anatomical location and morphological characteristics. Although a universally accepted assessment method has yet to be established, the following methods have been used to date.

1.) Pressure-Volume (Area) Diagram

The left atrial pressure curve is composed of an A-wave and a V-wave (Figure 1). The A-wave is recorded in left ventricular diastole after the P-wave showing atrial depolarization on electrocardiography. The rate of deceleration of the A-wave is an index of left atrial relaxation. On the other hand, the V-wave is formed in response to the left atrial pressure rise after pulmonary venous blood fills the left atrium. The V-wave is amplified during mitral regurgitation or reductions in left atrial compliance.

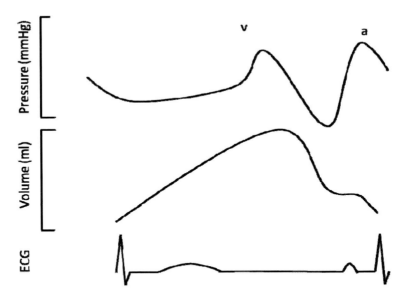

Figure 1. The changes of left atrial pressure and volume.

Measurement of atrial volume only in an anteroposterior direction is not sufficient, because the left atrium when loaded is apparently enlarged in a lateral direction. Thus, it is difficult to estimate left atrial volume by M-mode transthoracic echocardiography. Transesophageal echocardiography allows such estimation, and Toma et al determined the left atrial volume by measuring atrial septal motion with transesophageal M-mode echocardiography[17]. Non-invasive measurement of left atrial volume has been attempted using two- or three-dimensional echocardiography with automated boundary detection, tissue

Doppler echocardiography, computed tomography, magnetic resonance imaging, etc. Combining the left atrial pressure curve and determinations of left atrial volume allows the assessment of left atrial function employing a pressure–volume phase diagram.

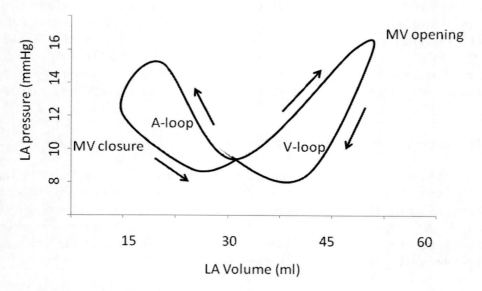

Figure 2. Left atrial pressure-volume relationship.

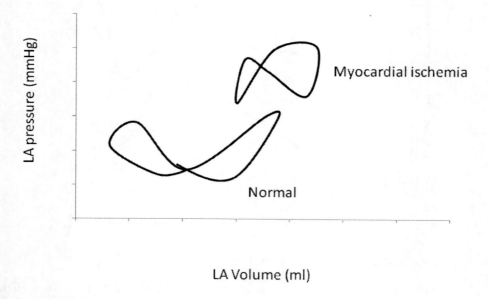

Figure 3. Left atrial pressure-volume diagram in a patient with myocardial ischemia

An atrial pressure-volume (area) diagram consists of an 'A-loop' representing booster pump function in atrial systole and a 'V-loop' representing reservoir function caused by active expansion (Figure 2). The area of the A loop represents atrial stroke work, and the slope of the line between minimal atrial pressure in the A-loop and maximal atrial pressure in the V-loop reflects atrial compliance (i.e., reservoir function). Decreased compliance, such as in myocardial ischemia or severe left ventricular dysfunction, increases the slope of this relation [3] (Figure 3). The atrial conduit function is defined as being between mitral valve opening and left atrial end-diastole, and the volume is calculated as the difference between maximum and end-diastolic volumes[18].

Left atrial end-systole marks the end of atrial contraction, and is often defined by minimal left atrial volume or maximal left atrial elastance. The elastance at end-systole of the left atrium is expressed as the pressure change (mm Hg) per unit of left atrial volume change (mL). End-systolic elastance (Ees) is calculated employing the slope (Figure 4)[4]. Maximal left atrial volume is obtained immediately before opening of the mitral valve and corresponds to the end of the T-wave on electrocardiography. Minimal left atrial volume is obtained at closure of the mitral valve and corresponds to the QSR-wave on the electrocardiography [18]. The Frank-Starling law can also be applied to the left atrium, and left atrial stroke work (corresponding to the area of A-loop, i.e., left atrial end-diastolic volume [EDV] – left atrial end-systolic volume [ESV]) correlates closely with preload of the left atrium [4].

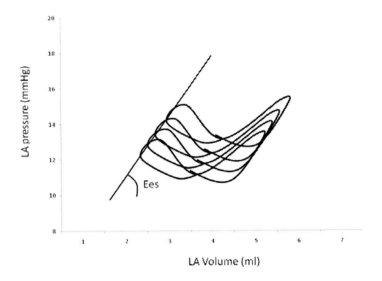

Figure 4. The elastance at end-systole of the left atrium is expressed as the pressure change (mm Hg) per unit of volume change (mL). End-systolic elastance (Ees) is calculated as the slope of end-systolic pressure volume relationship.

Left atrial stroke work is reduced in patients with heart failure, and left atrial compliance is lower in patients with heart failure and those with atrial fibrillation (AF) than in normal subjects. In addition, the increased inotropic state after dobutamine administration results in improved left atrial pump function (stroke work index) as well as increased Ees, reflecting the slope of the linear relation between end-systolic pressure and volume[3]. Reduced left atrial function increases left atrial volume and pressure, shifts the pressure-volume curve to the lower right, and reduces stroke work.

However, a non-invasive method for assessing left atrial volume has not yet been established. Due to this limitation in assessing left atrial volume, Doppler blood flow or tissue Doppler echocardiography is widely used in clinical practice.

2.) Doppler Blood Flow Waveform

The following methods are applicable to assessing left atrial function.

a.) Transmitral Flow (TMF)

The transmitral flow waveform consists of an early-diastolic E-wave and an atrial systolic A-wave. The E-wave is caused by left ventricular early-diastole, and the A-wave by atrial systole (Figure 5). The A-wave and E-wave reflect mainly booster pump and conduit functions, respectively, but it is important to note that these waveforms also result from other factors such as preload, afterload and heart rate (Table1) [19, 20]. In the case of left ventricular dysfunction, the E-wave usually falls, and if left atrial contraction is normal, the A-wave rises in compensation. The A-wave falls when left ventricular end-systolic pressure increases, but shows a similar waveform when left atrial contractile performance is reduced. Hence, these two waveforms must be distinguished from each other.

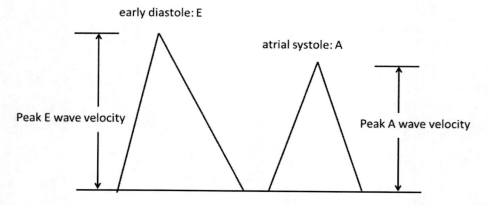

Figure 5. Transmitral pulsed Doppler flow velocity. A = flow velocity curve at atrial contraction, E = early diastolic flow velocity curve.

Table 1. Echocardiographic parameters of left atrial function

Parameters		Function	Normal values
TMF	Peak A	booster pump	0.44 ± 0.12 m/s (middle-aged)
			0.67 ± 0.21 m/s (70-80 years decades)
	Peak E	conduit	0.81 ± 0.2 m/s (middle-aged)
			0.58 ± 0.21 m/s (70-80 years decades)
PVF	PVA	booster pump	0.2 ± 0.14 m/s
	PVS2	reservoir	0.42 ± 0.08 m/s (20-29 years decades)
			0.51 ± 0.08 m/s (70-80 years decades)
	PVD	conduit	0.57 ± 0.1 m/s (20-29 years decades)
			0.35 ± 0.08 m/s (70-80 years decades)

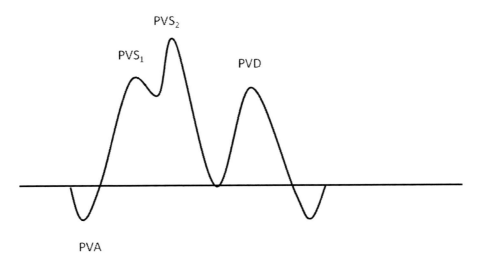

Figure 6. Pulsed Doppler pulmonary venous flow velocity curve. PVA = pulmonary venous reversal flow velocity at atrial contraction, PVS_1 = pulmonary systolic venous flow velocity 1, PVS_2 =pulmonary systolic venous flow velocity 2 and PVD = pulmonary venous diastolic flow velocity.

b.) Pulmonary Venous Flow (PVF)

To assess right atrial function, blood flow waveforms of the cervical or hepatic vein are used. The normal PVF consists of the first systolic wave (PVS1), second systolic wave (PVS2), early diastolic wave (PVD), and reversed flow wave when the left atrium contracts in late diastole (PVA). PVA reflects booster pump function of the left atrium and left ventricular distensibility. This wave is attributable to a portion of the ejected blood being regurgitated from the left atrium into the pulmonary vein due to the lack of a valve between these two organs. The proportion of ejected blood between the pulmonary vein and left ventricle is determined by left ventricular end-diastolic pressure. PVS2 and PVD mainly reflect reservoir and conduit functions, respectively, of the left atrium (Figure 6, Table1) [3].

c.) Left Atrial Appendage Flow (LAAF)

Since contraction of the left atrial appendage and left atrium correspond to the P-wave on electrocardiography, it can be used for assessing left atrial contractile performance. Normal LAAF typically consists of an early diastolic ejection wave (LAA-E), early diastolic inflow wave (LAA-Eb), atrial systolic ejection wave (LAA-A), and atrial systolic inflow wave (LAA-Ab). LAA-A reflects active contraction (booster pump function) and LAA-Ab active dilation (reservoir function), while both LAA-E (left ventricular relaxation) and LAA-Eb (blood inflow) reflect conduit function, of the left atrial appendage[21].

It is noteworthy that these waves do not precisely reflect left atrial functions because they vary according to heart rate, pre- and after-load, left ventricular function, mitral regurgitation, compliance of the left ventricular or pulmonary vein, etc. Tissue Doppler and strain-strain rate methods allow functions of the left atrium itself to be assessed under minimal left ventricle or hemodynamic influences as compared with existing methods, but are not yet in general use.

d.) Atrial Systolic Force

Atrial systolic force can be determined as follows based on Newton's Second Law of Motion (F = ma) as reported by Manning et al: [1, 18, 22]The force generated by contraction of the left atrium is proportional to the product of the mass of blood passing through the mitral valve during early atrial accelerated contraction and blood flow acceleration (formula 1). The mass of blood is the product of blood density (ρ = 1.06 g/cm^3) and the blood volume passing through the mitral valve, and can be obtained by the product of the mitral valve area and the area measured by Doppler Echo from the beginning of the atrial systolic A-wave to the Peak (formula 2). As the blood flow velocity almost linearly increases from the beginning of the A-wave to the Peak, the area can be approximated by half the product of A-wave maximal velocity and the time (ΔT) to attain the maximal velocity (formula 3). The blood flow acceleration is the slope of the line between the A-loop and the V-loop, and can also be approximated linearly, as mentioned above, giving formula 4. Left atrial systolic force (LASF) can be expressed as formula 5 derived from formula 1 after combining formulas 3 and 4. The mitral valve area, which is oval, can be calculated using a nearly circular aortic valve and equation of continuity from time integration and the mitral valve inflow waveform (the volume of blood passing through the aorta is equal to the volume of blood passing through the mitral valve) (formula 6).

LASF = mass of blood × blood flow acceleration （Newton's Second Law of Motion）   formula 1

Mass of blood = ρ × volume of blood passing through the mitral valve （ρ = 1.06 g/cm^3）   formula 2

= ρ × mitral valve area × 0.5 × A-wave maximal velocity × ΔT formula 3

Blood velocity = A-wave velocity/ΔT formula 4

LASF = 0.5 × ρ × mitral valve area × (left ventricular inflow A-wave maximal velocity)^2 formula 5

Aortic ejection waveform area × aortic valve area = mitral valve inflow waveform × mitral valve area   formula 6

The left atrial stroke work expressed as the A-loop in the pressure – volume diagram correlates closely with the motion energy of the left atrium.

3. Factors That Affect Atrial Function

Left atrial contraction increases according to the stiffness of the left ventricle, in association with aging. Although conduit function is reduced as left ventricular diastolic performance decreases with aging, reservoir function is unchanged[2]. With aging, left atrial ejection depends on left atrial active contraction. The pump function of the left atrium as well as that of the left ventricle rises with sympathetic nerve stimulation. Exercise induces sympathetic dominance, thereby increasing pump and reservoir, but not conduit, functions. Increased conduit function due to expansion of the left atrium is observed in athletes[23].

Several drugs are also known to affect atrial functions. Nitroprusside and dobutamine increase cardiac output in patients with congestive heart failure. Nitroprusside reduces left ventricular filling pressure and improves atrial pump function. Dobutamine increases both reservoir and conduit functions. Since vasodilators improve reduced compliance and systolic function of the left atrium, they may be useful for treating patients with chronic heart failure accompanied by limitations of ventricular filling. Volatile anesthetics (desflurane, sevoflurane, isoflurane) reduce left atrial pump function. Reservoir function is maintained at low doses and reduced at high doses of these drugs. However, propofol, an intravenous anesthetic, reduces the pump function of the left atrial muscle itself, while maintaining reservoir function[3, 24, 25].

4. Pathophysiological Conditions Associated with Atrial Dysfunction

Atrial functions play important roles in patients with left ventricular diastolic dysfunction or reduced compliance. In left ventricular relaxation abnormality, conduit function is reduced and reservoir and pump functions are increased [26]. Inflow from the pulmonary vein to the left atrium is limited during the reservoir period, leading to pulmonary edema. Left-ventricular-diastolic-heart failure can occur in conditions with significantly reduced left-ventricular compliance due to cardiac hypertrophy such as in hypertensive heart disease. In clinical conditions with reduced left-ventricular compliance, conduit function is reduced and there are compensatory increases in booster pump and reservoir functions of the left atrium. The enhanced booster pump function is due to increased preload (left atrial enlargement) according to the Frank-Starling Law and sympathetic dominance. However, if left-ventricular compliance is chronically reduced, left atrial hypertrophy occurs and left atrial compliance is reduced, leading to diminished reservoir and pump functions. Since left atrial functions play an important role in left ventricular inflow in such cases, if complicated by reduced left atrial functions or atrial fibrillation, exercise tolerance is markedly worsened by the loss of left-ventricular inflow associated with effective atrial contraction. Therefore, it is very important to understand atrial functions when discussing left ventricular diastolic performance.

In dilated cardiomyopathy, reservoir function is diminished due to reductions in pump function and left atrial compliance [27]. Effects on cardiac output or right ventricular function are balanced by compensatory conduit function. In cardiomyopathy associated with amyloidosis as well, reservoir function is diminished due to reductions in pump function and left atrial compliance, and there is a compensatory increase in conduit function. In hypertrophic heart disease, the stiffness of the left atrium is increased and reservoir function is reduced. Booster pump function is also reduced due to atrial afterload mismatch[28]. In stiff atrial syndrome, reservoir function is limited, and the V-wave rises in the left atrial pressure curve [3, 28]. This syndrome is associated with pulmonary hypertension, pulmonary edema, and heart failure. Atrial fibrillation causes loss of atrial coordination, reduces cardiac output, increases atrial pressure, reduces pump function, and results in loss of the A-loop. It also reduces reservoir function (left atrial compliance is diminished because relaxation does not occur after active contraction) and conduit function. After defibrillation aimed at eliminating atrial fibrillation and ablation therapy for paroxysmal atrial fibrillation, left atrial volume and functions show marked improvements [3].

In mitral valve disease, atrial functions are also changed [2, 28]. Mitral valve stenosis increases atrial afterload due to increased resistance. Because left atrial pump function cannot effectively overcome mechanical stenosis, the left atrium makes little contribution to the left ventricle. Long-term pressure load also reduces the unique pump function itself of the left atrium. Conduit function is also reduced. Reservoir function is reduced due to left atrial pressure being increased while compliance is reduced. Meanwhile, in acute mitral regurgitation, atrial contraction is significantly increased due to atrial enlargement (Frank-Starling law), and pump function is increased. Reservoir function is also increased due to enlargement of the left atrium. Progression of mitral regurgitation decreases the rate of atrial contraction and extension. Vasodilators like nitroprusside improve pump function by reducing left ventricular afterload.

In aortic valve stenosis, pump function is increased due to left atrial enlargement (Frank-Starling law) and reservoir function is decreased due to diminished left ventricular compliance (all three atrial functions are decreased in severe aortic valve stenosis) [28, 29]. Reservoir function is reduced due to diminished compliance (in the early stage, it is increased by compensatory pump function).

In myocardial infarction, if the atria are not affected by ischemia, atrial activity is enhanced, and in general, the ventricle and the atrium work in opposition to each other. Left atrial preload, booster pump function in left atrial descending artery stenosis, and both left atrial stroke work (A-loop area) and reservoir function (V-loop area) are increased. In cases with stenosis of the left common carotid artery, left atrial compliance is increased due to left atrial branching, while conduit function is increased. In heart failure, atrial functions (left atrial stroke work [A-loop area]) are enhanced in compensation in the early stage (reservoir function is increased, conduit function decreased), but stiffness of the left ventricle is increased and then afterload mismatch occurs. With further progression of left ventricular dysfunction, left ventricular compliance decreases, afterload on the left atrial muscle rises due to increased left ventricular diastolic wall stress, left atrial pump function diminishes due to energy depletion (reservoir function is reduced, conduit function predominates). The left atrium changes from a contraction chamber to a mere conduit tube. Reversible left atrial dysfunction is probably due to afterload mismatch rather than intrinsic left atrial disease. Therefore, coronary dilators can improve pump function by reducing afterload [28].

Conclusion

Assessment of atrial function is rather difficult as compared with that of the ventricle, and careful interpretation of results and observations is required. Hopefully, atrial function assessment will lead to early detection of disease states and treatment intervention. Establishment of reliable assessment methods for atrial function is anticipated to deepen understanding of atrial pathophysiology.

References

[1]   Manning WJ, Silverman DI, Katz SE, Douglas PS. Atrial ejection force: a noninvasive assessment of atrial systolic function. *Journal of the American College of Cardiology*. 1993;22(1):221-5. Epub 1993/07/01.

[2] Monica Ros,ca PL, Bogdan A Popescu, Luc A Pie'rard1. Left atrial function: pathophysiology, echocardiographic assessment, and clinical applications. *Heart.* 2011;Dec;97(23):1982-9.

[3] Pagel PS, Kehl F, Gare M, Hettrick DA, Kersten JR, Warltier DC. Mechanical function of the left atrium: new insights based on analysis of pressure-volume relations and Doppler echocardiography. *Anesthesiology.* 2003;98(4):975-94. Epub 2003/03/27.

[4] Stefanadis C. A clinical appraisal of left atrial function. *European Heart Journal.* 2000;0:1-15.

[5] Mitchell JH, Gupta DN, Payne RM. Influence of Atrial Systole on Effective Ventricular Stroke Volume. *Circulation research.* 1965;17:11-8. Epub 1965/07/01.

[6] Henderson Y SM, Chillingworth FP. The volume curve of the ventricles of the mammalian heart, and the significance of this curve in respect to the mechanics of the heart beat and the filling of the ventricles. *The American journal of physiology.* 1906;16:325–67.

[7] Suga H. Importance of atrial compliance in cardiac performance. *Circulation research.* 1974;35(1):39-43. Epub 1974/07/01.

[8] Ishida Y, Meisner JS, Tsujioka K, Gallo JI, Yoran C, Frater RW, et al. Left ventricular filling dynamics: influence of left ventricular relaxation and left atrial pressure. *Circulation.* 1986;74(1):187-96. Epub 1986/07/01.

[9] Grant C BI, Greene DG. The reservoir function of the left atrium during ventricular systole: An angiocardiographic study of atrial stroke volume and work. *The American journal of medicine.* 1964;37:36–43.

[10] Rahimtoola SH, Ehsani A, Sinno MZ, Loeb HS, Rosen KM, Gunnar RM. Left atrial transport function in myocardial infarction. Importance of its booster pump function. *The American journal of medicine.* 1975;59(5):686-94. Epub 1975/11/01.

[11] Appleton CP, Hatle LK, Popp RL. Relation of transmitral flow velocity patterns to left ventricular diastolic function: new insights from a combined hemodynamic and Doppler echocardiographic study. *Journal of the American College of Cardiology.* 1988;12(2):426-40. Epub 1988/08/01.

[12] Ito T, Suwa M, Kobashi A, Yagi H, Hirota Y, Kawamura K. Influence of altered loading conditions on left atrial appendage function in vivo. *The American journal of cardiology.* 1998;81(8):1056-9. Epub 1998/05/12.

[13] Piotrowski G, Goch A, Wlazlowski R, Gawor Z, Goch JH. Non-invasive methods of atrial function evaluation in heart diseases. *Medical science monitor : international medical journal of experimental and clinical research.* 2000;6(4):827-39. Epub 2001/02/24.

[14] Th M. Role of atrial natriuretic factor in volume control. *Kidney international.* 1996;49:1732-7.

[15] Ruskoaho H LH, Magga J. Mechanisms of mechanical load-induced atrial natriuretic peptide secretion: role of endothelin, nitric oxide, and angiotensin II. *J Mol Med.* 1997:876-85.

[16] de Bold AJ BB, Kuroski de Bold ML. Mechanical and neuroendocrine regulation of the endocrine heart. *Cardiovascular research.* 1996;31:7-18.

[17] Toma Y, Matsuda Y, Matsuzaki M, Anno Y, Uchida T, Hiroyama N, et al. Determination of atrial size by esophageal echocardiography. *The American journal of cardiology.* 1983;52(7):878-80. Epub 1983/10/01.

[18] Blume GG, McLeod CJ, Barnes ME, Seward JB, Pellikka PA, Bastiansen PM, et al. Left atrial function: physiology, assessment, and clinical implications. *European journal of echocardiography : the journal of the Working Group on Echocardiography of the European Society of Cardiology.* 2011;12(6):421-30. Epub 2011/05/14.

[19] Yamamoto K, Redfield MM, Nishimura RA. Analysis of left ventricular diastolic function. *Heart.* 1996;75(6 Suppl 2):27-35. Epub 1996/06/01.

[20] Rossvoll O, Hatle LK. Pulmonary venous flow velocities recorded by transthoracic Doppler ultrasound: relation to left ventricular diastolic pressures. *Journal of the American College of Cardiology.* 1993;21(7):1687-96. Epub 1993/06/01.

[21] Tabata T, Oki T, Iuchi A, Yamada H, Manabe K, Fukuda K, et al. Evaluation of left atrial appendage function by measurement of changes in flow velocity patterns after electrical cardioversion in patients with isolated atrial fibrillation. *The American journal of cardiology.* 1997;79(5):615-20. Epub 1997/03/01.

[22] Senzaki H, Kumakura R, Ishido H, Masutani S, Seki M, Yoshiba S. Left atrial systolic force in children: reference values for normal children and changes in cardiovascular disease with left ventricular volume overload or pressure overload. *Journal of the American Society of Echocardiography : official publication of the American Society of Echocardiography.* 2009;22(8):939-46. Epub 2009/06/26.

[23] Erol MK UM, Yilmaz M, Acikel M, Sevimli S, Alp N. Left atrial mechanical functions in elite male athletes. *The American journal of cardiology.* 2001;88:915–7, A9.

[24] Barbier P, Solomon SB, Schiller NB, Glantz SA. Left atrial relaxation and left ventricular systolic function determine left atrial reservoir function. *Circulation.* 1999;100(4):427-36. Epub 1999/07/27.

[25] Gelissen HP, Epema AH, Henning RH, Krijnen HJ, Hennis PJ, den Hertog A. Inotropic effects of propofol, thiopental, midazolam, etomidate, and ketamine on isolated human atrial muscle. *Anesthesiology.* 1996;84(2):397-403. Epub 1996/02/01.

[26] Prioli A, Marino P, Lanzoni L, Zardini P. Increasing degrees of left ventricular filling impairment modulate left atrial function in humans. *The American journal of cardiology.* 1998;82(6):756-61. Epub 1998/10/07.

[27] Paraskevaidis IA DT, Adamopoulos S. Left atrial functional reserve in patients with nonischemic dilated cardiomyopathy: an echocardiographic dobutamine study. *Chest.* 2002;122:1340-7.

[28] Stefanadis C, Dernellis J, Toutouzas P. A clinical appraisal of left atrial function. *Eur Heart J.* 2001;22(1):22-36. Epub 2001/01/03.

[29] O'Connor K MJ, Rosca M. Impact of aortic valve stenosis on left atrial phasic function. *The American journal of cardiology.* 2010;106:1157-62.

[30] Mantero A, Gentile F, Gualtierotti C, Azzollini M, Barbier P, Beretta L, et al. Left ventricular diastolic parameters in 288 normal subjects from 20 to 80 years old. *Eur Heart J.* 1995;16(1):94-105. Epub 1995/01/01.

[31] Gentile F, Mantero A, Lippolis A, Ornaghi M, Azzollini M, Barbier P, et al. Pulmonary venous flow velocity patterns in 143 normal subjects aged 20 to 80 years old. An echo 2D colour Doppler cooperative study. *Eur Heart J.* 1997;18(1):148-64. Epub 1997/01/01.

In: Hemodynamics: Monitoring, Theory and Applications
Editor: Hideaki Senzaki

ISBN: 978-1-62257-361-5
© 2013 Nova Science Publishers, Inc.

Chapter 9

Noninvasive Estimation of Central Venous Pressure by Measuring the Inferior Vena Cava Diameter Using Echography

Yoichi Iwamoto and Hideaki Senzaki[*]
Department of Pediatric Cardiology, Saitama Medical University,
Saitama, Japan

Keywords: central venous pressure, echocardiography, hemodynamics, inferior vena cava, respiration

Introduction

Assessment of the cardiac preload condition is a prerequisite for a better understanding and management of cardiovascular diseases. [1-5] Central venous pressure (CVP) is a simple yet useful index that denotes preload states in association with ventricular function and has been extensively used in a variety of clinical and experimental conditions. However, to measure the CVP, placement of a central venous catheter is required, thus limiting its use in routine clinical practice, especially in patients, due to the invasiveness of catheter insertion and the associated risk of complications. [6] Therefore, the development of noninvasive methods for estimating CVP would be of great clinical benefit.

The diameter of the inferior vena cava (IVCD) and its respirophasic variation (IVC collapsibility index: IVCCI) can be measured noninvasively by ultrasound, which reflect IVC volume and pressure status.

---

[*] Address for correspondence:Prof. Hideaki Senzaki, MD, FJCC, FACC, FAHA, Department of Pediatric Cardiology, Saitama Medical Center, Saitama Medical University, E-mail: hsenzaki@saitama-med.ac.jp.

The first article that mentioned ultrasonographic evaluation of the IVCD, its respiratory variation, and CVP was published in 1979. [7] Natori et al. have already demonstrated that the IVC lumen decreased in the early inspiratory phase, reached a minimum at the end of inspiration, and distended again during expiration in adult patients by using echography in the 1970s. [7]

They noticed that there was a significant correlation between CVP and IVCD or IVCCI. Since their article was published, many authors have tried to confirm their findings and disclose new facts concerning the relationship between CVP and IVCD or IVCCI. Therefore, the correlation between CVP and IVCD or IVCCI is well known.

Methods of Measurement of IVCD and IVCCI with Ultrasound

Almost all echography studies were performed with the patients in the supine position. [7-23] Measurements of IVCD were performed within 2.0 cm of the IVC-right atrial (RA) junction in almost all studies (Figure 1). In almost all studies, IVC imaging was obtained in subcostal sagittal view using echography; however, Chen et al. used a transverse view to measure the IVCD. [8] Though there is a discussion with regard to which is the correct view, ie, long axis view or short axis view, to obtain accurate data, Tamaki noted that the IVC moved caudally during inspiration and cranially during expiration, causing a shift of measurement points and, consequently, measurement errors. [9] Therefore, we recommend the subcostal sagittal view for imaging to acquire IVCD data. Natori et al. and Tamaki defined IVCCI as follows: $(IVCD_{in\ expiration} - IVCD_{in\ inspiration})/IVCD_{in\ expiration}$. [7,9] The authors of other studies defined IVVCI as: $(IVCD_{max} - IVCD_{min})/IVCD_{max}$. The latter definition is regarded to represent the same as the former one.

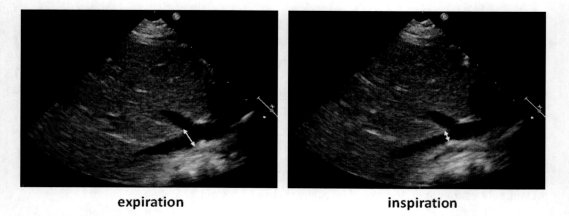

expiration   inspiration

Figure 1. Measurement of (Left) maximum and (Right) minimum diameters of the inferior vena cava (arrows) on echoghraphy (subcostal saggital view).

Usefulness of IVCCI Using Echography in Adult Patients

Tamaki et al. found that the correlation between CVP (mmHg) and IVCCI can be demonstrated by the following equation: $Y = 1.043 - 0.067X + 0.001X^2$ (Y = IVCCI, X = CVP) (Figure 2). [9] Capomolla et al. defined IVCCI as: $(IVCD_{max} - IVCD_{min})/IVCD_{max}$. They found that the right atrial pressure (RAP) can be calculated as $RAP = (6.4 \times IVCD_{min} + 0.04 \times IVCCI - 2)$ in all patients or as $RAP = (4.9 \times IVCD_{min} + 0.01 \times IVCCI - 0.2)$ in patients without tricuspid regurgitation. [10] However, these equations may vary. In general, a normal CVP is defined as ≤10 mmHg. Therefore, some authors used 10 mmHg as cutoff value of CVP in their studies. When using the previous 2 equations, Capomolla et al. found 81% or 93% agreement between invasive measurements of RAP in identifying patients with normal (≤5 mmHg), moderately increased (>5 mmHg and <10 mmHg), and markedly increased (≥10 mmHg) RAPrespectively. [10] Brennan et al. found that the IVCCI cutoff value was 0.4 with optimum predictive use for RAP ≥ 10 mmHg (sensitivity, 73% and specificity, 84%). [11] Kircher et al. found that 41 of 48 patients with an IVCCI of ≥0.5 had a RAP of <10 mmHg, and that 30 of 35 patients with an IVCCI of ≥0.5 had a RAP of <10 mmHg. [12]

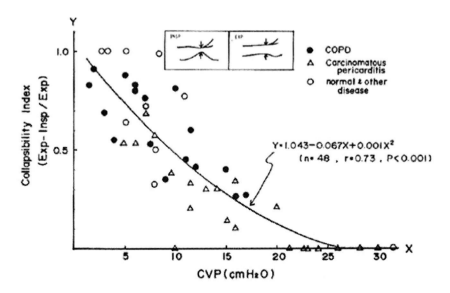

Figure 2. Relationship between collaspsibility index and CVP (Tamaki S, et al. Nihon Kyobu Shikkan Gakkai zasshi 1981;19:460-469).

Usefulness of IVCCI Using Echography in Pediatric Patients

There are only a few papers concerning the usefulness of noninvasive assessment of volume load or CVP by echography. [8, 13-15] Hruda et al. mentioned that only in spontaneously breathing neonates, a significant negative correlation between CVP and IVCCI was found (r = -0.631, P = 0.012). [14] We found that $IVCD_{max}$, $IVCD_{min}$, and IVCCI correlated significantly with CVP in spontaneously breathing children (R^2 = 0.26-0.47, $P <$ 0.05) (Figure 3). In addition, IVCCI under spontaneous breathing had the best area under the curve, with a sensitivity of 1.0 and a specificity of 0.98, for a cutoff value of 0.22 to predict elevated CVP (≥10 mmHg) in this analysis of receiver operator characteristic curve in pediatric patients with congenital heart disease. [15] Therefore, the usefulness of echographic measurement of IVCCI or IVCD to estimate CVP in pediatric patients has been proven.

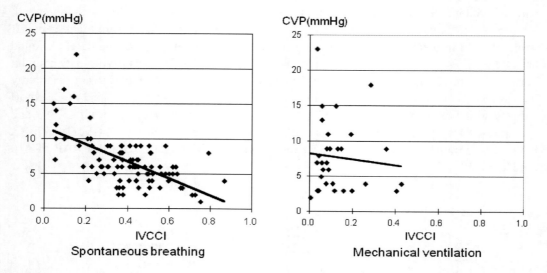

Figure 3. Relationship between IVCCI and CVP in pediatric patients with congenital heart disease.

Influence of Mechanical Ventilation on Measurement of IVCCI

The typical imaging of IVC in a patient with normal CVP under mechanical ventilation is displayed in Figure 4. Even during inspiratory phase, IVCD remains large. Therefore IVCCI is low despite the normal CVP. Because inspiration under mechanical ventilation results in an increase rather than a decrease in intra-thoracic pressure, and because basal IVCD is already increased by the positive intrathoracic pressure with mechanical ventilation, the respirophasic variation of IVCD should be minimized. [15] Actually the poor correlations between CVP (RAP) and IVCD or IVCCI of patients under mechanical ventilation were reported. Jue et al. found that the correlation between IVCD at expiration and mean RAP was only 0.58 and that the correlation between inspiratory change in IVCD and mean RAP was poor (r = 0.13) in patients receiving mechanical ventilation. [16] Hruda et al. found that the correlation between IVCCI and CVP was poor in neonates receiving conventional ventilation (r = -0.013, P = 0.963). [14] We also found that the correlation between IVCCI or IVCD and CVP was poor in pediatric patients with congenital heart disease under mechanical ventilation (R^2 = 0.02-0.08) (Figure 3). [15]

Despite these poor correlations, Jue et al. found that an IVCD of ≤12 mm predicted a RAP of ≤10 mmHg in 100% of cases (however, the sensitivity was only 25%). [16] Bendjeld et al. found that the IVCD at end-expiration and end-diastole with electrocardiogram (ECG) synchronization using the M-mode correlated linearly with the RAP (r = 0.81, $P < 0.0001$). [17] Thus, the possibility that IVCD with ECG synchronization is useful to estimate CVP cannot be denied.

Mechanical Ventilation

INSPIRATION   EXPIRATION

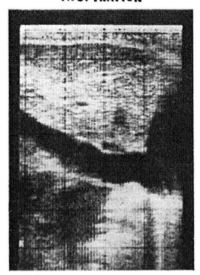 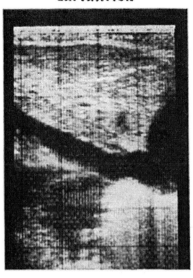

Figure 4. Respiratory change of IVC during mechanical ventilation. The left shows the IVC configuration when 400ml of air was introduced into the lung, and airway pressure readhed 23cmH$_2$O on inspiration. On the right, when positive pressure was cancelled, the airway pressure returned to 0cmH$_2$O on expiration. Although the IVC continuosly kept in a fully distened state through the entire ventilator phase, the diameter of IVC was rather greater on inspiration (left) than on expiration (right). (Tamaki S. et al. Nihon Kyobu Shikkan Gakkai zasshi 1981;19:460-460).

Conclusion

The usefulness of measuring IVCD or IVCCI to estimate CVP by echography has been proven. If physicians encounter a situation in which the CVP needs to be estimated without a central venous line, they may only have to bring an echo-machine to the patient.

References

[1] Senzaki H, Chen CH, Masutani S, Taketazu M, Kobayashi J, Kobayashi T, Sasaki N, Asano H, Kyo S, Yokote Y. Assessment of cardiovascular dynamics by pressure-area

relations in pediatric patients with congenital heart disease. *J Thorac Cardiovasc Surg* 2001;122:535-547.

[2] Senzaki H, Masutani S, Kobayashi J, Kobayashi T, Sasaki N, Asano H, Kyo S, Yokote Y, Ishizawa A. Ventricular afterload and ventricular work in Fontan circulation: comparison with normal two-ventricle circulation and single-ventricle circulation with blalock-taussig shunts. *Circulation* 2002;105:2885-2892.

[3] Seki M, Kato T, Masutani S, Matsunaga T, Senzaki H. Pulmonary arterial hypertension associated with gastroesophageal reflux in a 2-month-old boy with Down syndrome. Circ J. 2009;73:2352-2354.

[4] Masutani S, Iwamoto Y, Ishido H, Senzaki H. Relationship of maximum rate of pressure rise between aorta and left ventricle in pediatric patients. Implication for ventricular-vascular interaction with the potential for noninvasive determination of left ventricular contractility. Circ J. 2009;73:1698-1704.

[5] Ishido H, Masutani S, Senzaki H. Impaired pulmonary perfusion associated with thymus hyperplasia in an infant candidate for Fontan operation. *Circ J*. 2009;73:2348-2351.

[6] Senzaki H, Koike K, Isoda T, Ishizawa A, Hishi T, Yanagisawa M. Use of the internal jugular vein approach in balloon dilatation angioplasty of pulmonary artery stenosis in children. *Pediatr Cardiol* 1996;17:82-85.

[7] Natori H, Tamaki S, Kira S. Ultrasonographic evaluation of ventilatory effect on inferior vena caval configuration. *Am Rev Respir Dis* 1979;120;421-427.

[8] Chen L, Kim Y, Santucci KA. Use of ultrasound measurement of the inferior vena cava diameter as an objective tool in the assessment of children with clinical dehydration. *Acad Emerg Med* 2007;14:841-845.

[9] Tamaki S. Relationship between ventilatory change of the inferior vena cava and central venous pressure (author's translation). *Nihon Kyobu Shikkan Gakkai zasshi* 1981;19:460-469.

[10] Capomolla S, Febo O, Caporotondi A, Guazzotti G, Gnemmi M, Rossi A, Pinna G, Maesri R, Cobelli F. Non-invasive estimation of right atrial pressure by combined Doppler echogcardiographic measurements of the inferior vena cava in patients with congestive heart failure. *Ital Heart J.* 2000;Oct;1(10):684-90.

[11] Brennan JM, Blair JE, Goonewardena S, Ronan A, Shah D, Vasaiwala S, Kirkpatrick JN, Spencer KT. Reappraisal of the use of inferior vena cava for estimating right atrial pressure. *J Am Soc Echocardiogr* 2007;20:857-861.

[12] Kircher BJ, Himelman RB, Schiller NB. Noninvasive estimation of right atrial pressure from the inspiratory collapse of the inferior vena cava. *Am J Cardiol* 1990;66:493-496.

[13] Dönmez O, Mir S, Ozyürek R, Cura A, Kabasakal C. Inferior vena cava indices determine volume load in minimal lesion nephrotic syndrome. *Pediatr Nephrol.* 2001;16:251-255.

[14] Hruda J, Rothuis EG, van Elburg RM, Sobotka-Plojhar MA, Fetter WP. Echocardiographic assessment of preload conditions does not help at the neonatal intensive care unit. *Am J Perinatol* 2003;20:297-303.

[15] Iwamoto Y, Tamai A, Kohno K, Masutani S, Okada N, Senzaki H. Usefulness of respiratoty variation of inferior vena cava diameter for estimation of elevated central venous pressure in children with cardiovascular disease. *Circ J* 2011; 75:1209-12014.

[16] Jue J, Chng W, Schiller NB. Does inferior vena cava size predict right atrial pressures in patients receiving mechanical ventilation? *J Am Soc echocardiogr.* 1992 Nov-Dec;5(6):613-9. 15.

[17] Bendjelid K, Romand JA, Walder B, Suter PM, Fournier G. Correlation between measured inferior vena cava diameter and right atrial pressure depends on the echocardiographic method used in patients who are mechanically ventilated. *J Am Soc Echocardiogr* 2002;15;944-949

[18] Nagueh SF, Kopelen HA, Zoghbi WA. Relation of mean right atrial pressure to echocardiographic and Doppler parameters of right atrial and right ventricular function. *Circulation* 1996;93:1160-1169.

[19] Mintz GS, Kotler MN, Parry WR, Iskandrian AS, Kane SA. Real-time inferior vena caval ultrasonography: normal and abnormal findings and its use in assessing right-heart function. *Circulation* 1981;64:1018-1025.

[20] Moreno FL, Hagan AD, Holmen JR, Pryor TA, Strickland RD, Castle CH. Evaluation of size and dynamics of the inferior vena cava as an index of right-sided cardiac function. *Am J Cardiol* 1984;53:579-585.

[21] Avolio AP, Chen SG, Wang RP, Zhang CL, Li MF, O'Rourke MF. Effects of aging on changing arterial compliance and left ventricular load in a northern Chinese urban community. *Circulation* 1983;68:50-58.

[22] Kelley JR, Mack GW, Fahey JT. Diminished venous vascular capacitance in patients with univentricular hearts after the Fontan operation. *Am J Cardiol* 1995;76:158-163.

[23] Simonson JS, Schiller NB. Sonospirometry: a new method for noninvasive estimation of mean right atrial pressure based on two-dimensional echographic measurements of the inferior vena cava during measured inspiration. *J Am Coll Cardiol* 1988;11:557-564.

Chapter 10

Serological Monitoring of Hemodynamics

Masaya Sugimoto[1,2] *and Hideaki Senzaki*[1]
[1]Department of Pediatric Cardiology, Saitama Medical University, Saitama, Japan
[2]Department of Pediatrics, Asahikawa Medical University, Asahikawa, Japan

Introduction

In recent years, many advanced biomarkers have been developed and used both for the detection of cardiovascular disease and for pathological analyses. Biomarkers are not only used for acute-phase diagnosis of emergency cardiovascular disease and risk stratification but also for obtaining prognostic predictions in the chronic phase as well as for treatment evaluation. Thus far, several detection methods have been used for the treatment of cardiovascular disease, including electrocardiography, chest radiography (X-ray), echocardiography, radioisotope examinations, exercise tolerance tests, and catheterization studies. However, some of the advantages of using biomarkers are as follows: (1) an objective evaluation is possible using numerical values; (2) high level of reproducibility; (3) the ability to obtain repeated measurements; (4) mastering a testing technique is not required; (5) invasive or aggressive techniques, such as radiation exposure, are not required; and (6) measurements can be easily obtained without expensive specialist devices or equipment. The use of biomarkers makes objective evaluation possible by simply drawing a blood sample. However, the important factor is what is being observed in the obtained results, and serious mistakes can occur when results are wrongly interpreted. Therefore, diagnoses and prognostic evaluations should not be made using biomarkers alone, and it is important to draw comprehensive conclusions in conjunction with symptoms and findings of other investigations.

1. Basic Understanding of Serological Biomarkers

1.) Mechanisms of Heart Failure Progression

The pump function of the heart is regulated by heart rate, preload, afterload, and cardiac contractility. An objective understanding of these regulatory factors is imperative to the understanding of the pathology of heart failure and treatment progression. Three sequential myocardial mechanisms lead to heart failure: pressure overload, volume overload, and cardiomyopathy. In addition, the myocardium may be affected by the coronary artery disease that accompanies post-infarction myocardial remodeling. When the myocardium is subjected to any of these conditions, a number of compensatory mechanisms are initiated in order to maintain cardiac function. Such compensatory mechanisms are accompanied by accelerated neurohumoral factors and cardiac hypertrophy.

The body maintains homeostasis by ingeniously and intricately controlling various neurohumoral factors. Neurohumoral factors can be largely divided into 2 groups: the cardiac stimulant factors represented by the renin-angiotensin-aldosterone (RAA) system and the sympathetic nervous system; and the cardioprotective factors that promote vasodilation, inhibit myocardial hypertrophy, and suppress fibrosis. Cardiac stimulating factors are activated during the early stages of heart failure, resulting in increased cardiac output in order to maintain perfusion pressure to the vital organs, thereby compensating for the heart failure. However, if the activation of cardiac stimulation factors continues excessively over an extended period, a vicious cycle begins that eventually leads to chronic heart failure. The activation of neurohumoral factors in response to heart failure leads to heightened sympathetic nerve activity (according to the baroreceptor reflex) in association with increased renin and angiotensin II (AII) activity.

Vascular resistance subsequently results in an abnormal increase in afterload. Thus, the cardiac ventricles must perform work while resisting an even larger afterload, leading to further deterioration of ventricular function.

2.) Serological Markers in Cardiovascular Diseases

The fundamental concepts underlying the treatment of heart failure are appropriate and adequate control of the hyperactive active RAA and sympathetic nervous systems and improvement of the disrupted neurohumoral factor balance. To treat heart failure, it is important to first determine an indicator that can be used to ascertain whether to increase or decrease the dose of β-blockers and/or RAA system inhibitors. The most important indicators are patient symptoms and physical findings. It is important to first determine the amount of cardiac stress endured and the extent of myocardial damage and/or inflammatory changes. It is then important to determine how the neurohumoral factors have responded to these changes and to what extent self-repair has advanced. These questions can be answered by innovative utilization of cardiac biomarkers to determine the best possible treatment for the patient.

Cardiac biomarkers have been divided into the following 4 groups according to the objective:

a) related to myocardial stress and hypertrophy;
b) related to myocardial damage;
c) related to myocardial remodeling; and
d) related to inflammation.

The various types of cardiac biomarkers are shown in Figure 1. The representative objectives of these types will be explained in more detail below.

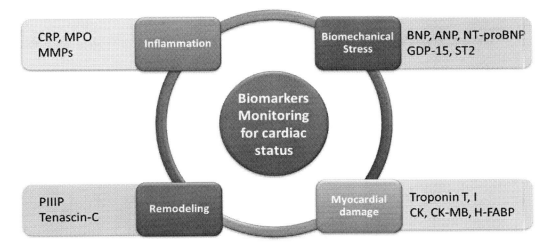

Figure 1. Biomarkers associated with various pathophysiological situation.

2. Details of Serological Markers

(a.) Related to Myocardial Stress and Hypertrophy

The following neurohumoral factors are activated during heart failure and play a vital role in the pathogenesis of the disease: noradrenalin, RAA, endothelin (ET-1), interleukin 6 (IL-6), tumor necrosis factor alpha (TNF-α), and others. However, these neurohumoral factors are interrelated; their blood concentrations change readily from moment to moment, and they are unstable substances. All these factors can cause problems with the measuring system. Therefore, monitoring the blood concentrations of such factors is not very practical during diagnosis and treatment.

1. Brain Natriuretic Peptide (BNP), N-Terminal ProBNP (NTproBNP)

BNP, a member of the natriuretic peptide family, was first isolated from a porcine brain in 1988 and has since been identified as a factor that is secreted from the heart. BNP is a powerful natriuretic, possesses vasodilator effects, and regulates the homeostasis of bodily fluids and electrolytes in conjunction with the central nervous system and peripheral tissues

[1]. BNP inhibits strain on sympathetic nerves, activation of the RAA system, and the synthesis of vasoconstrictive factors including catecholamines, AII, aldosterone, and ET-1. BNP increases the glomerular filtration rate and sodium excretion. Furthermore, BNP improves cardiac function by controlling hypertrophy in cardiomyocytes, fibroblast growth, and compensatory cardiac hypertrophy.

The predominant source of circulating BNP is the ventricles. BNP is released into the circulation when cardiomyocytes are subjected to various stressors, resulting in physiological activities such as diuretic and vasodilator actions and suppression of cardiac remodeling [2]. Several BNP molecular structures can be found in the circulation. NTproBNP is an *N*-terminal protein that originates from proBNP and is released from the myocardial cellular membrane when BNP is broken down by a protein known as furin [3]. NTproBNP, which has no known physiological function, is excreted in its original form from the kidney. Moreover, it has a longer half-life than BNP in the peripheral blood, can be measured in plasma as well as in serum, and is stable at normal temperatures, thus allowing for easy storage. Because of these characteristics, NTproBNP has recently received much attention as a useful cardiac biomarker for evaluation of heart failure in place of BNP.

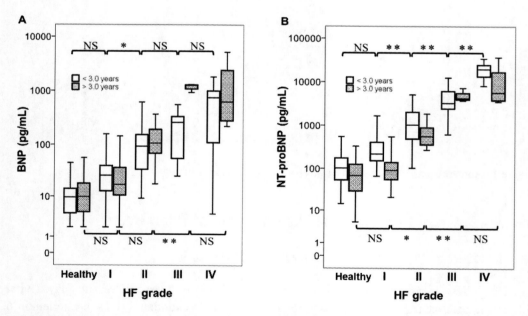

Figure 2. The (A) BNP and (B) NTprpBNP levels in the healthy group and 4 heart failure (HF) grades on a logarithmic scale. In each of the HF grades, the left boxes indicate below 3 years of age and the right boxes indicate 3 years of age or older respectively. Bars represent the media, 5th, 25th 75th and 95th percentiles. *P<0.05; **P<0.01. NS, not significant; BNP, B-type natriuetic peptide; CHF, congestive heart failure; NTproBNP, N-terminal pro-BNP.

The New York Heart Association (NYHA) functional classification, in which heart failure is classified according to severity and activity, is widely used in adults. Pfister et al. reported that BNP and NTproBNP values increase as the NYHA classification deteriorates [4]. Even in children, hemodynamics, including volume and/or pressure loading, corresponding to heart failure are experienced in conjunction with the anatomical abnormalities found in congenital heart disease (CHD). In our research, we have measured the BNP and NTproBNP values within the blood of children and compared these values with heart failure scores that are based on symptoms [5]. We have also reported the usefulness of using BNP and NTproBNP in evaluating the severity of heart failure (Figure 2).

Furthermore, BNP is an independent regulatory factor that reflects the end diastolic pressure and is reportedly more useful than ANP and other neurohumoral factors in the prognostic evaluation of chronic heart failure patients. In addition, BNP values increase according to both systolic and diastolic heart failure [6]. Currently, BNP is being widely utilized globally for the diagnosis of heart failure and the evaluation of disease severity in addition to a determinant of treatment effectiveness and an objective prognostic indicator [7, 8]. Several factors are known modifiers of BNP and NTproBNP values. Obesity decreases BNP and NTproBNP values whereas atrial fibrillation, aging, female sex, and renal dysfunction notably increase NTproBNP values.

(b.) Related to Myocardial Damage

Among the cardiac stimulation factors, high concentrations of noradrenalin, which are found in chronic heart failure, are cardiotoxic and cause myocardial necrosis. AII and TNF-α also cause myocardial necrosis and induce apoptosis. The known biomarkers used to diagnose myocardial damage include creatine kinase (CK), creatine kinase MB isoenzyme (CK-MB), myoglobin, and heart-type fatty acid-binding proteins (H-FABP), which are located in cytoplasm-soluble fractions. In addition to these, other markers such as troponin T, troponin I, and myosin light chains. Troponin T, troponin I, and H-FABP are muscle fiber-forming proteins that are located within cardiomyocytes and are released into the circulation when cardiomyocytes are damaged. A rapid measurement kit has been developed and has been utilized clinically in the diagnosis of acute coronary syndrome (ACS). In the ACC/AHA and ESC diagnosis guidelines for acute myocardial infarction (AMI) announced in 2010, the importance of rising troponin was emphasized and replaced the previously utilized CK and CK-MB [9].

1. Troponin T and Troponin I

Troponin, a structural protein found on the actin filaments of the myocardium, forms the complexes of troponin T (cTnT), I (cTnI), C, and tropomyosin. Troponin complexes regulate calcium-mediated muscle contractions, which take place between the actin and myosin of striated muscles in both skeletal and cardiac muscles. Over 90% of cTnT and cTnI are located on the structural myocardial filaments, with a small percentage found in the myocardial cytoplasm. Consequently, the efflux mechanism for troponin functions where myocardial apoptosis has occurred; this mechanism is also thought to function in areas that are damaged and therefore have abnormalities in membrane permeability. Because this efflux mechanism functions in areas of both apoptosis and abnormal membrane permeability, the release of troponin into the blood is bimodal. cTnT and cTnI increase from the third and fourth hour of onset in AMI patients, and is therefore useful in the detection of myocardial damage from the early stages of onset. This also allows for the diagnosis of minor myocardial damage that could not be detected using CK and CK-MB [10]. Furthermore, a correlation has been found between serum troponin values and the degree of severity in heart failure patients. However, the first-generation troponin assay has several limitations including antibody non-specificity, assay imprecision, lack of standardization, and the relatively late increase in circulating troponin levels after the onset of ischemia. Recently, a second-generation troponin assay (hsTnT, hsTnI) has become available. According to this highly sensitive troponin assay, it is now possible to evaluate myocardial ischemia at early stages. In a study of 5284 patients with chronic heart failure, the highly sensitive hsTnT was found to be a better prognostic factor of cardiovascular events than NTproBNP [11]. Serum hsTnI values even increased in patients without AMI or heart failure and increased in 75% of patients receiving intensive care unit treatment for septicemia or systemic inflammatory response syndrome [12]. It has been suggested that elements of systemic inflammation, including TNF-α, IL-6, and reactive oxygen species, induce myocardial damage [13]. In addition, an increase in hsTnI values can be seen in 40% of patients with acute pulmonary embolisms. Right ventricle pressure overload caused by sudden increases in pulmonary vascular resistance and hypoxia is also presumed to bring about myocardial damage [14]. Furthermore, significantly higher hsTnI values have been reported in HCM patients with thicker myocardial walls [15].

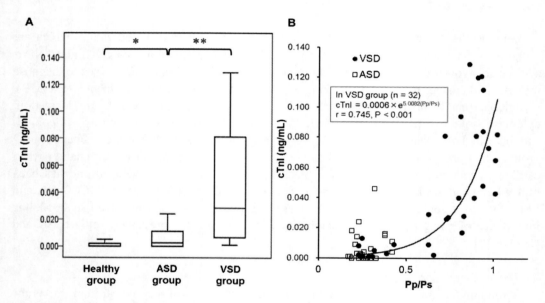

Figure 3. cTnI levels in the healthy, ASD, and VSD groups (A). The bars represent the median and the 5th, 25th, 75 and 95 percentiles. Relationship between cTnI levels and Pp/Ps (B) in VSD (closed circles, n=32) and ASD groups (open boxes, n=30). *P<0.05; **P<0.01. cTnI, cardiac troponin l; ASD, atrial septal defect; VSD, ventricular septal defect Pp/Ps, ratio of pulmonary to systemic arterial pressure.

Our pediatric study showed that the hsTnI cutoff level in children was 0.014 ng/mL, which was much lower than the cutoff level in adults (0.04 ng/mL). In addition, hsTnI values were significantly increased in children with CHD and atrial septal defect or ventricle septal defect, and a significant correlation with pulmonary blood pressure ratios was observed (Figure 3) [16]. Although the highly sensitive troponin measurement system did not only allow for early diagnosis of AMI, it was considered a beneficial tool in understanding myocardial damage that is currently progressing.

2. Heart-Type Fatty Acid-Binding Protein (H-FABP)

Cardiomyocytes use free fatty acids as an energy source under normal aerobic conditions. Free fatty acids that have been incorporated into cardiomyocytes from the circulation are β-oxidized within the mitochondria, producing ATP. H-FABP is a low molecular weight protein involved in the transport and buffering of fatty acids. Although it is located in skeletal muscles, it is found in overwhelming quantities within the myocardium. Because large quantities of cytoplasmic H-FABP are present and since it has a molecular weight of approximately 15 kDa, it is easily released into the circulation when the cell membrane is damaged. Therefore, speculation exists that the sensitivity of H-FABP in the detection of myocardial damage is better than troponin [17]. However, a study in which H-FABP was used independently in the early-stage diagnosis of AMI yielded disappointing results [18]. Arimoto et al. showed a strong correlation between H-FABP and severity of heart failure according to the NYHA functional classification, and reported that H-FABP is useful in the early diagnosis of heart failure [19]. Although very few reports have described pediatric H-FABP, a study measuring H-FABP in 238 children with CHD showed an increase in H-FABP values and an increase in the severity of heart failure according to the NYHA functional classification [20]. Furthermore, significant increases in H-FABP values were seen in the group with cyanosis.

(c.) Related to Myocardial Remodeling

The activation of the body's RAA system plays a central role in maintaining water and electrolyte balance and maintaining blood volume. The localized RAA system, however, plays a pivotal role in causing chronic heart failure. Renin is secreted from juxtaglomerular cells chiefly in response to a decrease in renal blood flow or the activation of sympathetic nerves. Angiotensinogen is converted by renin into angiotensin I and angiotensin I is, in turn, converted to AII by angiotensin-converting enzyme (ACE). This stimulates the production of aldosterone from the adrenal cortex. Renin acts as a rate-determining step in the RAA system, and the degree of RAA activation can be assessed on the basis of renin activation in the blood plasma and aldosterone concentrations. Because renin activation may be increased or decreased according to the use of drug treatments, the RAA system is presumably better represented by concentrations of aldosterone in the blood. According to Weber et al., aldosterone causes myocardial fibrosis independently of both myocardial hypertrophy and increases in blood pressure [21]. Myocardial fibrosis is controlled by spironolactone, an aldosterone antagonist. Myocardial hypertrophy and myocardial fibrosis cause remodeling of the ventricles, ultimately leading to decreased systolic and diastolic function, and ultimately heart failure.

1. Procollagen Type III N-Terminal Amino Peptide (PIIIP)

Fibroblasts begin to multiply when ischemic necrosis or apoptosis occurs in cardiomyocyte as a result of functional proinflammatory cytokines and tissue growth factors, subsequently resulting in collagen activation [22]. Furthermore, even when the cardiomyocyte is subjected to physical stimulation such as pressure or stretch loading, fibroblastic growth still occurs via the AT1 receptors produced by AII [23]. PIIIP flows from the tissues into the circulation, reflecting the metabolism of tissue collagen, and to date has been a useful indicator of hepatic collagen metabolism. In recent years, studies of myocardial infarction, hypertension, and DCM have suggested that PIIIP also reflects collagen metabolism in cardiac muscle and therefore also reflects remodeling [24-26]. Furthermore, hypoxia is responsible for activating collagen metabolism in fibroblasts. Where other indicators fail, PIIIP is proving to be useful as a myocardial remodeling indicator and is therefore beneficial in determining treatment results and prognoses [27, 28].

In a study of 170 children with CHD, we were able to prove for the first time that significant increases in PIIIP occurred in relation to CHD [29]. The high serum PIIIP levels observed in patients with pressure overload, volume overload, or cyanosis suggests accelerated collagen metabolism in the myocardium of children with CHD, signifying the occurrence of myocardial fibrosis (Table 1). Furthermore, the suppression of PIIIP levels during ACE inhibitor use suggests the involvement of the RAA system. At this point, the measurement of serum PIIIP is thought to be the most beneficial tool in understanding the state of myocardial remodeling. It may also be beneficial for the development of new treatment strategies and in aiding our understanding of cardiovascular disease.

Table 1. Serum PIIIP levels in each group

	Control	VSD	COA/AS	ASD	PS	TOF
Mean±SD (U/ml)	1.09±0.29	2.60±1.66	1.60±0.84	1.34±0.6	2.33±2.82	2.83±1.36
p value vs. control		<0.001	0.007	0.021	0.005	<0.001
age-included analysis by multiple regression		<0.001	<0.001	0.001	0.002	<0.001

Age-included analysis shows the results of multiple regression analysis with age as well as group included as independent variables.

VSD; ventricular septal defect (n=42; representing left ventricular (LV) volume overload), COA/AS; coarctation of the aorta (n=19 or aortic stenosis (n=7; representative of LV pressure overload), ASD; atrial septal defect (n=36; representative of right ventricular (RV) volume overload), PS; pulmonary stenosis (n=39; representative of RV pressure overload), TOF; tetralogy of Fallot (n=20; representative of RV pressure overload and hypoxemia.

(d.) Related to Inflammation

1. Pentraxin 3 (PTX3)

PTX3 belongs to the same pentraxin super family as CRP, an acute inflammatory response protein. PTX3 responds to inflammation signals such as IL-1, TNF-α, and lipopolysaccharides and is produced from somatic cells, including vascular endothelial, fibroblast, adipose, cartilage, periosteal, and epithelial cells [30]. In contrast to CRP, which is produced in the liver and predominantly in response to IL-6 stimuli, PTX3 is directly produced by cells throughout the body in response to pathogen-recognizing cells and their membrane toll-like receptors. PTX3 is barely detectable under normal conditions, but sudden increases are seen in patients with ailments such as AMI, infections, and autoimmune diseases. As a result, PTX3 is considered a more sensitive reflector of infection and inflammation in localized vessels than CRP.

Latini et al. suggested that PTX3 is useful as a new biomarker for the diagnoses and prognoses of AMI and heart failure [31]. In AMI patients, the plasma concentration of PTX3 increased early after disease onset [32]. Because PTX3 peaks faster than CRP, this protein has a possible use in early detection. Many cases of death have been reported in patients with high PTX3 concentrations, suggesting the use of PTX3 as a marker for severity and prognosis. Furthermore, significantly high PTX3 levels were observed in patients with normal cardiac contractility but failing dilation according to echocardiograms [33], and significantly high levels of PTX3 were reported in aortic stenosis patients [34]. In children, Leizo et al. utilized PTX3 with the aim of assessing the effectiveness of dexamethasone administered to reduce the body's inflammatory response after open-heart surgery. PTX3 has recently been the focus of attention as a new inflammation marker, and its wide use in various disease assessments is expected in the future.

2. Matrix metalloproteinase (MMP)-9

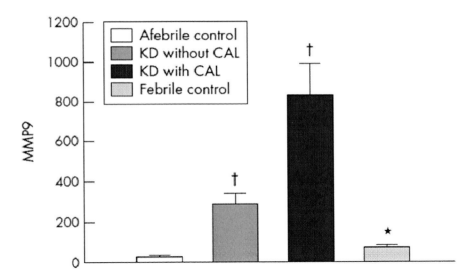

Figure 4. Comparison of MMP levels between Kawasaki disease (KD) patients with or without coronary artery lesions (CALs), afebrile healthy controls, and febrile disease controls. *Statistical significance v afebrile controls; †statistical significance v febrile controls. Data for MMP-9 are pregammaglobulin therapy.

MMPs are enzymes that break down the extracellular matrix (ECM). MMPs change the diameter and structure of blood vessels and play a vital role in the destabilization and breakdown of endothelial plaque. These enzymes are regulated by tissue inhibitors of metalloproteinases (TIMPs). MMPs break down the ECM of the cardiomyocyte and may be the cause of left ventricular dilatation and heart failure. Among the MMPs, MMP-9 damages fibrous capsules within endothelial plaques and is involved in the thinning of capsules and plaque rupture. The significance of measuring MMP-9 levels in relation to AMI was reported by Kai et al. in 1998 [35]. Current research shows that more cardiac deaths after ACS occurred in a group with higher levels of MMP-9 than in a group with lower levels [36]. Furthermore, MMP-9 has proven to be a useful prognostic factor because of its close correlation with post-AMI left-ventricular failure and with remodeling echo-evaluations in patients with heart failure [37]. Kawasaki disease is characterized by systemic vasculitis in which critical complications such as coronary artery dilation and aneurysm formation occur. Senzaki et al. found an increase in MMP/TIMP in the wall of dilated coronary arteries, suggesting that MMPs play a fixed role in the prevention and treatment of these complications (Figure 4) [38, 39].

3. Myeloperoxidase (MPO)

MPO is produced in association with the activation or degradation of leukocytes. MPO is found in abundance in neutrophilic leukocytes and macrophages that are involved in the breakdown of plaque and thinning of the fibrous capsule that envelopes plaque. The MPO enzyme is also related to the oxidation of lipids along the vascular wall. The high frequency of infiltration of MPO-positive neutrophilic leukocytes into the culprit lesions of ACS has been recognized [40]. MPO is thought to be useful as a pure plaque-destabilizing marker because it is not influenced by fibrinolytic therapy and has no correlation to heart failure. In 2001, Zhang et al. determined that levels of MPO were higher in patients with coronary artery disease than in healthy individuals [41]. During the CAPTURE trial with ACS patients as subjects, MPO levels exceeding 350 μg/L (measured during the hospital visit) were associated with a high incidence rate of cardiac death or myocardial infarction occurring after 6 months in a group of troponin-negative ACS patients where myocardial necrosis was not found, and the MPO measurement was considered an independent prognosis factor [42].

3. Multiple Biomarker Strategy

In recent years, the usefulness of cardiovascular biomarkers for detection and pathological analyses of patients with cardiovascular disease has been indicated. Thus far, heart failure has been diagnosed using a combination of subjective and objective symptoms, electrocardiograms, X-ray, and echocardiography. However, given the experience that is required to interpret the results, early diagnosis could be quite difficult, depending on the case. Biomarkers simply require procurement of a blood sample in order to obtain results, with the possibility of performing objective assessments for determining (1) diagnosis, (2) prognosis, and (3) treatment outcomes. Despite these advantages, it is difficult to imagine that a single biochemical indicator could be used to assess everything, particularly in syndromes with complex disease pathologies such as chronic heart failure. Therefore, a multi-biomarker strategy that is related to treatment and allows early diagnosis of cardiovascular disease through the skillful combination of numerous biomarkers, where each reflects a differing disease state, is currently receiving attention.

(a.) Biomarkers for Detecting AMI and ACS

AMI/ACS is a disease where a weak and unstable plaque that is surrounded by a thin fibrous capsule ruptures because of trauma such as damage to the vascular endothelium, stress to the vascular wall, or even inflammation. Rupture in turn triggers the formation of thrombosis in the surrounding regions, which leads to fatal myocardial ischemia or necrosis due to the sudden obstruction of the coronary artery lumen. The mechanism behind the onset of AMI can be divided into 7 steps: (1) plaque formation, (2) plaque destabilization, (3) plaque rupture, (4) thrombosis exacerbation, (5) myocardial ischemia, (6) myocardial necrosis, and (7) myocardial stress and ventricular remodeling [43].

The stratification of a detailed prognosis is possible by combining multiple biomarkers in which each reflects a different disease state. The combined use of H-FABP and BNP or the combined use of H-FABP, BNP, and PTX3 would be effective. These 3 markers can all be compared to normal conditions, where 1, 2, and 3 abnormalities reflect 5.4, 11.2, and 34.6 greater relative risks, respectively, of the onset of a cardiovascular event [44, 45].

(b.) Biomarkers for Detecting Heart Failure

Heart failure occurs when the myocardium is damaged due to myocardial infarction, high blood pressure, cardiomyopathy, or even valvular disease. Neurohumoral factors, including the RAA system, the sympathetic nervous system, ET-1, and the natriuretic peptide system, are activated as physiological compensatory mechanisms. These various neurohumoral factors can be divided into 2 groups: cardiac stimulation factors or cardioprotective factors. Heart failure develops as a result of a breakdown in the balance of these 2 groups. In cases of severe heart failure, the functions of natriuresis and vasodilation, which serve as cardioprotective compensatory mechanisms to reduce stress on the heart, are surpassed by cardiac stimulating factors such as the RAA system, sympathetic nervous system, and ET-1. Cardiac stimulating factors exacerbate peripheral vasoconstriction and hemodynamics. The progression of compensatory mechanisms, via cardiac stimulating factors, causes structural and electrical remodeling of the heart. In addition to causing increased cardiac loading, this also leads to further deterioration of ventricular function. Thus far, the importance of cytokines in the myocardium has not been completely determined. On the other hand, it is known that increased TNFα production in the heart and increase in TNFα concentration within the circulation is cardiotoxic. This type of TNFα overexpression promotes apoptosis, further aggravating the severity of heart failure.

The stratification of a detailed prognosis is possible by combining multiple biomarkers in which each reflects a different disease state, such as BNP and troponin. Although these are prognostic factors for all heart failure patients, BNP can theoretically show the current state of cardiac loading, whereas troponin is thought to show the myocardial damage that caused the heart failure. Therefore, these markers can be interpreted as opposing indicators. Many accounts describe the joint use of troponin with BNP or NTproBNP as useful in the determination of a heart failure prognosis [8, 46, 47].

Conclusion

There has been an explosive development of cardiac biomarkers, which can sometimes replace traditional methods of diagnosis and assessment such as echocardiograms. A deeper understanding of disease states is expected to be gained through the combined use of these markers. It is, however, important to note that diagnoses and prognoses should never be determined using biomarkers alone; comprehensive assessments should be conducted. We anticipate that suitable measurements and assessments will lead to better cardiac treatments in the future.

References

[1] de Lemos JA, McGuire DK, Drazner MH. B-type natriuretic peptide in cardiovascular disease. *Lancet*. 2003;362:316-322

[2] Levin ER, Gardner DG, Samson WK. Natriuretic peptides. *N Engl J Med*. 1998;339:321-328

[3] Hall C. Essential biochemistry and physiology of (nt-pro)bnp. *Eur J Heart Fail*. 2004;6:257-260

[4] Pfister R, Scholz M, Wielckens K, Erdmann E, Schneider CA. Use of nt-probnp in routine testing and comparison to bnp. *Eur J Heart Fail*. 2004;6:289-293

[5] Sugimoto M, Manabe H, Nakau K, Furuya A, Okushima K, Fujiyasu H, Kakuya F, Goh K, Fujieda K, Kajino H. The role of n-terminal pro-b-type natriuretic peptide in the diagnosis of congestive heart failure in children. - correlation with the heart failure score and comparison with b-type natriuretic peptide. *Circ J*. 2010;74:998-1005

[6] Watanabe S, Shite J, Takaoka H, Shinke T, Imuro Y, Ozawa T, Otake H, Matsumoto D, Ogasawara D, Paredes OL, Yokoyama M. Myocardial stiffness is an important determinant of the plasma brain natriuretic peptide concentration in patients with both diastolic and systolic heart failure. *Eur Heart J*. 2006;27:832-838

[7] Hartmann F, Packer M, Coats AJ, Fowler MB, Krum H, Mohacsi P, Rouleau JL, Tendera M, Castaigne A, Anker SD, Amann-Zalan I, Hoersch S, Katus HA. Prognostic impact of plasma n-terminal pro-brain natriuretic peptide in severe chronic congestive heart failure: A substudy of the carvedilol prospective randomized cumulative survival (copernicus) trial. *Circulation*. 2004;110:1780-1786

[8] Tang WH, Francis GS, Morrow DA, Newby LK, Cannon CP, Jesse RL, Storrow AB, Christenson RH, Apple FS, Ravkilde J, Wu AH. National academy of clinical biochemistry laboratory medicine practice guidelines: Clinical utilization of cardiac biomarker testing in heart failure. *Circulation*. 2007;116:e99-109

[9] Thygesen K, Mair J, Katus H, Plebani M, Venge P, Collinson P, Lindahl B, Giannitsis E, Hasin Y, Galvani M, Tubaro M, Alpert JS, Biasucci LM, Koenig W, Mueller C, Huber K, Hamm C, Jaffe AS. Recommendations for the use of cardiac troponin measurement in acute cardiac care. *Eur Heart J*. 2010;31:2197-2204

[10] Antman EM, Tanasijevic MJ, Thompson B, Schactman M, McCabe CH, Cannon CP, Fischer GA, Fung AY, Thompson C, Wybenga D, Braunwald E. Cardiac-specific troponin i levels to predict the risk of mortality in patients with acute coronary syndromes. *N Engl J Med*. 1996;335:1342-1349

[11] Masson S, Anand I, Favero C, Barlera S, Vago T, Bertocchi F, Maggioni AP, Tavazzi L, Tognoni G, Cohn JN, Latini R. Serial measurement of cardiac troponin t using a highly sensitive assay in patients with chronic heart failure: Data from 2 large randomized clinical trials. *Circulation*. 2012;125:280-288

[12] John J, Woodward DB, Wang Y, Yan SB, Fisher D, Kinasewitz GT, Heiselman D. Troponin-i as a prognosticator of mortality in severe sepsis patients. *J Crit Care.* 2010;25:270-275

[13] Korff S, Katus HA, Giannitsis E. Differential diagnosis of elevated troponins. *Heart.* 2006;92:987-993

[14] Meyer T, Binder L, Hruska N, Luthe H, Buchwald AB. Cardiac troponin i elevation in acute pulmonary embolism is associated with right ventricular dysfunction. *J Am Coll Cardiol.* 2000;36:1632-1636

[15] Petersen SE, Jerosch-Herold M, Hudsmith LE, Robson MD, Francis JM, Doll HA, Selvanayagam JB, Neubauer S, Watkins H. Evidence for microvascular dysfunction in hypertrophic cardiomyopathy: New insights from multiparametric magnetic resonance imaging. *Circulation.* 2007;115:2418-2425

[16] Sugimoto M, Ota K, Kajihama A, Nakau K, Manabe H, Kajino H. Volume overload and pressure overload due to left-to-right shunt-induced myocardial injury. - evaluation using a highly sensitive cardiac troponin-i assay in children with congenital heart disease. *Circ J.* 2011;75:2213-2219

[17] Seino Y, Ogata K, Takano T, Ishii J, Hishida H, Morita H, Takeshita H, Takagi Y, Sugiyama H, Tanaka T, Kitaura Y. Use of a whole blood rapid panel test for heart-type fatty acid-binding protein in patients with acute chest pain: Comparison with rapid troponin t and myoglobin tests. *Am J Med.* 2003;115:185-190

[18] Bruins Slot MH, Reitsma JB, Rutten FH, Hoes AW, van der Heijden GJ. Heart-type fatty acid-binding protein in the early diagnosis of acute myocardial infarction: A systematic review and meta-analysis. *Heart.* 2010;96:1957-1963

[19] Arimoto T, Takeishi Y, Niizeki T, Nozaki N, Hirono O, Watanabe T, Nitobe J, Tsunoda Y, Suzuki S, Koyama Y, Kitahara T, Okada A, Takahashi K, Kubota I. Cardiac sympathetic denervation and ongoing myocardial damage for prognosis in early stages of heart failure. *J Card Fail.* 2007;13:34-41

[20] Hayabuchi Y, Inoue M, Watanabe N, Sakata M, Ohnishi T, Kagami S. Serum concentration of heart-type fatty acid-binding protein in children and adolescents with congenital heart disease. *Circ J.* 2011;75:1992-1997

[21] Weber KT, Brilla CG. Pathological hypertrophy and cardiac interstitium. Fibrosis and renin-angiotensin-aldosterone system. *Circulation.* 1991;83:1849-1865

[22] de Almeida A, Mustin D, Forman MF, Brower GL, Janicki JS, Carver W. Effects of mast cells on the behavior of isolated heart fibroblasts: Modulation of collagen remodeling and gene expression. *J Cell Physiol.* 2002;191:51-59

[23] Schnee JM, Hsueh WA. Angiotensin ii, adhesion, and cardiac fibrosis. *Cardiovasc Res.* 2000;46:264-268

[24] Klappacher G, Franzen P, Haab D, Mehrabi M, Binder M, Plesch K, Pacher R, Grimm M, Pribill I, Eichler HG, et al. Measuring extracellular matrix turnover in the serum of patients with idiopathic or ischemic dilated cardiomyopathy and impact on diagnosis and prognosis. *Am J Cardiol.* 1995;75:913-918

[25] Jensen LT, Horslev-Petersen K, Toft P, Bentsen KD, Grande P, Simonsen EE, Lorenzen I. Serum aminoterminal type iii procollagen peptide reflects repair after acute myocardial infarction. *Circulation.* 1990;81:52-57

[26] Diez J, Laviades C, Mayor G, Gil MJ, Monreal I. Increased serum concentrations of procollagen peptides in essential hypertension. Relation to cardiac alterations. *Circulation.* 1995;91:1450-1456

[27] Host NB, Jensen LT, Bendixen PM, Jensen SE, Koldkjaer OG, Simonsen EE. The aminoterminal propeptide of type iii procollagen provides new information on prognosis after acute myocardial infarction. *Am J Cardiol.* 1995;76:869-873

[28] Poulsen SH, Host NB, Jensen SE, Egstrup K. Relationship between serum amino-terminal propeptide of type iii procollagen and changes of left ventricular function after acute myocardial infarction. *Circulation.* 2000;101:1527-1532

[29] Sugimoto M, Masutani S, Seki M, Kajino H, Fujieda K, Senzaki H. High serum levels of procollagen type iii n-terminal amino peptide in patients with congenital heart disease. *Heart.* 2009;95:2023-2028

[30] Bottazzi B, Garlanda C, Salvatori G, Jeannin P, Manfredi A, Mantovani A. Pentraxins as a key component of innate immunity. *Curr Opin Immunol.* 2006;18:10-15

[31] Latini R, Maggioni AP, Peri G, Gonzini L, Lucci D, Mocarelli P, Vago L, Pasqualini F, Signorini S, Soldateschi D, Tarli L, Schweiger C, Fresco C, Cecere R, Tognoni G, Mantovani A. Prognostic significance of the long pentraxin ptx3 in acute myocardial infarction. *Circulation.* 2004;110:2349-2354

[32] Peri G, Introna M, Corradi D, Iacuitti G, Signorini S, Avanzini F, Pizzetti F, Maggioni AP, Moccetti T, Metra M, Cas LD, Ghezzi P, Sipe JD, Re G, Olivetti G, Mantovani A, Latini R. Ptx3, a prototypical long pentraxin, is an early indicator of acute myocardial infarction in humans. *Circulation.* 2000;102:636-641

[33] Matsubara J, Sugiyama S, Nozaki T, Sugamura K, Konishi M, Ohba K, Matsuzawa Y, Akiyama E, Yamamoto E, Sakamoto K, Nagayoshi Y, Kaikita K, Sumida H, Kim-Mitsuyama S, Ogawa H. Pentraxin 3 is a new inflammatory marker correlated with left ventricular diastolic dysfunction and heart failure with normal ejection fraction. *J Am Coll Cardiol.* 2011;57:861-869

[34] Naito Y, Tsujino T, Akahori H, Ohyanagi M, Mitsuno M, Miyamoto Y, Hao H, Hirota S, Masuyama T. Increase in tissue and circulating pentraxin3 levels in patients with aortic valve stenosis. *Am Heart J.* 2010;160:685-691

[35] Kai H, Ikeda H, Yasukawa H, Kai M, Seki Y, Kuwahara F, Ueno T, Sugi K, Imaizumi T. Peripheral blood levels of matrix metalloproteases-2 and -9 are elevated in patients with acute coronary syndromes. *J Am Coll Cardiol.* 1998;32:368-372

[36] Blankenberg S, Rupprecht HJ, Poirier O, Bickel C, Smieja M, Hafner G, Meyer J, Cambien F, Tiret L. Plasma concentrations and genetic variation of matrix metalloproteinase 9 and prognosis of patients with cardiovascular disease. *Circulation.* 2003;107:1579-1585

[37] Kelly D, Khan SQ, Thompson M, Cockerill G, Ng LL, Samani N, Squire IB. Plasma tissue inhibitor of metalloproteinase-1 and matrix metalloproteinase-9: Novel indicators of left ventricular remodelling and prognosis after acute myocardial infarction. *Eur Heart J.* 2008;29:2116-2124

[38] Senzaki H, Masutani S, Kobayashi J, Kobayashi T, Nakano H, Nagasaka H, Sasaki N, Asano H, Kyo S, Yokote Y. Circulating matrix metalloproteinases and their inhibitors in patients with kawasaki disease. *Circulation.* 2001;104:860-863

[39] Senzaki H. The pathophysiology of coronary artery aneurysms in kawasaki disease: Role of matrix metalloproteinases. *Arch Dis Child.* 2006;91:847-851

[40] Naruko T, Ueda M, Haze K, van der Wal AC, van der Loos CM, Itoh A, Komatsu R, Ikura Y, Ogami M, Shimada Y, Ehara S, Yoshiyama M, Takeuchi K, Yoshikawa J, Becker AE. Neutrophil infiltration of culprit lesions in acute coronary syndromes. *Circulation*. 2002;106:2894-2900

[41] Zhang R, Brennan ML, Fu X, Aviles RJ, Pearce GL, Penn MS, Topol EJ, Sprecher DL, Hazen SL. Association between myeloperoxidase levels and risk of coronary artery disease. *JAMA*. 2001;286:2136-2142

[42] Baldus S, Heeschen C, Meinertz T, Zeiher AM, Eiserich JP, Munzel T, Simoons ML, Hamm CW. Myeloperoxidase serum levels predict risk in patients with acute coronary syndromes. *Circulation*. 2003;108:1440-1445

[43] Vasan RS. Biomarkers of cardiovascular disease: Molecular basis and practical considerations. *Circulation*. 2006;113:2335-2362

[44] Niizeki T, Takeishi Y, Arimoto T, Takahashi T, Okuyama H, Takabatake N, Nozaki N, Hirono O, Tsunoda Y, Shishido T, Takahashi H, Koyama Y, Fukao A, Kubota I. Combination of heart-type fatty acid binding protein and brain natriuretic peptide can reliably risk stratify patients hospitalized for chronic heart failure. *Circ J*. 2005;69:922-927

[45] Ishino M, Takeishi Y, Niizeki T, Watanabe T, Nitobe J, Miyamoto T, Miyashita T, Kitahara T, Suzuki S, Sasaki T, Bilim O, Kubota I. Risk stratification of chronic heart failure patients by multiple biomarkers: Implications of bnp, h-fabp, and ptx3. *Circ J*. 2008;72:1800-1805

[46] Horwich TB, Patel J, MacLellan WR, Fonarow GC. Cardiac troponin i is associated with impaired hemodynamics, progressive left ventricular dysfunction, and increased mortality rates in advanced heart failure. *Circulation*. 2003;108:833-838

[47] Sato Y, Kita T, Takatsu Y, Kimura T. Biochemical markers of myocyte injury in heart failure. *Heart*. 2004;90:1110-1113

Chapter 11

Red Blood Cell Distribution Width as a Monitoring Tool for Cardiovascular Diseases

Takuro Kojima and Hideaki Senzaki
Department of Pediatric Cardiology,
Saitama Medical University, Saitama, Japan

Introduction

Red blood cell distribution width (RDW) is a numerical measure of the variability of circulating erythrocytes, and this parameter is routinely reported as part of the complete blood cell count. Because anemia accelerates erythropoiesis, which increases the variability of circulating erythrocytes, RDW has been used for the differential diagnosis of anemia. However, the variability of erythrocytes also alters in response to several pathophysiological stimuli and thus may serve as a useful tool for monitoring several pathophysiological conditions, including cardiovascular diseases. In this chapter, we will discuss this topic by summarizing currently available data on RDW in cardiovascular disease.

1. What is RDW?

There are 2 types of RDW: standard deviation of RDW (RDW-SD) and coefficient of variation of RDW (RDW-CV). RDW-SD indicates 20% levels of RDW when the peak level is assigned as 100% (Figure 1). On the other hand, RDW-CV is defined by assuming a normal distribution of RDW (Figure 2) and is derived from the following equation:

RDW-CV (%) = (L2 - L1)/(L2 + L1) × 100, where L1 and L2 are points representing 68.26% of the total area under the curve.

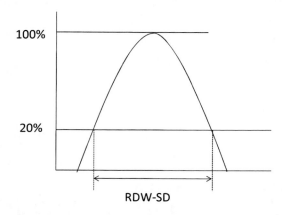

Figure 1.

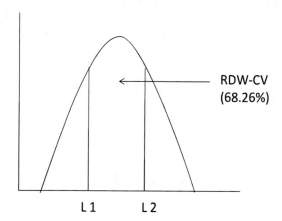

Figure 2.

Because RDW-CV depends on the mean corpuscular volume (MCV), RDW-CV is calculated as follow: RDW-CV = (SD/MCV) × 100 and was historically used for the differential diagnosis of anemia. On the other hand, RDW-SD is a quantitative index of anisocytosis and is not routinely used in the clinical setting. Therefore, in this chapter, we focus only on RDW-CV.

The normal range for RDW-CV is between 11.4% and 14.5%, but this range is age dependent and slightly higher in older people and neonates. Because a high RDW indicates greater heterogeneity of the size of circulating erythrocytes, ineffective erythropoiesis or increased destruction results in a higher RDW. Thus, RDW typically increases in patients with anemia because of iron and vitamin B12 deficiency, nutritional impairment, bone marrow dysfunction, or systemic inflammation.

2. RDW and Cardiovascular Disease

Here, we discuss the usefulness of RDW as a monitoring tool for cardiovascular diseases and conditions.

2.1. RDW as a Powerful Predictor of the Outcome of Cardiovascular Diseases

Recently, a strong association between elevated RDW and adverse outcome has been identified in patients with cardiovascular diseases. A subanalysis of the cardiovascular health and age-related maculopathy (CHARM) study and Duke Databank conducted by Felker et al. suggested that elevated RDW is a strong predictor for cardiovascular death and heart failure during hospitalization in chronic heart failure patients, and it showed a stronger statistical association than other traditional measures of risk, such as the New York Heart Association (NHYA) functional class, and ejection fraction. [1] After this early report, many studies reported RDW as a powerful prognostic marker in other forms of cardiovascular diseases. For example, RDW is reported to be a good predictor of mortality in patients with chronic heart failure as well as acute heart failure. RDW predicts the 1-year mortality in patients with acute heart failure. [2] In addition, there is a graded independent relation between higher levels of RDW and risk of death and cardiovascular events, eg, the development of new heart failure and coronary events, in patients with prior myocardial infarction. [3] Moreover, it has been reported that an increase in RDW during hospitalization is associated with a markedly increased mortality after hospital discharge in patients with acute myocardial infarction. [4]

The usefulness of RDW as a prognostic marker is also reported in patients with pulmonary hypertension. [5] The baseline RDW seems to be higher in patients with hemodynamically significant pulmonary hypertension than in those with other cardiovascular diseases. In patients with pulmonary hypertension, there is a graded increase in the mortality rate with increasing RDW levels. In addition, RDW outperforms N-terminal-pro B-type natriuretic peptide (NT-pro BNP) as a prognostic indicator in patients with pulmonary hypertension, suggesting that using RDW may be a cost-effective alternative compared to the more expansive NT-pro BNP. Thus, RDW has the potential to be a powerful prognostic indicator in various cardiovascular diseases, independent of other biomarkers.

2.2. RDW as a Biomarker in Heart Failure

As discussed above, RDW appears to be a useful predictive marker for heart failure. Thus, we further discuss the features of RDW in heart failure monitoring in comparison/association with other biomarkers.

a.) BNP/NT-Pro BNP and RDW

Of the commercial natriuretic peptide assays currently available, those for the measurements of BNP and its biologically inactive metabolite, NT-pro BNP, are considered the strongest prognostic markers for monitoring heart failure. However, these assays are relatively expensive and an excessive amount of blood sample is required. On the other hand, RDW is more cost-effective and a component of the complete blood count. In addition, RDW predicts mortality in patients with acute heart failure as good as BNP or NT-pro BNP and is independent of the prognostic value of these 2 measures. [2, 6] RDW may provide a valuable alternative biomarker for risk stratification in patients with heart disease, and the use of RDW together with BNP or NT-pro BNP may represent a powerful prognostic tool. [2, 6, 7]

b.) RDW and Inflammatory Cytokines in Heart Failure

It is well known that inflammatory cytokines play important roles in the progression of heart failure, and RDW may correlate with inflammation in heart failure. For example, inflammatory cytokines have been found to inhibit erythropoietin-induced erythrocyte maturation, which is reflected, in part, by an increase in RDW. [1] In addition, interleukin (IL)-1, IL-6, and tumor necrosis factors (TNFs) play important roles in the progression of heart failure, and RDW correlates with these cytokines; [8, 9] high RDW strongly correlates with elevated IL-6 and TNF receptor levels, and the IL-1β level inversely correlates with RDW.

c.) RDW and Anemia Status in Heart Failure

Traditionally, RDW was used for the differential diagnosis of anemia. Iron deficiency anemia and thalassemia were diagnosed by using RDW and MCV. As RDW is a quantitative measure of anisocytosis, it is clear that RDW is a hallmark of ineffective red blood cell production (such as in iron deficiency, B12 or folate deficiency, and hemoglobinopathies) and/or increased red blood cell destruction (such as hemolysis or after blood transfusion). Serum iron levels and MCV values decrease at higher RDWs, and erythropoietin levels increase with increasing RDW.

Anemia is common in patients with heart failure, but RDW predicts mortality in patients with heart failure regardless of their anemia status. [10] This means that RDW may be an earlier marker of prognosis than hemoglobin, as it may reflect early steps in the complex processes of anemia in heart failure, when ineffective production and increased destruction of red blood cells occur, but the hemoglobin level is still within the normal range.

2.3. Potential Mechanisms of RDW Elevation in Heart Failure

The reason for the association of RDW and outcome in acute and chronic cardiac conditions is not fully understood. RDW is an integrative correlate of ineffective red blood cell production, bone marrow function, inflammation, impaired renal function, and malnutrition. In addition, these factors correlate in a complicated way with each other and contribute to the progression of heart failure. For example, anemia (impaired iron mobilization) in patients with heart failure is mediated in part by overexpression of hepcidin, a peptide hormone which acts as regulator of human iron metabolism.[8] Hepcidin is upregulated by inflammation, and IL-6 plays a important role as powerful inducer. As described above, IL-6 strongly correlates with RDW. Furthermore, total cholesterol and glomerular filtration rate are reportedly decreased in patients with heart failure and high levels of RDW, indicating the close association between RDW and malnutrition/renal dysfunction in heart failure. [9] Inflammation is closely linked with anemia by regulating the iron metabolism in heart failure patients. In addition, the relationship of decreased erythropoietin secretion with impaired renal function is well known, and inflammatory cytokines directly affect erythropoietin production. Thus, an elevated RDW in patients with heart failure might reflect complex pathologic processes, such as impaired iron metabolism, nutritional status, renal function, and inflammation.

3. Future Perspective

Although mounting evidence suggests the usefulness of RDW as a monitoring tool for cardiovascular diseases, further studies are required in order to establish the routine utilization of RDW in the management of patients with cardiovascular diseases. First, it is unclear whether RDW reflects the therapeutic effectiveness in these conditions, ie, whether RDW can be a therapeutic target. Second, it is also unclear whether RDW follows relatively short-term cardiovascular fluctuations. Finally, there are not sufficient data about the relationship between RDW and congenital heart diseases. Because heart failure in patients with congenital heart disease is not the same as that in patients with myocardial infarctions or valvular diseases, further studies are needed in this particular area.

In conclusion, RDW provides a widely available, inexpensive, and good prognostic value in acute and chronic cardiovascular conditions. RDW may integrate complex interactions in cardiovascular conditions into single biomarker.

References

[1] G. Michael Felker, Larry A. Allen, Stuart J. Pocock, Linda K. Shaw, John J. V. McMurray, Marc A. Pfeffer, Karl Swedberg, Duolao Wang, Salim Yusuf, Eric L. Michelson, Christopher B. Granger; Red Cell Distribution Width as a Novel Prognostic Marker in Heart Failure. Data From the CHARM Program and the Duke Databank. *J Am Coll Cardiol* 2007; 50: 40-7

[2] Roland R.J. van Kimmenade, Asim A. Mohammed, Shanmugam Uthamalingam, Peter van der Meer, G. Michael Felker, and James L. Januzzi Jr.; Red boold cell distribution width and 1-year mortality in acute heart failure. *Eur J Heart Fail* (2010) 12, 129-136

[3] Marcello Tonelli, Frank Sacks, Malcolm Arnold, Lemuel Moye, Barry Davis, Marc Pfeffer ; Relation Between Red Blood Cell Distribution width and Cardiovascular Event Rate in People With Coronary Disease. *Circulation*. 2008; 117:163-168.

[4] Saleem Dabbah, Haim Hammerman, Walter Markiewicz, Doron Aronson; Relation Between Red Cell Distribution Width and Clinical Outcomes After Acute Myocardial Infarction. *Am J Cardiol* 2010; 105: 312-317

[5] Chetan V. Hampole, Amit K. Mehrotra, Thenappan Thenappan, Mardi Gomberg-Maitland, and Sanjiv J. Shah; Usefulness of Red Cell Distribution Width as a Prognostic Marker in Pulmonary Hypertension. *Am J Cardiol* 2009; 104: 868-872.

[6] Yahya Al-Najjar, Kevin M. Goode, Jufen Zhang, John G.F. Cleland, and Andrew L. Clark; Red cell distribution width: an inexpensive and powerful prognostic marker in heart failure. *Eur J Heart Fail* (2009) 11, 1155-1162.

[7] Colette E. Jackson, Jonathan R. Dalzell, Vladimir Bezlyak, Ioannis Tsorlalis, Rachel C. Myles, Richard Spooner, Ian Ford, Mark C. Petrie, Stuart M. Cobbe, John J. V. McMurray; Red Cell distribution width has incremental prognostic value to B-type natriuretic peptide in acute heart failure. *Eur J Heart Fail* (2009) 11, 1152-1154

[8] Larry A. Allen, G. Michael Felker, Mandeep R. Mehra, Jun R. Chiong, Stephanie H. Dunlap, Jalal K. Ghali, Daniel J. Lenihan, Ron M. Oren, Lynne E. Wagoner, Todd A. Schwartz, and Kirkwood F. Adams Jr.; Validation and Potential Mechanisms of Red

Cell Distribution width as a Prognostic Marker in Heart Failure. *J Card Fail* vol.16 No.3 2010.

[9] Zsolt Förhécz, Tímea Gombos, Gábor Borgulya, Zoltán Pozsonyi, Zoltán Prohászka, and Lívia Jánoskuti; Red cell distribution width in heart failure: Prediction of clinical events and relationship with markers of ineffective erythropoiesis, inflammation, renal function, and nutritional state. *Am heart J* 2009; 158: 659-66.

[10] Domingo A. Pascual-Figal, Juan C. Bonaque, Belen Redondo, Cesar Caro, Sergio Manzano-Fernandez, Jesús Sánchez-Mas, Iris P. Garrido, and Mariano Valdes; Red blood cell distribution width predicts long-term outcome regardless of anemia status in acute heart failure patients. *Eur J Heart Fail* (2009) 11, 840-846.

Chapter 12

Computer Simulation of Hemodynamics in Children with Congenital Heart Disease

Ryo Inuzuka and Hideaki Senzaki
Department of Pediatric Cardiology,
Saitama Medical University, Saitama, Japan

Introduction

Addressing the influence of a single parameter of the cardiovascular system on the total circulation is very important for better understanding the pathophysiology of cardiovascular disease. However, this is almost impossible *in vivo* because of the complex interrelationships existing among pressure, flow, resistance, and capacitance, and these are further complicated by the actions of reflex regulatory mechanisms. Mathematical models and computer simulations of the cardiovascular system can provide valid support in analyzing this problem. A computer model allows the hemodynamic effects of individual parameter changes to be investigated in rigorously quantitative terms.

In this chapter, we will discuss the basic theory of computer models of the cardiovascular system, built using standard components such as transmission lines, restrictors, capacitors, and a time-varying elastance model of the four pumping chambers of the heart with check valves. We will also present some simulation data for congenital heart disease.

1. Modeling of Heart Chambers

The time-varying elastance model describes the instantaneous relationship between chamber pressure and volume. When this model is coupled to a model of the circulation, one can simulate the heart response to various preloads and afterloads.

Suga and Sagawa et al. showed that the end-systolic pressure–volume relation (ESPVR) was linear and provided a measure of the chamber contractile state that was largely independent of loading conditions. [1, 2] ESPVR linearity enables a simple description of ventricular contraction using a time-varying elastance model in terms of the slope (elastance; E(t)) and the volume-axis intercept (Vd).

$$P(t) = E(t) \times (V(t) - Vd)$$

Suga and Sagawa et al. also demonstrated that when E(t) is normalized with respect to both its maximal amplitude (En = E/Emax) and the time at which the maximum occurs (tn = t/Tmax), this normalized curve (En(tn)) was fairly independent of loading conditions, contractile state, and heart rate in isolated canine hearts. [1, 2]

$$E(t) = Emax \times En(\frac{t}{Tmax})$$

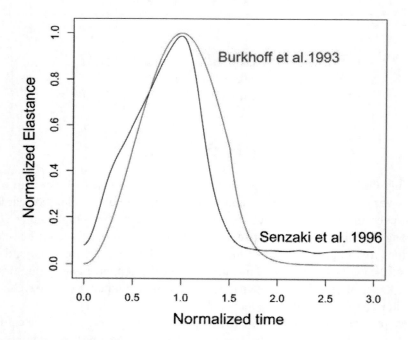

Figure 1. Normalized elastance curves used in previous studies. [3, 4]

Senzaki et al. confirmed that the normalized elastance curves are uniform, even in human left ventricles, and expressed this as a Fourier series, which is plotted in Figure 1. [3] There are numerous modifications of the time-varying elastance model to incorporate ventricular relaxation (τ) and diastolic properties of the ventricle (i.e., end-diastolic pressure–volume relationship) using sine and exponential curves. The following is an example of the time-varying elastance model for the left ventricle, proposed by Burkhoff et al. [4]

$$P(t) = En(t) \times (Pes(V) - Ped(V)) + Ped(V)$$

where

$$En(t) = 0.5 \times \left\{\sin\left[\pi(\frac{t}{Tmax} - 0.5)\right] + 1\right\} \quad \text{for } t < 1.5Tmax$$

$$En(t) = 0.5 * \exp(\frac{-t + 1.5Tmax}{\tau}) \quad \text{for } t \geq 1.5Tmax$$

$$Pes(V) = Emax \times (V - Vd)$$

$$Ped(V) = A \times \{\exp[B \times (V - Vd)] - 1\}$$

For atrial chambers, simpler curves (e.g., sine curves) are commonly used for the time-varying elastance model: [5–7]

$$P(t) = E(t) \times (Pes(V) - Ped(V)) + Ped(V)$$

where

$$E(t) = 0.5 \times \left[1 - \cos\left(\pi \times \frac{t}{Tmax}\right)\right]$$

$$Pes(V) = Emax \times (V - Vd)$$

$$Ped(V) = Emin \times (V - Vd)$$

Emin = the minimal amplitude of elastance

2. Modeling of Heart Valves

The simplest model of a heart valve in the electrical analog of the cardiovascular system is a diode, which allows an electrical current to pass in one direction, while blocking the current in the opposite direction. However, real valve motion is a more complex process than a simple change of status between open and closed, as in the diode model. Heart valves close and open passively under various external effects, such as a pressure gradient across the valve, vortex flow near the valve, and shear force acting on the valve leaflet surfaces, but the precise mechanisms remain difficult to characterize. [8, 9]

A pressure gradient across a cardiac valve is a major driving force of blood flow through the valve. There are three factors which relate flow rate and pressure drop across cardiac valves: viscous resistance (Rcv), Bernoulli resistance (Bcv), and inductance (Lcv). [10] Thus, the pressure drop (ΔP) across a cardiac valve can be expressed using the flow rate (Q) by

$$\Delta P = \text{Rcv} \times Q + \text{Bcv} \times Q \times |Q| + \text{Lcv} \times \frac{dQ}{dt}$$

where

Rcv = the coefficient of the viscous resistance

Bcv = the coefficient of flow separation

Lcv = the coefficient of inertial term

Models using these parameters have successfully simulated transvalvular flow under both normal and pathological conditions. [10, 11]

3. Modeling of Vascular System

In many ways, blood flow and electrical conduction behave similarly. Thus, by representing the blood pressure and flow by a voltage and a current, describing the effects of friction and inertia in blood flow by a resistance (R) and inductance (L), and the effect of vessel elasticity by a capacitance (C), the well-established methods for analyzing electrical circuits can be applied to cardiovascular simulation. [12] The simplest description is the two-element Windkessel model, consisting of a resistance and a compliance element (Figure 2A). [13] Poiseuille's law states that resistance is inversely proportional to the fourth power of the blood vessel radius. The resistance to flow in the arterial system is therefore mainly found in the peripheral vessels. The systemic arterial resistance (Rao) can simply be calculated as:

$$\text{Rao} = \frac{\text{mean aortic pressure} - \text{mean venous pressure}}{\text{cardiac output}}$$

The compliant element is mainly determined by the elasticity of the large vessels. It can be obtained by addition of the compliances of all vessels, and is therefore called total vascular compliance. The value of the total vascular compliance, C, is the ratio of a volume change (ΔV) and the resulting pressure change (ΔP):

$$C = \Delta V / \Delta P$$

An extended three-element Windkessel model was later developed by Westerhof et al.; [14] this model improved the high-frequency performance of the model in the input impedance analysis. This model has an extra resistance (Rc) connected in series with the RC Windkessel model, representing the characteristic impedance of the arterial network (Figure 2B). The characteristic impedance in the three-element Windkessel model can be seen as a link between the lumped Windkessel model and wave travel aspects of the arterial system since the characteristic impedance equals wave speed times blood density divided by (aortic) cross-sectional area. [12, 15]

Computer Simulation of Hemodynamics in Children with Congenital Heart Disease 147

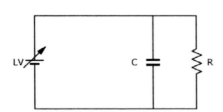
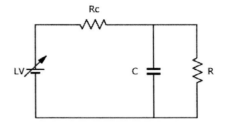

Figure 2. The Windkessel models. C = compliance, R = resistance, LV = left ventricle and Rc = characteristic impedance.

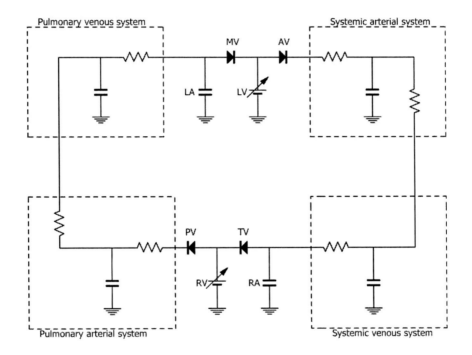

Figure 3. A multi-compartment model for the whole vascular network. Three-element Windkessel models for arterial systems and two-element Windkessel models for venous systems are used. AV = aortic valve, RA = right atrium, RV = right ventricle, LA = left atrium, LV = left ventricle, MV = mitral valve, PV = pulmonary valve, T = tricuspid valve.

Multi-compartment models have been developed for computing the internal distribution of pressure and flow in the different segments of the vessel network. In these models, the whole vascular network is described as a connected system of small segments (e.g., arterial and venous systems), and each segment consists of an RLC circuit that reflects the local vessel properties. The vascular network can be segmented further, depending on the accuracy required. Examples of vascular models and normal values used in previous studies are shown in Figure 3.

Lumped parameter models (electrical analog) assume a uniform distribution of pressure and flow within any compartment of the model, and thus are unable to account for wave propagation. The propagation of pressure and flow waves in the vessel network significantly affects cardiovascular physiology, especially in the aorta and larger systemic arteries. To account for wave propagation and reflection, one-dimensional models are required. These include anatomical information on the vessels, such as the distribution of cross-sectional areas and branching of the vessels. Two- and three-dimensional models can reveal more detailed and precise pressure and flow distributions in the vessel network, but the relatively high demands on computational resources have limited their use. [15]

4. Modeling of Autonomic Functions

The autonomic nervous system is one of the most important mechanisms in achieving rapid circulatory control aimed at maintaining blood pressure. When the blood pressure is outside the normal ranges, baroreceptors trigger circulatory regulation by redistributing blood to different areas of the body through sympathetic and/or parasympathetic nerves. This baroreflex occurs via changes in systemic arterial resistance, systemic venous unstressed volume, systemic venous compliance, and heart rate. Whether baroreflexes have a significant effect on cardiac contractility is still controversial. Arterial baroreceptors, which are the most sensitive receptors, are located in the carotid sinuses, aortic arch, and at the origin of the right subclavian artery.

Autonomic function is often modeled as a feedback regulatory system in response to arterial baroreceptors (Pa). Ursino et al. have developed an analytical model of neuro-regulation, using the sigmoid function ($\sigma(Pa)$) to describe the nonlinear static gain. [16] An example of regulation for a variable X (e.g., systemic arterial resistance, systemic venous unstressed volume, systemic venous compliance, and heart period) and a target arterial pressure Pt is as follows:

$$\frac{dX}{dt} = \frac{-X+\sigma}{t1}$$

$$\sigma = \frac{Xmax + Xmin \times \exp\left(\frac{Pa-Pt}{r1}\right)}{1+\exp\left(\frac{Pa-Pt}{r1}\right)}$$

where

Xmax and Xmin = the upper and lower saturation values of the variable

t1 = the time constant of the regulatory action

r1 = the constant parameter related to the central slope of the sigmoidal curve.

5. Simulation of the Whole Cardiovascular System

Connecting each component of the cardiovascular system, such as heart chambers, valves, and vessels, and simulating the cardiovascular system corresponds to solving a set of equations with the initial conditions. Lumped parameter models are described by a set of simultaneous ordinary differential equations based on conservation of mass and momentum, and the higher-dimensional models produce a series of partial differential equations obtained using the Navier–Stokes equations.

Recently, several researchers have developed multi-scale models that integrate a one-dimensional or higher-dimensional arterial network model into a lumped parameter model of the entire system, [10] and thus are able to account for global hemodynamics and arterial wave propagation simultaneously.

6. Congenital Heart Diseases

Congenital heart diseases contain anatomically heterogeneous populations. Studying the influence of a single hemodynamic parameter on the cardiovascular system in congenital heart disease is important as it may vary depending on the anatomy. Once the cardiovascular model for normal biventricular circulation has been completed, the construction of hemodynamic models for congenital heart diseases is relatively straightforward.

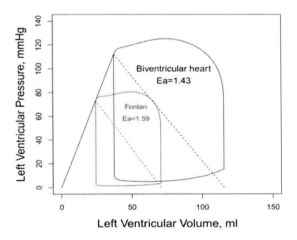

Figure 4. Simulated pressure–volume relationship in Fontan circulation compared with left ventricle in normal biventricular circulation.

Here we present an example of simulation of Fontan circulation. The effective arterial elastance, which is measured as the ratio of ventricular end-systolic pressure to stroke volume, reflects the ventricular afterload. [17] As is shown in Figure 4, Fontan circulation is characterized by reduced preload and increased afterload, which results in reduction in stroke volume compared with normal biventricular circulation. The results are very similar to those of clinical studies of patients with this unique circulation. [18]

Conclusion

Based on the similarity between blood flow and electric conduction, the cardiovascular system can be simulated as an electric analogue. By changing the structure of an electric circuit, various types of congenital heart disease can be modeled flexibly. When the time-varying elastance model, which represents cardiac chambers, is coupled to a model of the circulation, one can characterize the heart response to various preload and afterload, which may vary depending on the anatomy in congenital heart disease.

The slopes of the dotted line represent the effective arterial elastance (Ea). The same parameters for the ventricular, valvular, and vascular properties were assumed in the analysis.

References

[1] Suga H, Sagawa K, Shoukas AA. Load independence of the instantaneous pressure-volume ratio of the canine left ventricle and effects of epinephrine and heart rate on the ratio. *Circ Res*.32(3):314-322 1973.

[2] Suga H, Sagawa K. Instantaneous pressure-volume relationships and their ratio in the excised, supported canine left ventricle. *Circ Res*.35(1):117-126 1974.

[3] Senzaki H, Chen CH, Kass DA. Single-beat estimation of end-systolic pressure-volume relation in humans. A new method with the potential for noninvasive application. *Circulation*.94(10):2497-2506 1996.

[4] Burkhoff D, Tyberg JV. Why does pulmonary venous pressure rise after onset of LV dysfunction: a theoretical analysis. *Am J Physiol*.265(5 Pt 2):H1819-1828 1993.

[5] Thomas JD, Zhou J, Greenberg N, Bibawy G, McCarthy PM, Vandervoort PM. Physical and physiological determinants of pulmonary venous flow: numerical analysis. *Am J Physiol*.272(5 Pt 2):H2453-2465 1997.

[6] Lau VK, Sagawa K, Suga H. Instantaneous pressure-volume relationship of right atrium during isovolumic contraction in canine heart. *Am J Physiol*.236(5):H672-679 1979.

[7] Alexander J, Jr., Sunagawa K, Chang N, Sagawa K. Instantaneous pressure-volume relation of the ejecting canine left atrium. *Circ Res*.61(2):209-219 1987.

[8] Yacoub MH, Kilner PJ, Birks EJ, Misfeld M. The aortic outflow and root: a tale of dynamism and crosstalk. *Ann Thorac Surg*.68(3 Suppl):S37-43 1999.

[9] Korakianitis T, Shi Y. Numerical simulation of cardiovascular dynamics with healthy and diseased heart valves. *J Biomech*.39(11):1964-1982 2006.

[10] Liang F, Takagi S, Himeno R, Liu H. Multi-scale modeling of the human cardiovascular system with applications to aortic valvular and arterial stenoses. *Med Biol Eng Comput*.47(7):743-755 2009.

[11] Sun Y, Sjoberg BJ, Ask P, Loyd D, Wranne B. Mathematical model that characterizes transmitral and pulmonary venous flow velocity patterns. *Am J Physiol*.268(1 Pt 2):H476-489 1995.

[12] Westerhof N, Lankhaar JW, Westerhof BE. The arterial Windkessel. *Med Biol Eng Comput*.47(2):131-141 2009.

[13] Sagawa K, Lie RK, Schaefer J. Translation of Otto Frank's paper "Die Grundform des Arteriellen Pulses" Zeitschrift fur Biologie 37: 483-526 (1899). *J Mol Cell Cardiol.*22(3):253-254 1990.

[14] Westerhof N, Elzinga G, Sipkema P. An artificial arterial system for pumping hearts. *J Appl Physiol.*31(5):776-781 1971.

[15] Shi Y, Lawford P, Hose R. Review of zero-D and 1-D models of blood flow in the cardiovascular system. *Biomed Eng Online.*10:33

[16] Ursino M, Cavalcanti S, Bertuglia S, Colantuoni A. Theoretical analysis of complex oscillations in multibranched microvascular networks. *Microvasc Res.*51(2):229-249 1996.

[17] Kelly RP, Ting CT, Yang TM, Liu CP, Maughan WL, Chang MS, Kass DA. Effective arterial elastance as index of arterial vascular load in humans. *Circulation.*86(2):513-521 1992.

[18] Senzaki H, Masutani S, Ishido H, Taketazu M, Kobayashi T, Sasaki N, Asano H, Katogi T, Kyo S, Yokote Y. Cardiac Rest and Reserve Function in Patients with Fontan Circulation. *J Am Coll Cardiol.* 2006;47:2528-35.

In: Hemodynamics: Monitoring, Theory and Applications
Editor: Hideaki Senzaki
ISBN: 978-1-62257-361-5
© 2013 Nova Science Publishers, Inc.

Chapter 13

Applications of Computational Fluid Dynamics in Abdominal Aortic Aneurysms

Zhonghua Sun[*]

Discipline of Medical Imaging, Department of Imaging and Applied Physics,
Curtin University, Perth, Australia

Abstract

Abdominal aortic aneurysm is a common vascular disease that affects elderly population. Currently, open surgery still remains as the gold standard technique for treatment of abdominal aortic aneurysm. However, endovascular aneurysm repair, as a less invasive technique, has become widely used in many clinical centres and its effectiveness has been confirmed by many studies when compared to open surgery. Computed tomography (CT) angiography has been regarded as the preferred imaging modality for both pre-operative planning and post-procedure follow-up. However, CT is limited to the visualization of anatomical details, thus it fails to provide information about the hemodynamic effects caused by the implanted endovascular stent grafts. Computational fluid dynamics (CFD) is increasingly used to study the fluid phenomena inside the human vascular system. Applications of CFD in the abdominal aortic aneurysm include assisting in developing better stent graft design; lowering the chances of procedure-related complications such as renal dysfunction or stent graft migration, and providing a good understanding of the fluid-stent graft interaction based on aortic models. This book chapter provides an overview of the abdominal aortic aneurysm and treatment options, with a focus on the endovascular stent graft repair, and the applications of CFD in the abdominal aortic aneurysm pre- and post-stent graft repair.

---

[*] Corresponding author: Associate Professor Zhonghua Sun, Discipline of Medical Imaging, Department of Imaging and Applied Physics, Curtin University, GPO Box, U1987, Perth, Western Australia 6845, Australia, Tel +61-8-9266 7509, Fax: +61-8-9266 2377, Email: z.sun@curtin.edu.au.

Introduction

Abdominal aortic aneurysm (AAA) occurs when the aortic wall becomes weakened, resulting in focal enlargement of the blood vessel. An AAA is defined as an enlargement of the aorta of at least 1.5 times its normal aortic diameter or greater than 3 cm diameter in the maximum transverse dimension (Fig 1). Most of the AAAs (>80%) are located in an infrarenal position (aneurysm extends cranially more than 15 mm below the renal arteries) (Fig 2A), while only a small percentage of them belong to juxtarenal (Fig 2B) (origin of aneurysm less than 15 mm below the renal arteries) or suprarenal AAAs (dilatation of the infrarenal aorta up to or above the level of renal artery ostium) (Fig 2C). Common risk factors attributable to the development of AAAs include increased age, smoking, atherosclerosis and hypertension [1]. AAAs are about three to four times more common in men than in women.

Most people with AAAs do not have aneurysm-related symptoms and the diagnosis therefore mainly depends on incidentally clinical investigation for other conditions (e.g. physical examination or ultrasound or X-ray examination). Because most AAAs are asymptomatic, it is difficult to estimate their prevalence, but screening studies in the UK have reported a prevalence of 1.3-12.7% depending on the age group studied [2]. The incidence of symptomatic AAAs in men is approximately 25 per 100,000 at age 50, increasing to 78 per 100,000 in those older than 70 years [2]. The implementation of a national screening program for AAA is recommended with the aim of reducing the aneurysm-associated mortality [3].

Once an aneurysm has been detected by routine physical exam and radiographic studies, the risk of rupture is weighed against the risk of surgical repair for each individual patient. Among patients with ruptured AAA the mortality rate is about 80% which increases up to 90% when in-hospital deaths are included [4]. The major determinant for risk of rupture is aneurismal diameter. In the absence of natural history data concerning patients with aortic aneurysms the risk of rupture is estimated from the respective diameters of the abdominal aorta. The risk of operative complications is determined not only by age, cardiac and pulmonary function, but by the extent of aorta involved.

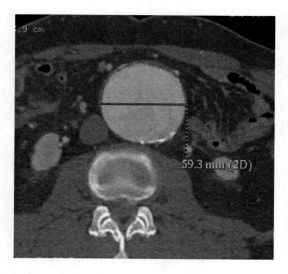

Figure 1. 2D axial image shows measurement of an abdominal aortic aneurysm (AAA) based on maximal transverse diameter (5.9 cm).

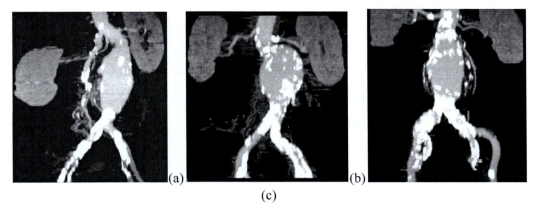

Figure 2. Coronal maximum-intensity projection (MIP) images show an infrarenal AAA (A), juxtarenal AAA (B) and suprarenal AAA (C).

1. Abdominal Aortic Aneurysm: Treatment Options

Definitive therapy for AAAs is aimed towards prevention of aneurysm rupture, i.e by placement of the dilated segment of aorta with a prosthetic graft. To determine whether an individual patient is a candidate for graft replacement, many factors need to be considered, including the risk of aneurysm rupture, life expectancy, anticipated quality of life after the operation, and the risk of surgical therapy [5].

Patients can be treated by conventional open surgical repair which involves laparotomy and insertion of a prosthetic graft to replace the aneurismal aorta. Open surgical repair is considered the gold standard to treat AAAs. However, open aneurysm repair is a major operation, and it is associated with peri-procedure or postprocedure-related complications. Population-based studies report the morbidity and mortality rates are significant. Mortality may be as high as 8%, and 10% may suffer cardiac complications [6].

In an attempt to reduce the surgical risk in patients with accompanied medical conditions less invasive methods of aneurysm repair have been considered. AAAs can also be treated by a minimally invasive approach which involves placement of an endoluminal stent–graft through the transfemoral approach. This procedure called as endovascular aneurysm repair (EVAR) has revolutionized the treatment of AAAs in the last two decades.

2. Endovascular Aneurysm Repair

Instead of graft replacement via an extensive procedure through abdominal or flank incision under general anesthesia, EVAR involves the process with a thin-walled prosthesis being compressed into a catheter, introduced into the femoral artery via a limited groin incision under local anesthesia, and advanced into the abdominal aorta to exclude the aneurysm from the systemic circulation.

Since Dotter first described coiled stainless steel wire stents in 1969 [7], many types of endovascular stents and grafts have been developed [8-10]. More than two decades ago, Parodi et al [11] introduced a minimally invasive, endovascular device to repair AAA. Subsequently, a variety of endovascular devices have undergone clinical evaluation in the hope of achieving satisfactory results compared to open surgical repair [12-15]. These devices differ from one another with respect to design features, including modularity; metallic composition and structure of the stent (nitinol, stainless steel); the thickness, porosity, and chemical composition of the graft material (synthetic versus biological); the method of attaching the fabric to the stent (endo or exostent configurations); and the presence or absence of a penetrating method of fixing the device to the aortic wall with barbs and hooks, and creation of an opening in the graft fabric to accommodate the orifice of the vessel targeted for preservation [16-21]. Of these devices, suprarenal and fenestrated stent grafts represent the two major technological developments in EVAR with more patients with AAA benefiting from these two types of endovascular devices.

2.1. Suprarenal Stent Grafting

One of the most important modifications in aortic stent-grafts was the development of suprarenal fixation, which was originally proposed by Lawrence et al in experimental animal studies using Gianturco stents [22, 23]. Placement of an uncovered stent over the renal artery orifices was reported to improve the proximal fixation of stent-grafts in AAAs [24, 25]. Deployment of a bare proximal stent across the aortic branches serves dual functions: prevention of stent-graft migration and optimization of the hemostatic seal at the cephalad end of the device by using the available length of the infrarenal neck (Fig 3). Failure of either of these functions precludes successful endovascular repair. However, attachment may be improved by adding hooks and barbs to the proximal stent [22, 23]. Malina et al reported that stronger fixation can be provided by barbs that perforate the entire aortic wall, enhancing the strength of stent-graft fixation by at least 10 fold [26]. Suprarenal fixation also provides a platform for the development of fenestrated or branched stent-grafts that extend across and above the renal arteries to exclude thoracoabdominal aneurysms.

Theoretically, the suprarenal stent-graft technique can extend the applicability of endovascular aortic repair to more complex AAAs. However, although suprarenal fixation may improve sealing and facilitate durable exclusion of aneurysms without device migration, there is obvious concern that crossing the renal ostia with stents may have a deleterious effect on renal blood flow. Short to medium-term results of suprarenal fixation have been satisfactory; according to reports from various centres [27-31], no significant impact has been observed on renal perfusion or renal function.

Nonetheless, there are still concerns about the safety of suprarenal fixation in the long term [32, 33]. The consequences of stent strut coverage of the renal ostium and the hemodynamic consequences can manifest in various ways, e.g., interference with renal blood flow or renal function, decreased cross-sectional area of the renal ostium, or a biological response of the aorta to the stent struts, resulting in myointimal proliferation around the stents [34-36]. A better understanding of these issues is of paramount importance to both clinicians and manufacturers, as they are directly related to the application of appropriate surveillance protocols and stent-graft designs.

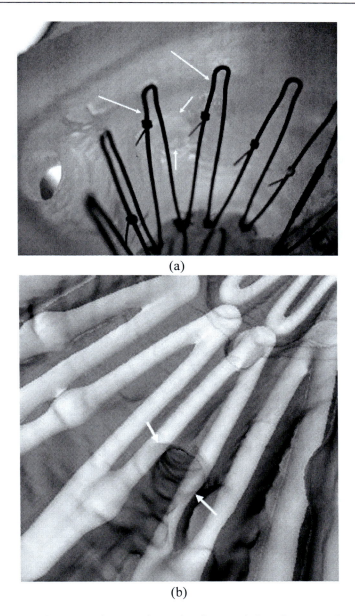

Figure 3. A photograph of an aorta phantom shows that the actual size of suprarenal stents with stent wires crossing the right renal ostium (short arrows in A). Virtual endoscopic view generated with computed tomography image shows that right renal ostium is covered by two stent wires (arrows in B). Long arrows refer to the suprarenal stent wires.

2.2. Fenestrated Stent Grafting

Although suprarenal stent grafting has been employed with apparent success, there are instances in which satisfactory endovascular exclusion of an aortic aneurysm cannot be obtained without sacrificing important side branches. Fenestrated stent-grafts were developed to preserve blood flow to the visceral arteries and enhance stability by inserting stents into the side branches to produce a durable relationship between the graft fenestration and the branch ostium [37, 38].

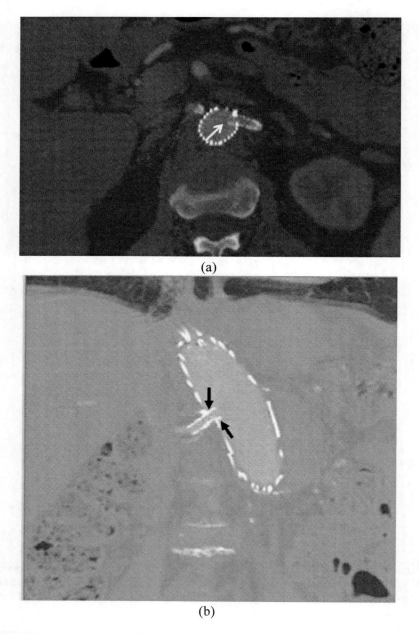

Figure 4. 2D axial image shows a small intra-aortic portion of a fenestrated left renal stent (arrow in A). Coronal reformatted image in another patient reveals the fenestrated right renal stent with intra-aortic protrusion (arrows in B). As shown in these images, most of the fenestrated renal stents remain in the renal arteries with only a small part protruding into the abdominal aorta.

The stent graft fenestration involves creating an opening in the graft fabric to accommodate the orifice of the vessel targeted for preservation. The fenestration can be secured to the renal and other visceral arteries such as celiac axis or superior mesenteric artery by implantation of bare or covered stents across the graft-ostium interface so that a portion of the stent protrudes into the aortic lumen. The principles of fenestration are to preserve blood flow to renal or visceral vessels and enhance stability by inserting stents into side branches to produce a durable relationship between the stent graft fenestration and the branch ostium. The initial animal feasibility study of a fenestrated endovascular graft was reported in 1999 [21], which led to successful implantation in human subjects [39-42]. Today, the primary use of a fenestrated stent-graft is to treat infrarenal aneurysms that have infrarenal necks <10 mm long, or juxtarenal or suprarenal aneurysms with unfavourable aneurysm necks. Fenestrated stent grafts have concerns similar to those that apply to conventional endovascular repair, i.e., structural durability, endoleaks, renal dysfunction, and stent graft migration.

A systematic review of the literature from 1999 to 2006 showed that short-term results of fenestrated stent grafting are encouraging [43]. Perioperative target vessel patency rate was 97% (95% CI, 92%–100%) and 90% (85%–95%) during follow-up. No conversions to open surgery were required. Perioperative mortality was 1.1% (0.4% – 2.7%) and the endoleak rate after 30 days was 9.4% (2.6%–16.3%). However, long-term data are limited, with only four studies reporting more than 12 months' mean follow-up.

Despite advances in endovascular technology, there is the potential loss of the target vessel resulting from the fenestrated technique. Normally, a stent protrudes into the aortic lumen by ~5 mm (Fig 4) [44, 45]. In some cases, an extended portion of the renal stent is placed inside the aorta through fenestrated stent grafting. Thus, it could be expected that blood flow will be affected to some extent in patients treated with fenestrated stent grafts, and this requires further investigation to ensure the long-term safety of this technique.

3. Medical Image Visualization of Abdominal Aortic Aneurysms

Unlike open surgical repair of AAA, successful completion of EVAR largely depends on medical imaging, and spiral CT angiography (CTA) has been confirmed to be the preferred modality in both preoperative planning and postoperative follow-up of endovascular aneurysm repair [46-48].

The development of multislice CT (MSCT) has provided important advantages over single slice CT with regard to CT angiography of the aorta and aortic stent grafts [49, 50]. MSCT enables faster scans than single slice CT by providing high-volume coverage and thin-section image within a single breath hold, resulting in improved spatial resolution in the longitudinal plane. MSCT has been reported to be superior to single slice CT in nearly all clinical applications [49]. Spiral CTA in imaging aorta and stent grafts has been complemented by a series of 3D postprocessing reconstructions, including multiplanar reformation (Fig 5), surface shaded display (Fig 6), maximum-intensity projection (Fig 7), volume rendering (Fig 8) and virtual intravascular endoscopy (Fig 9). These 3D reconstructions have been reported to offer additional information when compared to 2D axial images in both pre-operative planning and post-operative follow-up of aortic stent grafting [44, 45, 51-55].

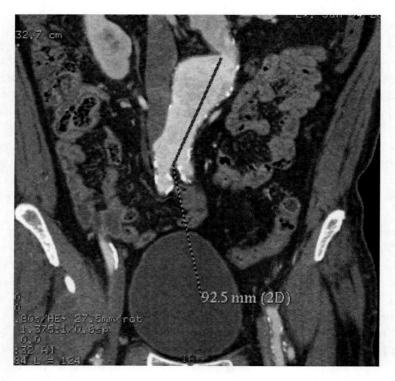

Figure 5. Coronal multiplanar reformatted image shows an infrarenal AAA with measurement of the aneurysm length extending from the infrarenal position to the common iliac arteries.

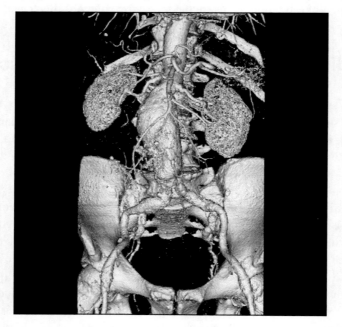

Figure 6. 3D surface shaded display demonstrates an infrarenal AAA with involvement of bilateral common iliac arteries.

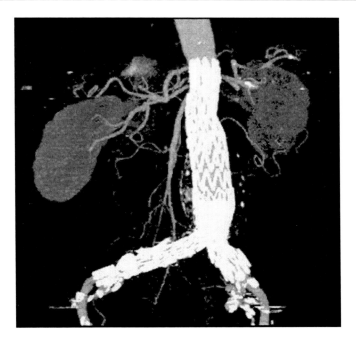

Figure 7. Coronal MIP shows patent renal arteries in a patient treated with suprarenal stent graft. High density suprarenal stents are implanted above the renal arteries with good perfusion to renal arteries and kidneys.

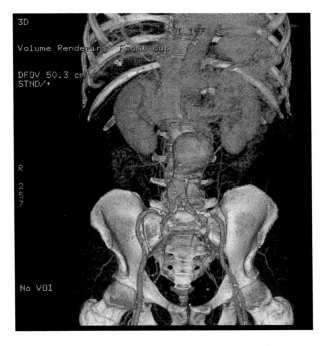

Figure 8. 3D volume rendering shows an infrarenal AAA in relation to the common iliac arteries, kidneys and pelvic bony structures.

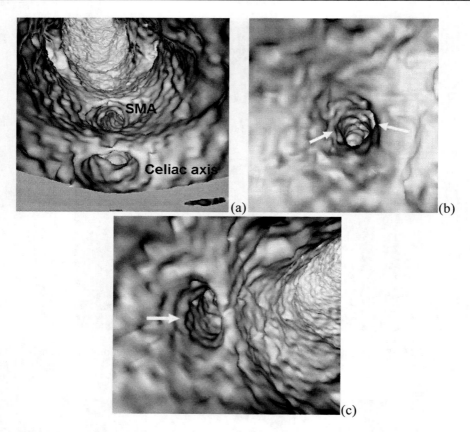

Figure 9. Virtual intravascular endoscopy demonstrates intraluminal appearances of the celiac axis and superior mesenteric ostia (A), left renal ostium (arrows in B) and right renal ostium (arrow in C). SMA- superior mesentery artery.

4. Computational Fluid Dynamics in Endovascular Aneurysm Repair

CT angiography provides excellent anatomical details of abdominal aorta and stent-grafts, thus enabling assessment of the diameter of aneurysms and stent-grafts relative to the aortic branches. Despite these advantages, CT angiography is limited to the image visualization and lacks providing information about hemodynamic changes to the abdominal aorta and renal arteries following implantation of stent-grafts. Although mechanisms are unknown, stent placement may alter local hemodynamcis, which might lead to the dispersion of late multiple emboli when coupled with wall movement [56]. Thus, studies based on computer modeling of AAA pre-and post-stent grafting will assist analysis of hemodynamic changes of the blood vessel, even before the morphological changes such as stenosis or occlusion to the renal or other visceral arteries are actually formed.

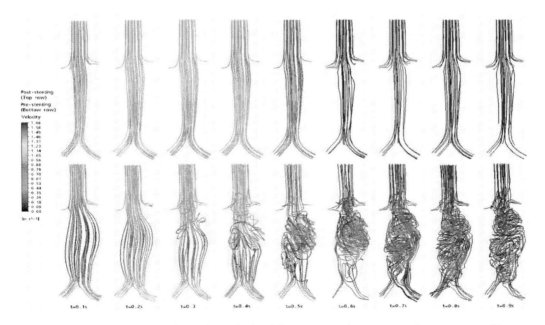

Figure 10. Computational fluid dynamic analysis of flow pattern change pre-and post-stent grafting. The flow recirculation was absent and flow pattern became more smooth and laminar following placement of endovascular stent grafts (t=0.1-0.9s, top row images) than that observed in pre-stent grafting (t=0.1-0.9s, bottom row images). Flow recirculation was more obvious (t=0.6-0.9s) in late diastolic phase than that in systolic phase (t=0.1-0.5s).

In recent years, computational fluid dynamics (CFD) techniques have been increasingly used by researchers seeking to understand vascular hemodynamics. CFD is a numerical method that can provide valuable information that is extremely difficult to be obtained experimentally. CFD methods possess the potential to enhance the data obtained from *in vivo* methods by providing a complete characterization of hemodynamic conditions (blood velocity and pressure as a function of space and time) under precisely controlled conditions. Rigorous CFD analysis is increasingly performed to study the fluid phenomenon inside the human vascular system. Different experimental and numerical studies have focused on the hemodynamic changes in AAA with and without a stent-graft [57-63]. These studies either computed wall stresses or simulated the interaction between blood flow and aneurysm wall in order to assess prognostic factors for aneurysm rupture risk, or measured the flow pattern in stented AAA (Fig 10), or investigated the forces on bifurcated stent-grafts. Only a few studies focused on determining the changes of blood flow after stent-graft implantation by application of coupled fluid structure interaction dynamics [61-63].

4.1. Simulation of Normal Physiological Hemodynamics

In order to ensure that CFD analysis reflects the realistic environment of human blood vessel, normal physiological hemodynamics should be considered for the 3D numerical simulations. This allows studying the aneurismal fluid mechanics by taking into account the instantaneous fluid forces acting on the wall and the effect of the wall motion on the fluid dynamic field. The fluid and materials properties for different entities are referenced from a previous study [62]. The boundary conditions are time-dependent [64]. The velocity inlet (abdominal aorta at the level of celiac axis) boundary conditions (Fig 11) are taken from the referenced value showing measurement of the aortic blood velocity and Reynolds number (Fig 12). A time-dependent pressure is also imposed at the outlets (Fig 13).

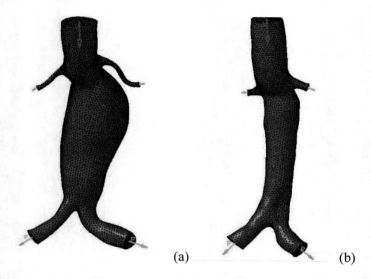

(a)   (b)

Figure 11. An aortic mesh model prior to (A) and post-stent graft implantation (B). Arrows point to the inlet and outlet of blood flow through the abdominal aorta and its branches.

The fluid (blood) is assumed to behave as a Newtonian fluid, as this is well known for the larger vessels of the human body. The implanted stent within the blood is set as a non-fluid material as it is solid and non-elastic. The fluid density is set to 1060 kg/m^3 and a viscosity of 0.0027 Pa s, corresponding to the standard values cited in the literature [64]. The flow is assumed to be incompressible and laminar. Given these assumptions, the fluid dynamics of the system is fully governed by the Navier-Strokes equations.

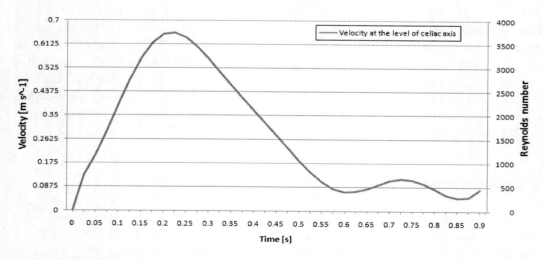

Figure 12. Flow pulsatile at the celiac axis. Flow pulsatile is applied in different cardiac cycles at the celiac axis.

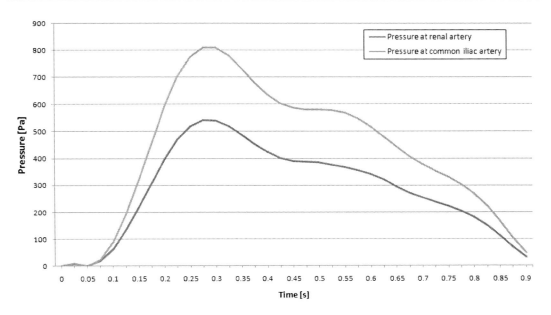

Figure 13. Time-dependent pressure at the main aortic arteries. A time-dependent pressure is applied in different cardiac cycles at the renal and common iliac arteries.

Based on the above parameters, the CFD analysis is performed with the blood flow simulated at different cardiac phases (systolic and diastolic cycles) and calculated in the aortic aneurysm, renal arteries and common iliac arteries in terms of flow pattern, wall pressure and wall shear stress pre-and post-stent grafting.

4.2. Computational Fluid Dynamics in Suprarenal Stent Grafting

The concern of long-term outcomes of suprarenal stent grafting or suprarenal fixation is manifested in two folds: first, the long-term safety of placing the suprarenal stents across the renal arteries is not confirmed with regard to its effect on the renal arteries or renal function; second, the interference of suprarenal stent struts/wires with the renal artery ostium in terms of morphological changes in relation to the configuration/number of stent wires crossing the renal artery ostium is not fully understood. It has been reported that the renal artery ostium demonstrated morphological changes following suprarenal fixation [65], while the effect of stent wires on renal blood flow has not been systematically studied.

Liffman et al in their experimental study using computational fluid dynamics analysis concluded that no significant reduction of renal blood flow was observed when the renal artery ostia (independent of the diameter of renal artery ostia, 3 mm vs 7 mm; or the number of stent wires, single vs multiple) were crossed by stent wires [34]. Our previous report using CFD to analyse the effects of suprarenal stent wires on renal blood flow is consistent with their findings to some extent [63]. Our analysis showed that reduction of flow velocity was independent of the diameter of renal ostium and the number of stent wires. However, our results demonstrated findings different from others as the type of stent struts encroaching the renal ostium and stent wire thickness determined the renal blood flow, with single wire centrally crossing producing more than 20% reduction of flow velocity.

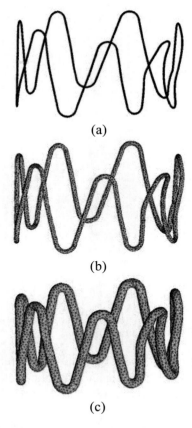

Figure 14. Meshing models of the suprarenal stent wires with a diameter of 0.4 mm, 1.0 mm and 2.0 mm, respectively (A-C).

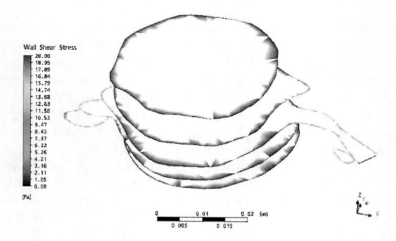

Figure 15. (Continued).

Applications of Computational Fluid Dynamics in Abdominal Aortic Aneurysms 167

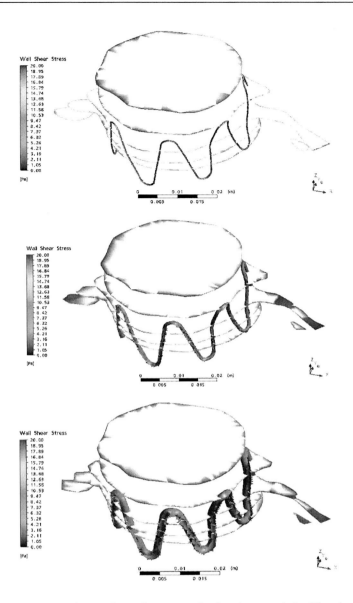

Figure 15. Wall shear stress at the renal arteries was noticed to decreased significanly when the stent wires crossed the renal artery ostia, especially apparent in the presence of stent wires with a diameter of 1.0 mm and 2.0, as shown in Fig 15 C and D, compared to that observed with a wire thickness of 0.4 mm (B) and non-wire crossing (A).

Since it is possible for the blood material to adhere to the wires and thus may affect the flow of blood into the renal artery. This was confirmed by a previous experimental study showing that small bits of materials were deposited onto the wire, leading to the increase of cross-sectional area of the stent wire [34]. Thus, simulation of a stent wire thickness larger than the original diameter of 0.4 mm is necessary to reflect this situation (Fig 14).

The wall shear stress at the renal arteries was found to decrease significantly following suprarenal stent grafting, according to CFD analysis of realistic aortic models (Fig 15) [63], and this should arise clinical awareness, as low wall shear stress is associated with neointimal hyperplasia in either bypass graft or stent [66]. Thus, a low shear stress could lead to reduction of the cross-sectional area of renal ostium owing to presence of stent wires (because of formation of neointimal hyperplasia on the stent surface). It has been reported that augmentation of wall shear stress is accompanied by a local reduction in neointimal hyperplasia [67]. Another potential risk of a low shear stress is the formation of artery plaque or atherosclerosis in the aortic branches [68]. Therefore, from a clinical point of view, hemodynamic analysis of the interference of stent struts with renal arteries is important for understanding the long-term safety of the suprarenal stent grafting, although this needs further studies to confirm it.

4.3. Computational Fluid Dynamics in Fenestrated Stent Grafting

Fixation of the fenestration to the renal and other visceral arteries can be provided by implantation of bare or covered stents across the graft-artery ostia interfaces so that a portion of the fenestrated stents protrudes into the aortic lumen. Short to mid-term outcomes of fenestrated stent grafting are satisfactory [39-41, 69], however, there are concerns about the patency of fenestrated vessels and interference of fenestrated stents with hemodynamics, as normally about one-third of the fenestrated stents protrudes into the aorta after implantation [44, 45]. Although the exact mechanisms are not known, it has been reported that the placement of stents alters the hemodynamics and this coupled with wall movement may lead to the dispersion of late multiple emboli [56]. The complex structures that are introduced into the blood flow (renal blood flow in the fenestrated repair) may enhance biochemical thrombosis cascade [70, 71], as well as directly affect the local hemodynamics.

The purpose of implantation of a stent-graft is to exclude the aneurysm from systemic blood circulation so that the aneurysm gradually shrinks and becomes smaller while the blood flows through the new conduit, which is produced by the stent graft. For this purpose of treatment, there is no difference between conventional endovascular aneurysm repair and fenestrated stent grafting. The unique characteristics of fenestrated stent grafting involve creating an opening in the graft material with insertion of fenestrated stents into the fenestrated vessels, mainly the renal arteries. In addition, a fenestrated stent normally protrudes into the aortic lumen by less than 5 mm, as reported in previous studies (Fig 16) [44, 45]. Therefore, there is a potential risk for fenestrated stents to interfere with renal blood flow. However, this was not observed in a recent study as the calculated velocity to the renal arteries did not show significant changes following implantation of fenestrated stents, indicating the safety of placing fenestrated stents into the renal arteries, even if in the presence of a certain length of stent protrusion (Fig 17) [72].

Realistic AAA models generated from patients treated with fenestrated stent grafts were used to simulate the blood flow patterns and velocity changes, according to our previous study [72]. Moreover, the actual intraluminal appearance of fenestrated renal stents was simulated to reflect the real patients' treatment. It is within expectation that flow recirculation or vortex was observed at the proximal renal arteries because of intra-aortic protruded stents (Fig 17), however, the effect of fenestrated stents on renal velocity was minimal.

CFD analysis of aortic models with simulated fenestrated renal stents showed that the reduced wall shear stress was present in the renal arteries following insertion of fenestrated renal stents, indicating the potential risk of interference with renal hemodynamics or development of stenosis (Fig 18) [72]. From a clinical point of view, hemodynamic analysis of the interference of renal stents is considered important for understanding the long-term safety of the fenestrated stent grafting, although this needs further studies to confirm it.

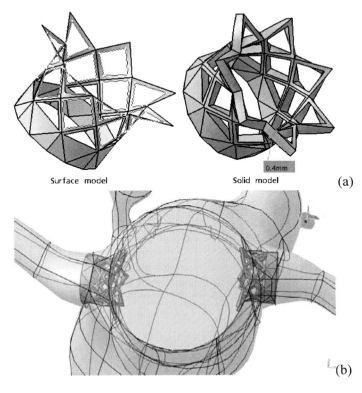

Figure 16. Simulation of intraluminal appearance of fenestrated renal stents. Figure 16A shows the simulated surface and solid models of the fenestrated renal stent, while figure 16B is the appearance of the simulated stent inside the renal arteries with a protruding length of 5-7 mm into the abdominal aorta.

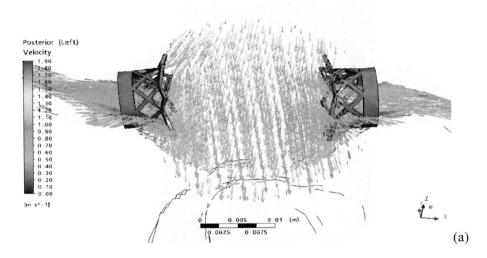

Figure 17. (Continued).

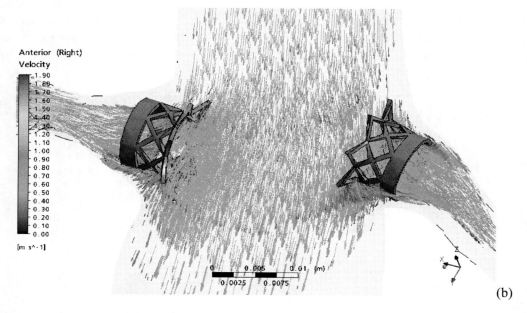

Figure 17. Flow velocity in a realistic aortic model with simulation of fenestrated renal stents. Flow velocity calculated in a patient after placement of fenestrated stents at bilateral renal arteries. Flow recirculation was apparently seen in the proximal parts of the renal arteries due to stent protrusion (A). Flow velocity was slightly decreased in the presence of stent protrusion (7.0 mm) (B), although this did not reach significant difference.

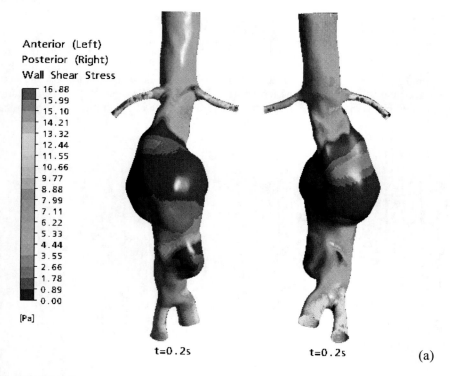

Figure 18. (Continued).

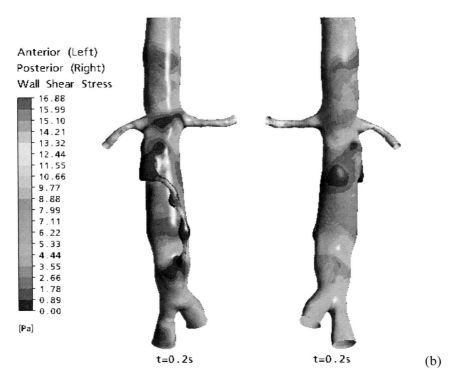

Figure 18. Wall shear stress at pre-and post-fenestration. Wall shear stress was significantly higher inside the aneurysm following fenestration (B) when compared to pre-fenestration (A). Wall shear stress was reduced at the proximal and distal aneurysm necks and renal arteries following fenestrated stent grafting when compared to the pre-stent grafting simulation.

5. Current Status and Future Directions

The large multicenter randomized trials have demonstrated that EVAR is a viable alternative to open repair for the majority of patients presenting with AAA. It has been reported that a clear short-term benefit of EVAR, with 1.7% of patients dying by 30 days compared with 4.7% of those treated with open surgery [73, 74]. In addition, EVAR had at least two-thirds lower 30-day and in-hospital mortality compared with open repair. The randomized trial comparing open and endovascular repair of AAA concluded that endovascular repair is preferable to open repair over the first 30 days after the procedure [74]. These randomized controlled trials indicated that in patients who are candidates for both open surgery and EVAR, endovascular repair leads to lower rates of operative mortality and complications and the significant reduction in the rate of systemic complications, thus it is a preferable approach in these patients.

While open surgery still remains the gold standard for treatment of patients with AAA, there is no doubt that EVAR has been confirmed to be an effective alternative to open surgery. EVAR continues to benefit more patients and it will become more applicable and durable with technical improvements. New stent-graft technology such as fenestrated and branched grafts makes this technique available to more patients, especially in those with unsuitable or complicated aneurysm necks [19, 20, 39-41], although long-term follow-up is needed to prove the stability and patency of fenestrated vessels.

Lifelong surveillance is necessary after EVAR, and there is increasing evidence of a trend from using conventional CT follow-up to ultrasound monitoring [75]. Recent data suggest that EVAR is most beneficial in the fittest patients, who may survive longer [76]. Thus, the long-term risk of radiation-induced cancer needs to be considered when choosing CT as the method of choice for routine follow-up. Optimization of CT scanning protocols is of paramount importance to provide diagnostic images with minimal radiation exposure to patients, as CT is associated with high radiation dose.

Traditional imaging-based surveillance restricted to the monitoring of changes in AAA morphology and the detection of endoleaks has proven unreliable in preventing aneurysm rupture [76]. Accurate endoleak detection and classification is essential following EVAR because an endoleak is evidence of flow, which produces a pressure gradient. Endoleak is the most common complication associated with endovascular aneurysm repair. It is defined as persistent blood flow outside the graft and within the aneurysm sac. Endoleak, regardless of size or type, can transmit systemic pressure to the aneurysm sac, leading to continued expansion of the aneurysm or increased risk for rupture. Researchers using the method of fluid-structure interaction in realistic AAA models evaluated sac pressure, impact of endoleaks on AAA rupture risk, and potential stent-graft migration [77-79]. These analyses indicated that endoleaks may increase sac pressure to near the systemic pressure levels, which could cause more clinical concern.

Liffman et al showed that a transverse oscillating movement of a curved stent-graft system was a function of the pressure difference between the stent-graft and aneurysm [80]. This may be a useful visual diagnostic tool for a vascular surgeon to indicate an endoleak in curved stent-graft systems. If the curved stent-graft oscillates transversely, then there is an insufficient pressure seal (no differential or only a small pressure difference between the stent-graft lumen and aneurysm sac), indicating an endoleak. However, if the curved stent-graft system does not oscillate transversely, then this is consistent with an acceptable pressure seal.

Quantitative hemodynamic changes of flow rate and flow pattern caused by stent-graft implantation can be analysed with CFD, thus allowing more accurate assessment of treatment outcomes. CFD is a highly promising technique and improves our understanding of the local structural and fluid dynamic conditions in patients with AAA after stent-graft placement. The future development of more realistic, patient-specific models will demonstrate potential to assist stent-graft design and improve success rate of EVAR.

Summary and Conclusion

The past decades have witnessed a remarkable evolution and transformation in our approach to the treatment of aortic aneurysms. EVAR has gained wide acceptance in selected patients as an effective alternative to traditional open surgery of abdominal aortic aneurysm. We can expect continuing improvements in endovascular device design to include the treatment of suprarenal and thoracoabdominal aneurysms. The role of open surgical repair will diminish but not disappear. As more experience and skill in endovascular aneurysm repair is gained, vascular specialists will be challenged to maintain their skills in open repair.

EVAR is associated with a lifetime risk of rupture because most patients will live for years after the procedure. Purpose of future research should be improving the efficiency of the follow-up methods after EVAR and evaluation of new stent graft designs to prevent graft-related complications. While medical imaging techniques still play a key role in the routine follow-up of EVAR, use of CFD in the evaluation of treatment outcomes is recommended in patients treated with suprarenal and fenestrated stent grafts. CFD analysis provides insight into the hemodynamic effects of stents wires on the renal arteries, therefore, improving understanding of the interference of implanted stent grafts with blood flow. CFD could be used as a complementary tool to medical image visualization in the efficient follow-up of endovascular aneurysm repair.

References

[1] Alcorn HG, Wolfson SK Jr, Sutton-Tyrell K. Risk factors for abdominal aortic aneurysms in older adults enrolled in Cardiovascular Health Study. *Arterioscler Thromb Vasc Biol* 1996; 16:963–970.

[2] Endovascular stent–grafts for the treatment of abdominal aortic aneurysms. NICE technology appraisal guidance 167. *www.nice.org.uk*.

[3] Desai M, Eaton-Evans J, Hillery C, et al. AAA stent-grafts: past problems and future prospects. *Ann Biomed Eng* 2010; 38: 1259-1274.

[4] Krupski WC, Rutherford RB. Update on open repair of abdominal aortic aneurysms: the challenges for endovascular repair. *J Am Coll Surg* 2004; 199:946–960.

[5] Norrgard O, Angqvist K-A, Johnson O. Familial aortic aneurysms: serum concentrations of triglyceride, cholesterol, HDL-cholesterol and (VLDL+LDL)-cholesterol. *Br J Surg* 1985; 72: 113-116.

[6] Blankensteijn JD, Lindenburg FP, Van der Graaf Y, Eikelboom BC. Influence of study design on reported mortality and morbidity rates after abdominal aortic aneurysm repair. *Br J Surg* 1998; 85:1624–1630.

[7] Dotter CT. Transluminally placed coilspring endarterial tube grafts. Long-term patency in canine popliteal artery. *Invest Radiol*. 1969;4:329-332.

[8] Dotter CT, Buschmann RW, McKinney, MK, et al. Transluminal expandable nitinol coil stent grafting: preliminary report. *Radiology* 1983;147:259-260.

[9] Maass D, Zollikofer CL, Largiader F, et al. Radiological follow-up of transluminally inserted vascular endoprostheses: an experimental study using expanding spirals. *Radiology* 1984;152:659-663.

[10] Duprat G, Wright KC, Charnsangavej C, et al. Flexible balloon-expanded stent for small vessels. Work in progress. *Radiology* 1987;162:276-278.

[11] Parodi JC, Palmaz JC, Barone HD. Transfemoral intraluminal graft implantation for abdominal aortic aneurysms. *Ann Vasc Surg* 1991;5:491-499.

[12] Moore WS, Vescera CL. Repair of abdominal aortic aneurysm by transfemoral endovascular graft placement. *Ann Surg* 1994;220:331-341.

[13] Moore WS, Rutherford RB. Transfemoral endovascular repair of abdominal aortic aneurysm: results of the North American EVT phase 1 trial. *J Vasc Surg* 1996;23:543-553.

[14] Chuter TAM, Wendt G, Hopkinson BR, et al. Bifurcated stent-graft for abdominal aortic aneurysm. *Cardiovasc Surg* 1997;5:388-392.

[15] Blum U, Voshage G, Beyerdorf F, et al. Two-center German experience with aortic endografting. *J Endovasc Surg* 1997;4:137-146.

[16] Marin ML, Parsons RE, Hollier LH, et al. Impact of transrenal aortic endograft placement on endovascular graft repair of abdominal aortic aneurysms. *J Vasc Surg* 1998;28:638-646.

[17] Birch PC, Start RD, Whitbread T, et al. The effects of crossing porcine renal artery ostia with various endovascular stents. *Eur J Vasc Endovasc Surg* 1999;17:185-190.

[18] Malina M, Lindh M, Ivancev K, et al. The effect of endovascular aortic stents placed across the renal arteries. *Eur J Vasc Endovasc Surg* 1997;13:207-213.

[19] Ferko A, Krajina A, Jon B, et al. Juxtarenal aortic aneurysm: endoluminal transfemoral repair? *Eur Radiol* 1997;7:703-707.

[20] Stanley BM, Semmens JB, Lawrence-Brown MMD, et al. Fenestration in endovascular grafts for aortic aneurysm repair: new horizons for preserving blood flow in branch vessels. *J Endovasc Ther* 2001;8:16-24.

[21] Browne TF, Hartley D, Purchas S, et al. A fenestrated covered suprarenal aortic stent. *Eur J Vasc Endovasc Surg* 1999;18:445-449.

[22] Lawrence DD, Charnsangavej C, Wright KC, et al. Percutaneous endovascular graft: experimental evaluation. *Radiology* 1987;163:357-360.

[23] Yoshioka T, Wright KC, Wallace S, et al. Self-expanding endovascular graft: an experimental study in dogs. *AJR Am J Roentgenol* 1988;151:673-676.

[24] Gordon MK, Lawrence-Brown MMD, Hartley D, et al. A self-expanding endoluminal graft for treatment of aneurysms: results through the development phase. *Aust NZ J Surg* 1996;66:621-625.

[25] Lawrence-Brown M, Hartley D, MacSweeney STR, et al. The Perth endoluminal bifurcated graft system - development and early experience. *Cardiovasc Surg* 1996;4:706-712.

[26] Malina M, Lindblad B, Ivancev K, et al. Endovascular AAA exclusion: will stents with hooks and barbs prevent stent-graft migration? *J Endovasc Surg* 1998;5:310-317.

[27] Lobato AC, Quick RC, Vaughn PL, et al. Transrenal fixation of aortic endografts: intermediate follow-up of a single-center experience. *J Endovasc Ther* 2000;7:273-278.

[28] Bove PG, Long GW, Zelenock GB, et al. Transrenal fixation of aortic stent-grafts for the treatment of infrarenal aortic aneurysmal disease. *J Vasc Surg* 2000;32:697-703.

[29] Alric P, Hinchliffe RJ, Picot MC, et al. Long-term renal function following endovascular aneurysm repair with infrarenal and suprarenal aortic stent-grafts. *J Endovasc Ther* 2003;10:397-405.

[30] Izzedine H, Koskas F, Cluzel P, et al. Renal function after aortic stent-grafting including coverage of renal arterial ostia. *Am J Kidney Dis* 2002;39:730-736.

[31] O'Donnell, Sun Z, Winder J, Lau LL, Ellis PK, Blair PH. Suprarenal fixation of endovascular aortic stent grafts: assessment of medium-term to long-term renal function by analysis of juxtarenal stent morphology. *J Vasc Surg* 2007; 45: 694-700.

[32] Burks JA, Faries PL, Gravereaux EC, et al. Endovascular repair of abdominal aortic aneurysms: stent-graft fixation across the visceral arteries. *J Vasc Surg* 2002;35:109-113.

[33] Cayne NS, Rhee SJ, Veith FJ, et al. Does transrenal fixation of aortic endografts impair renal function? *J Vasc Surg* 2003;38:639-644.

[34] Liffman K, Lawrence-Brown MMD, Semmens JB, et al. Suprarenal fixation: effect on blood flow of an endoluminal stent wire across an arterial orifice. *J Endovasc Ther* 2003;10:260-274.

[35] Desgranges P, Huntin E, Kedzia C, et al. Aortic stents covering the renal artery ostia: an animal study. *J Vasc Interv Radiol* 1997;8:77-82.

[36] Yee DC, Williams SK, Salzmann DL, et al. Stent versus endovascular graft healing characteristics in the porcine iliac artery. *J Vasc Surg* 1998;9:609-617.

[37] Anderson JL, Berce M, Hartley D. Endoluminal aortic grafting with renal and superior mesenteric artery incorporation by graft fenestration. *J Endovasc Ther* 2001;8:3-15.

[38] Park JH, Chung JW, Choo IW, et al. Fenestrated stent-grafts for preserving visceral arterial branches in the treatment of abdominal aortic aneurysms: preliminary experience. *J Vasc Interv Radiol* 1996;7:819-823.

[39] Muhs BE, Verhoeven EL, Zeebregts CJ, et al. Mid-term results of endovascular aneurysm repair with branched and fenestrated endografts. *J Vasc Surg* 2006;44:9-15.

[40] Verhoeven EL, Prins TR, Tielliu IF, et al. Treatment of short-necked infrarenal aortic aneurysms with fenestrated stent-grafts: short-term results. *Eur J Vasc Endovasc Surg* 2004;27:477-483.

[41] Greenberg RK, Haulon S, O'Neill S, et al. Primary endovascular repair of juxtarenal aneurysms with fenestrated endovascular grafting. *Eur J Vasc Endovasc Surg* 2004;27:484-491.

[42] Greenberg RK, Haulon S, Lyden SP, et al. Endovascular management of juxtarenal aneurysms with fenestrated endovascular grafting. *J Vasc Surg* 2004;39:279-287.

[43] Sun Z, Mwipatayi BP, Semmens JB, Lawrence-Brown MM. Short to midterm outcomes of fenestrated endovascular grafts in the treatment of abdominal aortic aneurysms: a systematic review. *J Endovasc Ther* 2006; 13:747–753

[44] Sun Z, Allen Y, Nadkarni S, Wright R, Hartley D, Lawrence-Brown M. CT virtual intravascular endoscopy in the visualization of fenestrated endovascular grafts. *J Endovasc Ther* 2008; 15:42-51.

[45] Sun Z, Allen Y, Mwipatayi B, Hartley D, Lawrence-Brown M. Multislice CT angiography in the follow-up of fenestrated endovascular grafts: Effect of slice thickness on 2D and 3D visualization of the fenestrated stents. *J Endovasc Ther* 2008; 15: 417- 426.

[46] Sun Z. Helical CT angiography of abdominal aortic aneurysms treated with suprarenal stent grafting. *Cardiovasc Intervent Radiol* 2003; 26: 290-295.

[47] Rydberg J, Kopecky KK, Lalka SG, et al. Stent grafting of abdominal aortic aneurysms: Pre- and postoperative evaluation with multislice helical CT. *J Comput Assit Tomgr* 2001; 25(4): 580-586.

[48] Armerding MD, Rubin GD, Beaulieu CF, Slonim SM, Olcott EW, Samuels SL, et al. Aortic aneurysmal disease: Assessment of stent-grafted treatment-CT versus conventional angiography. *Radiology* 2000; 215: 138-146.

[49] Hu H, He HD, Foley WD, Fox SH. Four multidetector-row helical CT: image quality and volume coverage speed. *Radiology* 2000; 215: 55-62.

[50] Rubin GD, Shiau MC, Leung AN, Kee ST, Logan LJ, Sofilos MC. Aorta and iliac arteries: single versus multiple detector-row helical CT angiography. *Radiology* 2000; 215: 670-676.

[51] Sun Z. 3D multislice CT angiography in post-aortic stent grafting: A pictorial essay. *Korean J Radiol* 2006; 7: 205-211.

[52] Sun Z, Allen Y, Mwipatayi B, Hartley D, Lawrence-Brown M. Multislice CT angiography of fenestrated endovascular stent grafting of abdominal aortic aneurysms: A pictorial review of 2D/3D visualizations. *Korean J Radiol* 2009; 10: 285-293.

[53] Sun Z, Squelch A, Bartlett A, Cunningham K, Lawrence-Brown M. 3D stereoscopic visualization in fenestrated stent grafts. *Cardiovasc Intervent Radiol* 2009; 32: 1053-1058.

[54] Sun Z, Winder J, Kelly B, Ellis P, Hirst D. CT virtual intravascular endoscopy of abdominal aortic aneurysms treated with suprarenal endovascular stent grafting. *Abdom Imaging* 2003; 28(4): 580-587.

[55] Sun Z, Winder J, Kelly B, Ellis P, Kennedy P, Hirst D. Diagnostic value of CT virtual intravascular endoscopy in aortic stent grafting. *J Endovasc Ther* 2004, 11: 13-25.

[56] Richter GM, Palmaz JC, Noeldge G, et al. Relationship between blood flow, thrombus, and neointima in stents. J Vasc Interv Radiol 1999; 10:598–604.

[57] Chong CK, How TV. Flow patterns in an endovascular stent-graft for abdominal aortic aneurysm repair. *J Biomech* 2004;37:89–97.

[58] Di Martino ES, Guadagni G, Fumero A, et al. Fluid–structure interaction within realistic three-dimensional models of the aneurysmatic aorta as a guidance to assess the risk of rupture of the aneurysm. *Med Eng Phys* 2001; 23:647–655.

[59] Wang DH, Makaroun MS, Webster MW, et al. Effect of intraluminal thrombus on wall stress in patient-specific models of abdominal aortic aneurysm. *J Vasc Surg* 2002; 36:598–604.

[60] Li Z, Kleinstreuer C. Fluid–structure interaction effects on sac blood pressure and wall stress in a stented aneurysm. *J Biomech Eng* 2005; 127:662–671.

[61] Li Z, Kleinstreuer C. Blood flow and structure interactions in a stented abdominal aortic aneurysm model. *Med Eng Phys* 2005; 27:369–382.

[62] Frauenfelder T, Lotfey M, Boehm T, Wildermuth S. Computational fluid dynamics: Hemodynamic changes in abdominal aortic aneurysm after stent-graft implantation. *Cardiovasc Intervent Radiol* 2006; 29: 613-623

[63] Sun Z, Chaichana T. Investigation of hemodynamic effect of stent wires on renal arteries in patients with abdominal aortic aneurysms treated with suprarenal stent grafts. *Cardiovasc Intervent Radiol* 2009; 32: 647-657.

[64] Borghi A, Wood N, Mohiaddin R., Xu X. Fluid-solid interaction simulation of flow and stress pattern in thoracoabdominal aneurysms: A patient-specific study. *J Fluids Structures* 2007; 2: 270-280.

[65] Sun Z, O'Donnell M, Winder R, Ellis P, Blair P. Effect of suprarenal fixation of aortic stent grafts on renal ostium: Assessment of morphological changes by virtual intravascular endoscopy. *J Endovasc Ther* 2007; 14: 650-660.

[66] Wentzel J, Krams R, Schuurbiers J, et al. Relationship between neointimal thickness and shear stress wall stent implantation in human coronary arteries. *Circulation* 2001; 103: 1740-1745.

[67] Carlier S, van Damme L, Blommerde C, et al. Augmentation of wall shear stress I inhibits neointimal hyperplasia after stent implantation: Inhibition through reduction inflammation? *Circulation* 2003; 107: 2741-2746.

[68] Prati F, Di Mario C, Moussa I, et al. In-stent neointimal proliferation correlates with the amount of residual plaque burden outside the stent: an intravascular ultrasound study. *Circulation* 1999; 99: 1011-1014.

[69] SemmensJB, Lawrence-Brown MD, Hartley DE, Allen YB, Green R, Nadkarni S. Outcomes of fenestrated endografts in the treatment of abdominal aortic aneurysms in Western Australia (1997-2004). *J Endovasc Ther* 2006; 13: 320-329.

[70] Beythien C, Gutensohn K, Bau J, et al. Influence of stent length and heparin coating on platelet activation: a flow cytometric analysis in a pulsed floating model. *Thrombosis Research* 1999; 94: 79-86.

[71] Peacock J, Hankins S, Jones T, Lutz R. Flow instabilities induced by coronary artery stents: assessment with an in vitro pulse duplicator. *J Biomech* 1995; 28: 17-26.

[72] Sun Z, Chaichana T. Fenestrated stent graft repair of abdominal aortic aneurysm: Hemodynamic analysis of effect of fenestrated stents on renal arteries. *Korean J Radiol* 2010; 11: 95-106.

[73] Greenhalgh RM, Brown LC, Kwong GP, et al. Comparison of endovascular aneurysm repair with open repair in patients with abdominal aortic aneurysm (EVAR trial1), 30-day operative mortality results: randomised controlled trial. *Lancet* 2004; 364: 843-848.

[74] Prinssen M, Verhoeven EL, Buth J, et al. A randomized trial comparing conventional and endovascular repair of abdominal aortic aneurysms. *N Engl J Med* 2004; 14 (351): 1607-1618.

[75] Lawrence-Brown MMD, Sun Z, Semmens JB, Liffman K, Sutalo ID, Hartley DB. Type II endoleaks: when is intervention indicated and what is the index of suspicion for types I or III? *J Endovasc Ther* 2009; 16 (Suppl I): I 106-I 118.

[76] Weerakkody RA, Walsh SR, Cousin C, et al. Radiation exposure during endovascular aneurysm repair. *Br J Surg* 2008;95:699–702.

[77] Li Z, Kleinstreuer C. Effects of major endoleaks on a stented abdominal aortic aneurysm. *ASME J Biomech Eng* 2006;128:59-68.

[78] Li Z, Kleinstreuer C. Computational analysis of type II endoleaks in a stented abdominal aortic aneurysm model. *J Biomech* 2006;39:2573-2582.

[79] Chong CK, How TV, Gilling-Smith GL, et al. Modeling endoleaks and collateral reperfusion following endovascular AAA exclusion. *J Endovasc Ther* 2003;10:424-432.

[80] Liffman K, Sutalo ID, Lawrence-Brown MM, et al. Movement and dislocation of modular stent-grafts due to pulsatile flow and the pressure difference between the stent-graft and the aneurysm sac. *J Endovasc Ther* 2006;13:51-61.

Chapter 14

Echocardiographic Evaluation of Fetal Hemodynamics

Mio Taketazu and Hideaki Senzaki
Saitama Medical University, Saitama, Japan

Introduction

Fetal hemodynamics differs considerably from postnatal hemodynamics, in the characteristics of the myocardium and specific channels of blood flow. The basic knowledge about mammalian fetal circulation has been derived from studies on sheep. With the recent development of fetal echocardiography, human fetal hemodynamics can be evaluated under normal and abnormal conditions. Since the relations between adult cardiovascular impairments and abnormal hemodynamics in utero have been studied for a long period[1, 2], it is now important to understand fetal cardiovascular physiology and the mechanism of cardiovascular disturbance after birth. This chapter outlines the hemodynamics of fetal circulation and in utero evaluation of cardiovascular physiology with fetal echocardiography.

1. Hemodynamics of Fetal Circulation

Fetal Circulation

In utero, oxygenation occurs in the placenta and the oxygenated blood returns to the fetus through the umbilical vein. After birth, oxygenation occurs in the lungs of the infant and pulmonary circulation is completely separated from systemic circulation. There is no mixing of oxygenated pulmonary venous blood and systemic venous blood. Studies on fetal lambs have shown that about half of the blood from the umbilical vein bypasses the hepatic circulation and directly enters the inferior vena cava via the ductus venosus [3]. Although well-oxygenated blood flow through the ductus venosus is confluent with the systemic venous blood flow of the abdominal inferior vena cava and hepatic vein, the ductus venosus blood flow is preferentially distributed through the foramen ovale into the left atrium and left ventricle, and the blood from the inferior and superior vena cava passes through the tricuspid valve and is distributed into the right ventricle [4] (Figure 1). The mechanisms for this selective streaming have not been fully defined. One of the possible mechanisms is that a part of the atrium septum overlies the inferior vena cava and directs the posterior left portion of the inferior vena caval blood into the left atrium. Another potential mechanism is the difference in the blood stream velocities between the abdominal inferior vena cava and the ductus venosus. The mean blood velocity in the ductus venosus is much higher than that in the abdominal inferior vena cava, which results in the difference between the velocities of the ductus venosus and abdominal vena caval stream [5]. After receiving poorly oxygenated blood from the superior vena cava and inferior vena cava, the right ventricle ejects the blood into the main pulmonary artery. Because both the right and left ventricles eject blood into systemic circulation in utero, fetal cardiac output is usually expressed as combined cardiac output (CCO) of the 2 ventricles. In chronically instrumented fetal lambs, the volume of blood ejected by the right ventricle is about two-thirds that of the CCO [6]. In humans, the ratio of right to left ventricular output is about 1.2-1.3 to 1 [7, 8], probably because of the differences in the blood distribution to the brain between human fetus and lamb fetus. Further, the right ventricular output is about 55% of CCO in the human fetus. Because of the high resistance of pulmonary arteries in utero, only 25% of CCO passes into the pulmonary circulation even in the late gestation period [6, 9]. The remaining blood is directed into the descending aorta via the ductus arteriosus, and there is no retrograde flow through the ductus arteriosus to the ascending aorta and its branches [4].

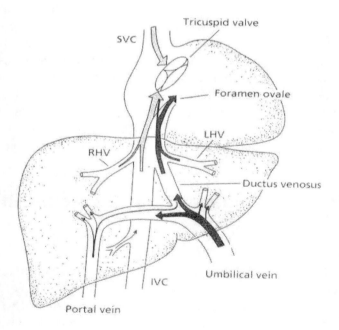

Figure 1. Venous flow distribution in a lamb fetus. Ductus venosus blood preferentially flows through the foramen ovale, while the inferior/superior vena caval blood is preferentially directed toward the tricuspid valve. SVC, superior vena cava; IVC, inferior vena cava; LHV, left hepatic vein; RVH, right hepatic vein [6].

The highly oxygenated blood from the foramen ovale and the blood from the pulmonary veins enters the left ventricle through the left atrium and is ejected into the ascending aorta. Most of the left ventricular output is distributed to the upper body, including the coronary and cerebral circulation, which is about 35% of CCO [4]. The remaining blood (10% of CCO) passes across the aortic isthmus into the descending aorta and mixes with the blood from the ductus arteriosus, which accounts for 40% of CCO distributing the lower body and placenta. Because of the low resistance of placenta, 26% of CCO is distributed in the placenta [4, 6] (Figure 2).

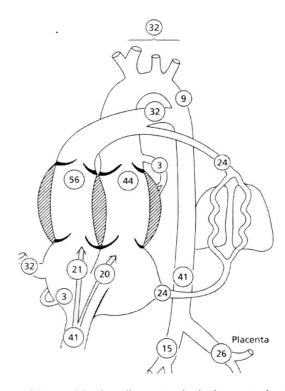

Figure 2. The percentages of the combined cardiac output in the late-gestation human fetus [6].

Fetal Vascular Pressures

Since the fetus is surrounded by amniotic fluid in the uterus, all fetal vascular pressures are affected by the pressure in the amniotic cavity. In ewe, intra-amniotic pressure is usually 8 to 10 mmHg and fetal venous pressures are supposed to be similar to amniotic pressure at the baseline [6].

The umbilical venous pressure is about 8 to 10 mmHg near the umbilical ring; normally, the pressure shows continuous flat waveform with no phase change during atrial systole. The effect of no pulsatile pressure extends into the portal vein, where the mean pressure is 5 to 6 mmHg. In contrast, the inferior and superior vena caval pressures show phasic waveforms with the cardiac cycle. The mean pressures in the superior and inferior vena cava and the right atrium are about 2 to 3 mmHg, and the mean left atrial pressure is 1 to 2 mmHg, which is lower than the right atrial pressure. The right and left systolic and end-diastolic ventricular pressures are similar because the ductus arteriosus connects the aortic artery and the main pulmonary artery. Aortic pressure increases with gestational age in the lamb fetus, from the mean level of 25 to 30 mmHg to 60 to 70 mmHg [6].

Oxygen Saturation in Blood

There is a large pO_2 gradient across the placenta; maternal arterial pO_2 is 90 to 100 mmHg in the pregnant ewe, while the pO_2 of umbilical venous blood is 32 to 35 mmHg. Since the P50 (the pO_2 at which hemoglobin is saturated by 50%) for fetal blood in the sheep is lower than that of adult blood, the oxygen saturation of umbilical venous blood is about 90% [6]. The blood in abdominal inferior vena cava, hepatic veins, and superior vena cava has an oxygen saturation of 35% to 40%. While the right ventricular oxygen saturation is 50%, the left ventricular and ascending aortic blood has oxygen saturation of about 55%.

Determinants of Fetal Cardiac Output

1.) Fetal Myocardium

Histologically, the fetal myocardium is composed of up to 60% of noncontractile elements, whereas the adult myocardium contains only 30% noncontractile elements [10]. The small number of sarcomeres and contractile units in the fetal myocardium reduce the contractile ability of fetal heart. The number of sarcomeres and the myofilament content of the cells change with maturation, with the acquisition of the transverse tubular system. Impaired calcium release process from troponin C in fetus has also been observed in experimental animal studies [11]. Sympathetic nerve endings are sparse or even absent in fetal myocardium [12-14], and the concentration of beta-adrenergic receptor, which influences the response to stress, is low in fetal heart [15]. These immaturities of fetal myocardium influence the contraction, stiffness, and relaxation of fetal heart.

Despite these immaturities, the fetal systolic performance estimated by fetal echocardiography appears to be similar to that of the adults in normal physiologic situations. There is only a small difference in the combined ventricular output, normalized for fetal body weight, between 18 weeks of gestation and full-term. The dp/dt max of the left ventricle of the fetal lamb is comparable to the values of the adult ewe [16]. The shortening fraction of the left ventricle measured by M-mode echocardiography is an average of 32% throughout the second and third trimester of pregnancy in the fetus [17]. In contrast, impaired relaxation of the fetal myocardium is observed in the Doppler velocity patterns through the atrioventricular valves. In the fetus, A wave is greater than E wave throughout the gestation period, indicating that passive early filling is impaired and active atrial contraction mainly contributes to empty the atrium [18].

2.) Heart Rate

The role of heart rate in regulating cardiac output is an area of controversy in fetal physiology. In the studies of fetal lamb, changes in the heart rate and not the Frank-Starling mechanism is the key determinant of cardiac output, since increases in preload result in only limited increases in stroke volume and cardiac output [19, 20]. However, in Doppler echocardiographic study of human fetus, increase in heart rate within a physiologic range results in a decrease in ventricular size and volume but it does not change the ventricular output [21].

3.) Preload

In newborn lambs, rapid intravenous infusions of 0.9% NaCl solution increased cardiac output with an increase in atrial pressure [22]. Cardiac output increased progressively with an elevation of atrial pressure to 15 mmHg. Similarly, fetal output increased when atrial pressure increased by 2 to 4 mmHg above resting levels with intravenous infusion of electrolyte solution; however, further increase in pressure does not result in greater output by the ventricle [6, 23, 24], suggesting that fetal heart normally operates near the peak of its ventricular function curve (Figure 3). Increased myocardial stiffness may explain this limitation in stroke volume augmentation in fetal heart. When end-diastolic diameter is used as a preload index, a positive relationship has been found between the diameter and stroke volume in fetal lamb [16]. A decrease in atrial pressure with the removal of fetal blood results in a reduction of cardiac output [23].

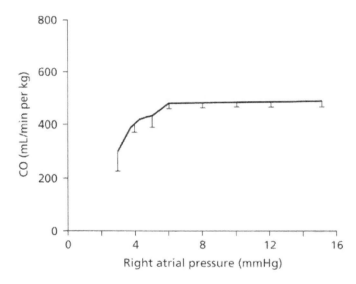

Figure 3. Changes in combined cardiac output with acute reduction of atrial pressure by blood removal and increase in atrial pressure by infusion of electrolyte solution in fetal lambs [6]. CO, cardiac output.

4.) Afterload

In studies of fetal lambs, arterial pressure elevation by balloon occlusion of aortic isthmus markedly reduced left ventricular stroke volume at constant atrial pressure levels [25] (Figure 4). In the fetal lamb, right ventricle exhibits greater sensitivity to changes in afterload than left ventricle [26]. Clinically, the ductus arteriosus is the communication between the aorta and pulmonary artery, which results in almost identical pressures in both ventricles. The main peripheral elements contributing to fetal ventricular afterload are the placental circulation to the right ventricle and the cerebral circulation to the left ventricle. Under high placental resistance in the case of uteroplacental insufficiency, selective changes in peripheral vascular resistances, the so-called brain-sparing effect, influence the fetal cardiac hemodynamics [27]. Cerebral vasodilation decreases left ventricular afterload and results in a relative increase in the left cardiac output together with decreased right cardiac output. These hemodynamic changes are compatible with the preferential shift of cardiac output to the left ventricle and improve the perfusion to the brain.

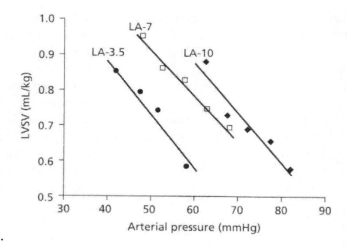

Figure 4. An increase in arterial pressure reduces the left ventricular volume at fixed atrial pressure. Further, at any level of arterial pressure, an increase in left atrial pressure increases the left ventricular stroke volume. LVSV, left ventricular stroke volume; LA, left atrial pressure [6].

Alteration of Blood Flow Distribution with Advancing Gestation

The proportion of the CCO distributed to the fetal organs and placenta changes with advancing gestation. The blood flow to placenta decreases gradually with gestational age, from 45% at midterm to 38% to 40% at term in lambs. Blood distribution of the brain increases progressively from 2.2% at midterm to 3% at term in lambs, and reaches 24% in human fetuses [6]. The percentages of CCO to the lungs and gastrointestinal tract increase rapidly at the end of gestation. The increase in flow to these organs could be related to increase in the size of the vascular bed, due to growth in new vessels or increased metabolic activity with vasodilatation.

2. Evaluation of Fetal Hemodynamics with Fetal Echocardiography

Many parameters have been proposed for quantitative evaluation of fetal cardiac function. Most parameters were first developed for adult heart evaluation and were then adapted to the fetus.

M-Mode Assessment

In the fetal examination, the M-mode cursor is placed perpendicular to interventricular septum at the level of mitral and tricuspid valves. Shortening fraction is one of the most frequently used parameters to represent fetal ventricular contraction. Shortening fraction and the mean velocity of circumferential fiber shortening (mean Vcf) are constant throughout the gestation period, with the level of shortening fraction of approximately 0.3 and the mean Vcf approximately 1.3 in both ventricles [17].

Recently, ventricular long-axis function, ie, the performance of the longitudinally oriented fibers, has been extensively studied in adults and children using conventional M-mode echocardiography [28-30] and has been adopted for fetal examination using free-angular M-mode[31]. This technique can be used to evaluate the right ventricular function, because of the longitudinal orientation of the deep right ventricular muscle fibers [32, 33], and for evaluating the fetal cardiac function that is mainly performed by the right ventricle. However, cardiac functional assessment in the fetus is yet to be fully performed.

Atrioventricular Flow

In the normal fetus, the A-wave is always greater than the E-wave, but the E/A ratio increases throughout the gestation period. The increase in E/A ratio is due to increasing E-wave velocity, while the A-wave remains constant throughout the gestation period [18]. The increase in E-wave might result from improved ventricular relaxation [34]. Alternatively, it may indicate changes in preload with advancing gestation. Although the fetal E/A ratio shows poor correlation with isovolumetric relaxation time [35] or venous flow patterns [36], monophasic A-V flow patterns, with the complete absence of normal biphasic morphology, indicate poor cardiac output state, such as aortic stenosis [37], twin-to-twin transfusion syndrome [38], and in cases of fetal growth, retardation with poor prognosis [39].

Myocardial Performance Index

In the fetus, left ventricular myocardial performance index (MPI) is obtained by simultaneous Doppler trace of the left ventricle outflow and inflow (Figure 5). Although alteration of fetal MPI is a controversial issue in normal conditions [40-42], the fetal MPI in abnormal conditions indicate the outcomes of impaired fetuses. In twin-to-twin transfusion syndrome, MPI of the recipient fetus correlates with pathologic severity [38, 43, 44]. MPI is also abnormal in fetuses with growth retardation [45, 46], suggesting the abnormal cardiac physiology in this condition. Left ventricular MPI might be an important index predicting poor outcome in fetuses with Epstein's anomaly [47, 48].

Doppler Flow Assessment of Fetal Peripheral Vessels

The fetal cardiac function is not only assessed based on the measurements of intracardiac function but also by Doppler assessment of the fetal circulation, which provides a complete evaluation of the effects of cardiac preload and afterload on fetal wellbeing. Doppler flow assessment of fetal peripheral vessels can give information about the alteration of flow distribution through the gestation period or the distribution under abnormal condition and their influence on fetal cardiac output or function.

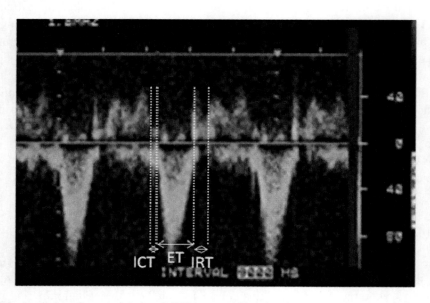

Figure 5. Myocardial performance index (MPI) measured by simultaneous Doppler trace at left ventricular outflow and inflow. ET, ventricular ejection time; ICT, isovolumetric contraction time; IRT, isovolumetric relaxation time. MPI = (ICT + IRT)/ET.

Analysis of Doppler flow within venous channels contiguous with the atriums provides a good approximation of the pressure within atrium itself (Figure 6). The normal waveforms of these veins are constructed by S-wave indicating the maximal forward flow corresponding to ventricular systole, D-wave corresponding to early ventricular diastole, and A-wave corresponding to atrial kick. Doppler indices of venous waveforms are used to evaluate the signs of fetal congestive heart failure, and the inferior vena cava and ductus venosus have been most intensively studied for this purpose. Preload index, which is the ratio between the peak velocity of A-wave and the peak velocity of S-wave in inferior vena cava velocity waveform, is one of the useful indices to predict fetal compromise [49]. Flow velocity wave form in the ductus venosus also changes significantly in cardiac dysfunction. Normally, the wave form is biphasic pattern with S-wave, D-wave, and a trough during atrial contraction. No reverse or cessation of flow during atrial systole is observed in the ductus venosus.

Because of the parallel arrangement of ventricles and the presence of shunts between right and left circulations, fetal blood distribution can change depending on the in utero environment. In fetal growth restriction due to uteroplacental insufficiency, selective changes in peripheral blood flow distribution, the so-called brain-sparing effect, may occur [27]. In this condition, umbilical artery resistance increases, and internal carotid and middle cerebral artery resistance reduces, resulting in an increase in the flow distribution to the brain and a decrease in flow to the descending aorta [50-52]. Cerebral vasodilatation decreases left ventricular afterload, and subsequently systemic and pulmonary vasoconstriction increases right ventricular afterload [53]. As a consequence, left cardiac output is relatively increased while right cardiac output is relatively decreased. These intracardiac hemodynamic changes improve the perfusion to the brain and myocardium and serve to maintain oxygen supply to the brain at near normal levels. However, in deteriorating fetuses, cardiac output gradually declines, suggesting that a progressive deterioration of cardiac function and cardiac filling is also progressively impaired. In these fetuses, ventricular filling properties are impaired with a lower E/A ratio at the atrioventricular valves, possibly due to myocardial impairment by hypoxemia 53. Increased A-wave reversal in the inferior vena cava occurs with progressive fetal deterioration, suggesting a high pressure in the right atrium [49].

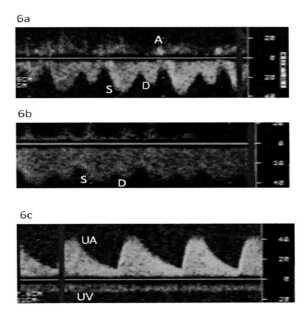

Figure 6. Venous velocity waveforms in a normal fetus. (6a) Velocity waveform from the inferior vena cava showing the systolic (S) and diastolic (D) waves and reverse flow during atrial contraction (A). (6b) Velocity waveform from the ductus venosus. (6c) Velocity waveforms from the umbilical artery (UA) and vein (UV). Note the continuous flow pattern in the umbilical vein.

Further deterioration extends the abnormal reverse flow in the inferior vena cava to the ductus venosus, and finally, the high venous pressure causes a reduction of velocity at end diastole in the umbilical vein, causing typical end-diastolic pulsations [54] (Figure 7). At this stage, intrauterine death may occur at a median of 3.5 days later [55]. Reversal of A-wave in the ductus venosus and pulsatile umbilical venous flow are also indicative of stage III in Quintero staging of twin-to-twin transfusion syndrome [56]. The waveforms of the inferior vena cava and ductus venosus can also indicate left heart failure because of the widely open foramen ovale in normal heart structure; however, while the pulmonary venous flow pattern does not significantly change the left heart failure in normally structured heart. Nevertheless, pulmonary venous waveforms are well correlated with high left atrium pressure in left heart obstruction [57]. Normally, pulmonary venous waveform is constructed with a forward S-wave, D-wave, and forward or small reverse flow during atrial contraction. In hypoplastic left heart syndrome, continuous forward S- and D-wave with a small A-wave reversal are observed when foramen ovale is wide open. However, the reverse A-wave increases in size with the obstruction of foramen ovale. The short, very pulsatile, to-and-fro flow pattern suggests critically high left atrial pressure and indicates critical outcome after birth (Figure 8).

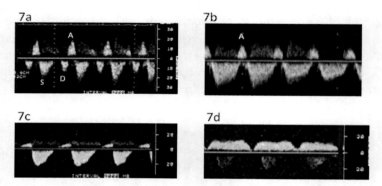

Figure 7. Venous velocity waveforms in a severely growth-restricted fetus. (7a) Velocity waveform from the inferior vena cava showing the systolic (S) and diastolic (D) waves and markedly increased reverse flow during atrial contraction (A). (7b) Velocity waveform from the ductus venosus. The large A-wave is reversed. (7c) Velocity waveform from the umbilical artery. Note the absence of end-diastolic velocities. (7d) Velocity waveform from the umbilical vein. A typical end-diastolic pulsation is observed.

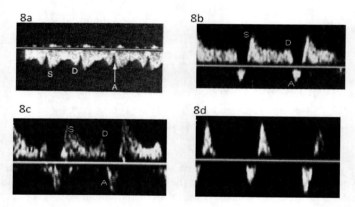

Figure 8. Pulmonary venous velocity waveforms in a normal fetus and in fetuses with hypoplastic left heart syndrome. (8a) Velocity waveforms in the normal fetus. S, forward wave during ventricular systole. D, forward wave during ventricular diastole. A, cessation of forward flow during atrial contraction. (8b). Velocity waveforms in a fetus with hypoplastic left heart syndrome and widely open foramen ovale. A small A-wave is observed. (8c), velocity waveform in a fetus with hypoplastic left heart syndrome and restrictive foramen ovale. A-wave is larger than that observed in 8b. (8d) The forward and reverse blood flow observed in a fetus with hypoplastic left heart syndrome and intact atrium septum.

3. Newly Advanced Techniques for Fetal Heart Evaluation

Three- and Four-Dimensional Ultrasonography

Three- and four-dimensional ultrasonography (3DUS/4DUS) technologies are used for fetal cardiac evaluation, mainly with the aid of spatiotemporal image correlation (STIC) [58].

This technique can deliver a volume dataset containing a complete reconstructed cardiac cycle, and an operator can measure the cardiac ventricle volume either manually or semi-automatically even if the shapes of ventricles are distorted. The studies of 3DUS/4DUS assessment of fetal cardiac function are based primarily on cardiac ventricular volumetry. Virtual Organ Computer-aided AnaLysis (VOCAL) is a new technique that measures the volume of a defined area automatically by reconstructing planes around a fixed central axis, and is applied to evaluate the normal or abnormal ventricular volume, fetal stroke volume, ejection fraction, or cardiac output [59, 60].

Tissue Doppler Imaging

While fetal tissue Doppler imaging (TDI) measurement is often technically difficult because of inadequate fetal position or low myocardial peak velocities, recent studies support the use of TDI as a sensitive tool for evaluating abnormal cardiac function in fetuses with growth restriction [45, 61, 62] or fetal hydrops [63]. Although there still have been conflicting reports about its usefulness in the assessment of fetal cardiac function, they have commonly revealed failed diastolic function (higher E/E' ratio or higher E'/A' ratio) or high myocardial performance index measured with TDI in affected fetuses.

Magnetic Resonance Imaging

Accurate delineation and functional assessment of the right ventricle are important in fetal circulation. Magnetic resonance imaging (MRI) is currently considered to be the reference standard for the right ventricle assessment after birth [64, 65]. The most important factor limiting the introduction of MRI in fetal cardiology is the lack of ECG-triggering method in utero. In an animal model, a novel triggering method involving MR-compatible cardiotocography allowed the assessment of fetal cardiac function [66]. Metric optimized gating in the absence of a gating signal can be another technique to evaluate fetal cardiac function with MRI. The technique was validated with pulsatile flow phantom in experiments with adults and in vivo application in the fetal population [67]. In the sheep model, fetal oxygen saturation in the carotid artery and both ventricles could be assessed with MR oximetry [68]. With these ongoing developments, fetal cardiac MRI will probably be technically feasible in the future.

Conclusion

Despite the limitation of a lack of pressure measurement, fetal echocardiography provides useful information about pathophysiology of fetal hemodynamics. Development of the newer mode of echo machines together with our incessant inquiring mind could further explore the mystery of fetal circulation.

References

[1] Barker DJ. The origins of the developmental origins theory. *Journal of internal medicine*. 2007;261:412-417

[2] Cheung YF, Wong KY, Lam BC, Tsoi NS. Relation of arterial stiffness with gestational age and birth weight. *Arch Dis Child*. 2004;89:217-221

[3] Edelstone DI, Rudolph AM. Preferential streaming of ductus venosus blood to the brain and heart in fetal lambs. *Am J Physiol*. 1979;237:H724-729

[4] Rudolph AM. Distribution and regulation of blood flow in the fetal and neonatal lamb. *Circ Res*. 1985;57:811-821

[5] Schmidt KG, Silverman NH, Rudolph AM. Assessment of flow events at the ductus venosus-inferior vena cava junction and at the foramen ovale in fetal sheep by use of multimodal ultrasound. *Circulation*. 1996;93:826-833

[6] Rudolph AM. *Congenital diseases of the heart: Clinical-physiological considerations.* . Wiley-Blackwell; 2009.

[7] Allan LD, Chita SK, Al-Ghazali W, Crawford DC, Tynan M. Doppler echocardiographic evaluation of the normal human fetal heart. *Br Heart J*. 1987;57:528-533

[8] De Smedt MC, Visser GH, Meijboom EJ. Fetal cardiac output estimated by doppler echocardiography during mid- and late gestation. *Am J Cardiol*. 1987;60:338-342

[9] Rasanen J, Wood DC, Weiner S, Ludomirski A, Huhta JC. Role of the pulmonary circulation in the distribution of human fetal cardiac output during the second half of pregnancy. *Circulation*. 1996;94:1068-1073

[10] Friedman WF. The intrinsic physiologic properties of the developing heart. *Prog Cardiovasc Dis*. 1972;15:87-111

[11] Mahony L. Calcium homeostasis and control of contractility in the developing heart. *Semin Perinatol*. 1996;20:510-519

[12] Lipp JA, Rudolph AM. Sympathetic nerve development in the rat and guinea-pig heart. *Biology of the neonate*. 1972;21:76-82

[13] Friedman WF, Pool PE, Jacobowitz D, Seagren SC, Braunwald E. Sympathetic innervation of the developing rabbit heart. Biochemical and histochemical comparisons of fetal, neonatal, and adult myocardium. *Circ Res*. 1968;23:25-32

[14] Lebowitz EA, Novick JS, Rudolph AM. Development of myocardial sympathetic innervation in the fetal lamb. *Pediatr Res*. 1972;6:887-893

[15] Birk E, Tyndall MR, Erickson LC, Rudolph AM, Roberts JM. Effects of thyroid hormone on myocardial adrenergic beta-receptor responsiveness and function during late gestation. *Pediatr Res*. 1992;31:468-473

[16] Anderson P. Myocardial development. *Fetal and neonatal cardiology*. 1990:17-38

[17] DeVore GR, Siassi B, Platt LD. Fetal echocardiography. Iv. M-mode assessment of ventricular size and contractility during the second and third trimesters of pregnancy in the normal fetus. *Am J Obstet Gynecol*. 1984;150:981-988

[18] Reed KL, Meijboom EJ, Sahn DJ, Scagnelli SA, Valdes-Cruz LM, Shenker L. Cardiac doppler flow velocities in human fetuses. *Circulation*. 1986;73:41-46

[19] Rudolph AM, Heymann MA. Cardiac output in the fetal lamb: The effects of spontaneous and induced changes of heart rate on right and left ventricular output. *Am J Obstet Gynecol*. 1976;124:183-192

[20] Rudolph AM, Heyman MA. Fetal and neonatal circulation and respiration. *Annual review of physiology*. 1974;36:187-207

[21] Kenny J, Plappert T, Doubilet P, Salzman D, Sutton MG. Effects of heart rate on ventricular size, stroke volume, and output in the normal human fetus: A prospective doppler echocardiographic study. *Circulation*. 1987;76:52-58

[22] Klopfenstein HS, Rudolph AM. Postnatal changes in the circulation and responses to volume loading in sheep. *Circ Res*. 1978;42:839-845

[23] Gilbert RD. Control of fetal cardiac output during changes in blood volume. *Am J Physiol*. 1980;238:H80-86

[24] Thornburg KL, Morton MJ. Filling and arterial pressures as determinants of left ventricular stroke volume in fetal lambs. *Am J Physiol*. 1986;251:H961-968

[25] Hawkins J, Van Hare GF, Schmidt KG, Rudolph AM. Effects of increasing afterload on left ventricular output in fetal lambs. *Circ Res*. 1989;65:127-134

[26] Reller MD, Morton MJ, Reid DL, Thornburg KL. Fetal lamb ventricles respond differently to filling and arterial pressures and to in utero ventilation. *Pediatr Res*. 1987;22:621-626

[27] Peeters LL, Sheldon RE, Jones MD, Jr., Makowski EL, Meschia G. Blood flow to fetal organs as a function of arterial oxygen content. *Am J Obstet Gynecol*. 1979;135:637-646

[28] Henein MY, Gibson DG. Normal long axis function. *Heart*. 1999;81:111-113

[29] Henein MY, Gibson DG. Long axis function in disease. *Heart*. 1999;81:229-231

[30] Jones CJ, Raposo L, Gibson DG. Functional importance of the long axis dynamics of the human left ventricle. *Br Heart J*. 1990;63:215-220

[31] Carvalho JS, O'Sullivan C, Shinebourne EA, Henein MY. Right and left ventricular long-axis function in the fetus using angular m-mode. *Ultrasound Obstet Gynecol*. 2001;18:619-622

[32] Ho SY, Nihoyannopoulos P. Anatomy, echocardiography, and normal right ventricular dimensions. *Heart*. 2006;92 Suppl 1:i2-13

[33] Gardiner HM, Pasquini L, Wolfenden J, Barlow A, Li W, Kulinskaya E, Henein M. Myocardial tissue doppler and long axis function in the fetal heart. *Int J Cardiol*. 2006;113:39-47

[34] Carceller-Blanchard AM, Fouron JC. Determinants of the doppler flow velocity profile through the mitral valve of the human fetus. *Br Heart J*. 1993;70:457-460

[35] Van Mieghem T, Dekoninck P, Steenhaut P, Deprest J. Methods for prenatal assessment of fetal cardiac function. *Prenat Diagn*. 2009

[36] Hecher K, Campbell S, Doyle P, Harrington K, Nicolaides K. Assessment of fetal compromise by doppler ultrasound investigation of the fetal circulation. Arterial, intracardiac, and venous blood flow velocity studies. *Circulation*. 1995;91:129-138

[37] Makikallio K, McElhinney DB, Levine JC, Marx GR, Colan SD, Marshall AC, Lock JE, Marcus EN, Tworetzky W. Fetal aortic valve stenosis and the evolution of hypoplastic left heart syndrome: Patient selection for fetal intervention. *Circulation*. 2006;113:1401-1405

[38] Rychik J, Tian Z, Bebbington M, Xu F, McCann M, Mann S, Wilson RD, Johnson MP. The twin-twin transfusion syndrome: Spectrum of cardiovascular abnormality and development of a cardiovascular score to assess severity of disease. *Am J Obstet Gynecol.* 2007;197:392 e391-398

[39] Makikallio K, Rasanen J, Makikallio T, Vuolteenaho O, Huhta JC. Human fetal cardiovascular profile score and neonatal outcome in intrauterine growth restriction. *Ultrasound Obstet Gynecol.* 2008;31:48-54

[40] Tsutsumi T, Ishii M, Eto G, Hota M, Kato H. Serial evaluation for myocardial performance in fetuses and neonates using a new doppler index. *Pediatr Int.* 1999;41:722-727

[41] Hernandez-Andrade E, Figueroa-Diesel H, Kottman C, Illanes S, Arraztoa J, Acosta-Rojas R, Gratacos E. Gestational-age-adjusted reference values for the modified myocardial performance index for evaluation of fetal left cardiac function. *Ultrasound Obstet Gynecol.* 2007;29:321-325

[42] van Splunder IP, Wladimiroff JW. Cardiac functional changes in the human fetus in the late first and early second trimesters. *Ultrasound Obstet Gynecol.* 1996;7:411-415

[43] Raboisson MJ, Fouron JC, Lamoureux J, Leduc L, Grignon A, Proulx F, Gamache S. Early intertwin differences in myocardial performance during the twin-to-twin transfusion syndrome. *Circulation.* 2004;110:3043-3048

[44] Stirnemann JJ, Mougeot M, Proulx F, Nasr B, Essaoui M, Fouron JC, Ville Y. Profiling fetal cardiac function in twin-twin transfusion syndrome. *Ultrasound Obstet Gynecol.* 2010;35:19-27

[45] Comas M, Crispi F, Cruz-Martinez R, Figueras F, Gratacos E. Tissue doppler echocardiographic markers of cardiac dysfunction in small-for-gestational age fetuses. *Am J Obstet Gynecol.* 2011;205:57 e51-56

[46] Cruz-Martinez R, Figueras F, Hernandez-Andrade E, Oros D, Gratacos E. Changes in myocardial performance index and aortic isthmus and ductus venosus doppler in term, small-for-gestational age fetuses with normal umbilical artery pulsatility index. *Ultrasound Obstet Gynecol.* 2011;38:400-405

[47] Chen Y, Lv G, Li B, Wang Z. Cerebral vascular resistance and left ventricular myocardial performance in fetuses with ebstein's anomaly. *Am J Perinatol.* 2009;26:253-258

[48] Inamura N, Taketazu M, Smallhorn JF, Hornberger LK. Left ventricular myocardial performance in the fetus with severe tricuspid valve disease and tricuspid insufficiency. *Am J Perinatol.* 2005;22:91-97

[49] Rizzo G, Capponi A, Talone PE, Arduini D, Romanini C. Doppler indices from inferior vena cava and ductus venosus in predicting ph and oxygen tension in umbilical blood at cordocentesis in growth-retarded fetuses. *Ultrasound Obstet Gynecol.* 1996;7:401-410

[50] Groenenberg IA, Wladimiroff JW, Hop WC. Fetal cardiac and peripheral arterial flow velocity waveforms in intrauterine growth retardation. *Circulation.* 1989;80:1711-1717

[51] Bilardo CM, Nicolaides KH, Campbell S. Doppler measurements of fetal and uteroplacental circulations: Relationship with umbilical venous blood gases measured at cordocentesis. *Am J Obstet Gynecol.* 1990;162:115-120

[52] Vyas S, Nicolaides KH, Bower S, Campbell S. Middle cerebral artery flow velocity waveforms in fetal hypoxaemia. *Br J Obstet Gynaecol.* 1990;97:797-803

[53] Rizzo G, Arduini D, Romanini C. Doppler echocardiographic assessment of fetal cardiac function. *Ultrasound Obstet Gynecol.* 1992;2:434-445

[54] Rizzo G, Capponi A, Soregaroli M, Arduini D, Romanini C. Umbilical vein pulsations and acid-base status at cordocentesis in growth-retarded fetuses with absent end-diastolic velocity in umbilical artery. *Biology of the neonate.* 1995;68:163-168

[55] Baschat AA, Gembruch U, Reiss I, Gortner L, Diedrich K. Demonstration of fetal coronary blood flow by doppler ultrasound in relation to arterial and venous flow velocity waveforms and perinatal outcome--the 'heart-sparing effect'. *Ultrasound Obstet Gynecol.* 1997;9:162-172

[56] Quintero RA, Morales WJ, Allen MH, Bornick PW, Johnson PK, Kruger M. Staging of twin-twin transfusion syndrome. *J Perinatol.* 1999;19:550-555

[57] Taketazu M, Barrea C, Smallhorn JF, Wilson GJ, Hornberger LK. Intrauterine pulmonary venous flow and restrictive foramen ovale in fetal hypoplastic left heart syndrome. *J Am Coll Cardiol.* 2004;43:1902-1907

[58] Yagel S, Cohen SM, Shapiro I, Valsky DV. 3d and 4d ultrasound in fetal cardiac scanning: A new look at the fetal heart. *Ultrasound Obstet Gynecol.* 2007;29:81-95

[59] Hamill N, Yeo L, Romero R, Hassan SS, Myers SA, Mittal P, Kusanovic JP, Balasubramaniam M, Chaiworapongsa T, Vaisbuch E, Espinoza J, Gotsch F, Goncalves LF, Lee W. Fetal cardiac ventricular volume, cardiac output, and ejection fraction determined with 4-dimensional ultrasound using spatiotemporal image correlation and virtual organ computer-aided analysis. *Am J Obstet Gynecol.* 2011;205:76 e71-10

[60] Messing B, Cohen SM, Valsky DV, Rosenak D, Hochner-Celnikier D, Savchev S, Yagel S. Fetal cardiac ventricle volumetry in the second half of gestation assessed by 4d ultrasound using stic combined with inversion mode. *Ultrasound Obstet Gynecol.* 2007;30:142-151

[61] Watanabe S, Hashimoto I, Saito K, Watanabe K, Hirono K, Uese K, Ichida F, Saito S, Miyawaki T, Niemann P, Sahn DJ. Characterization of ventricular myocardial performance in the fetus by tissue doppler imaging. *Circ J.* 2009;73:943-947

[62] Naujorks AA, Zielinsky P, Beltrame PA, Castagna RC, Petracco R, Busato A, Nicoloso AL, Piccoli A, Manica JL. Myocardial tissue doppler assessment of diastolic function in the growth-restricted fetus. *Ultrasound Obstet Gynecol.* 2009;34:68-73

[63] Aoki M, Harada K, Ogawa M, Tanaka T. Quantitative assessment of right ventricular function using doppler tissue imaging in fetuses with and without heart failure. *J Am Soc Echocardiogr.* 2004;17:28-35

[64] Mogelvang J, Stubgaard M, Thomsen C, Henriksen O. Evaluation of right ventricular volumes measured by magnetic resonance imaging. *Eur Heart J.* 1988;9:529-533

[65] Krishnamurthy R. The role of mri and ct in congenital heart disease. *Pediatr Radiol.* 2009;39 Suppl 2:S196-204

[66] Yamamura J, Kopp I, Frisch M, Fischer R, Valett K, Hecher K, Adam G, Wedegartner U. Cardiac mri of the fetal heart using a novel triggering method: Initial results in an animal model. *Journal of magnetic resonance imaging : JMRI.* 2012

[67] Jansz MS, Seed M, van Amerom JF, Wong D, Grosse-Wortmann L, Yoo SJ, Macgowan CK. Metric optimized gating for fetal cardiac mri. *Magnetic resonance in medicine : official journal of the Society of Magnetic Resonance in Medicine / Society of Magnetic Resonance in Medicine.* 2010;64:1304-1314

[68] Wedegartner U, Kooijman H, Yamamura J, Frisch M, Weber C, Buchert R, Huff A, Hecher K, Adam G. In vivo mri measurement of fetal blood oxygen saturation in cardiac ventricles of fetal sheep: A feasibility study. *Magnetic resonance in medicine : official journal of the Society of Magnetic Resonance in Medicine / Society of Magnetic Resonance in Medicine.* 2010;64:32-41

Chapter 15

Contribution of Renal or Glomerular Hemodynamic in Evaluating Renal Diseases and Drug Effects in the Kidney

Ana D. O. Paixão*, Bruna R. M. Sant'Helena and Leucio D. Vieira-Filho

Departamento de Fisiologia e Farmacologia, Universidade Federal de Pernambuco, Recife, PE, Brazil

Introduction

Renal hemodynamics refers to the forces or mechanisms involved in blood circulation through the kidney. When these forces are changed, fluid maintenance and renal integrity could be threatened. Blood pressure (BP) drives renal hemodynamics: it determines the status of glomerular capillary pressure (P_{GC}) and the glomerular filtration rate (GFR). The kidneys have autoregulatory mechanisms that protect the organism from unnecessary loss of fluid and maintain their structural integrity when BP is changed [1, 2]. Renal autoregulation consists of 2 synchronized mechanisms, known as myogenic and tubuloglomerular feedbacks (TGF), which are triggered when BP increases. The myogenic mechanism depends only on blood pressure-induced contractility on the afferent arteriole, while TGF involves the macula densa in the juxtaglomerular apparatus. These mechanisms regulate renal blood flow (RBF) by afferent arteriole vasoconstriction, and thus P_{GC} and GFR increments are prevented. In humans, the initial stage of diabetic nephropathy is frequently associated with loss of renal autoregulation and afferent arteriolar vasodilatation [3]. In hypertensive individuals, renal function depends on the stage of hypertension. When arteriolar disease is minimal, the arteriole autoregulate accordingly, while in conditions in which significant renal arteriolar

---

* Corresponding author: Ana D. O. Paixão, Departamento de Fisiologia e Farmacologia, Universidade Federal de Pernambuco, Av. Prof. Moraes Rego, s/n – Cidade Universitária, 50670-901, Recife, PE, Brazil.

disease develops, such as in the setting of severe hypertension, the autoregulatory response is impaired [4]. In experimental models, the fawn-hooded hypertensive rat is characterized by impairment of myogenic tone [5] and precocious renal end-organ damage, whereas the spontaneously hypertensive rat (SHR) is characterized by exaggerated pressure-induced afferent arteriolar constriction [6] and late occurrence of glomerulosclerosis [7]. The BP range for renal autoregulation varies among species, but it normally begins at 75-85 mmHg and ranges up to 160 mmHg [1]. Below and above the range of autoregulation, RBF is dependent on BP, leaving the kidney more vulnerable to structural adaptations that may develop with renal damage.

In this chapter, it will be briefly reviewed the importance of experimental evidence that show how whole renal and glomerular hemodynamic studies help to understand renal structural changes that could lead to chronic kidney disease (CKD) in hypertensive or diabetic rats.

1. Measurement of Whole Renal and Glomerular Hemodynamics

One current method to measure renal hemodynamics in humans or experimental animals depends on creatinine or inulin and para-aminohipuurate clearances for GFR and renal plasma flow (RPF), respectively. A hematocrit (Hct) reading is also needed, to calculate the RBF, when RBF = RPF/(1 − Hct). Other useful hemodynamic parameters are filtration fraction (FF), which is the ratio between GFR and RPF (FF = GFR/RPF), and renal vascular resistance (RVR), which is the ratio between mean arterial pressure (MAP) and RBF (RVR = MAP/RBF). Besides creatinine and inulin, the clearances of others substances such as ^{125}I-iothalamate can be useful in measuring GFR.

For experimental animals, apparatuses that measure RBF, such as flowmeters are available. RPF is calculated from RBF and Hct values. The method used in our Laboratory to measure renal hemodynamics in rats is given below.

Measurement of Renal Hemodynamics in Rats

Renal hemodynamics are measured under sodium pentobarbital (60 mg/kg i.p), anesthesia, as previously described [8-10]. Briefly, animals are tracheostomized using PE-240 polyethylene tubing. The left femoral artery and both jugular veins are catheterized with PE-50 polyethylene tubing, and the left ureter is catheterized with PE-10 polyethylene tubing. A flow probe (1.0 V, Transonic System) is placed around the left renal artery. Mean arterial pressure (MAP) and Hct are measured immediately after femoral artery catheterization (i.e. initial MAP and initial Hct, respectively). To assess GFR, 10% inulin in physiological saline is infused at 1.2 ml/h through the left jugular vein. To maintain euvolemia, iso-oncotic serum (20% v/w) is infused through the right jugular vein during surgery and throughout the evaluation of renal hemodynamics [11]. After the surgical procedure has been completed, anesthesia is supplemented (45 mg/kg i.p). Measurement of renal hemodynamics is initiated 1 h after completion of surgery, comprised of 2 x 20 min intervals during which 2 urinary samples and 3 blood samples are collected. MAP and RBF are continuously monitored during both periods using a BP transducer (Transpac) and a flow probe, respectively, the recordings being carried out with Windaq. Inulin is measured by the method of Fuhr [12]. Each renal hemodynamic parameter is corrected for the corresponding kidney weight (g).

Measurement of Glomerular Hemodynamics

In the first half of the twenty century, the micropuncture technique used in kidney of frog and *Necturus*, proved useful in identifying the nature of glomerular ultrafiltrate in the proximal tubule, as well as the fluid composition in other tubular segments [13]. At the beginning of second half of the century, micropuncture was used to identify renal autoregulation mechanisms [13], and in the early 1970s, when Munich-Wistar rats were identified, it was used to determine the physical forces driving the single nephron glomerular filtration rate (SNGFR) [14], once this strain had glomeruli on the kidney surface. Another novelty at that time was the direct measurement of P_{GC} using a servo-nulling pressure transducer. Some parameters of glomerular hemodynamics, such as SNGFR, hydrostatic pressure in the proximal tubule (P_T), efferent arteriolar filtration pressure (P_{EA}) and peritubular hydrostatic pressure (P_C) had been measured in Sprague-Dawley rats, as well as P_{GC}, but using an indirect method, the stop flow technique [15]. Other parameters were established at that time. They included the measurement of the unique ultrafiltration coefficient (K_f) and its independence from glomerular plasma flow (Q_A) in volume expanded rats [16], the Q_A dependence of SNGFR in euvolemic and expanded rats [17], the increased afferent (R_A) and efferent arteriolar (R_E) resistances during ischemia that prevents increment in P_{GC} [18], increased P_{GC} as the basis for renal structural injury in hypertension [19], and the role of increased oncotic pressure in efferent arteriole on glomerulotubular balance [20]. In the following two decades, glomerular hemodynamic studies defined some aspects of the correlation between hypertension and CKD, such as glomerular hypertension (i. e. increased P_{GC}) leads to susceptibility to progressive glomerular injury [21, 22].

2. Knowledge of Renal Hemodynamics in Hypertension

In the United States of America, hypertension is considered the second cause of CKD [23]. Changes in renal hemodynamics due to increased MAP are important causes of renal injury [7, 24]. Fawn-hooded rats are a genetic model of hypertension that leads to precocious albuminuria and glomerulosclerosis [22]. Early development of kidney disease is due to loss of myogenic tonus in afferent arterioles [5], as a consequence of increased production of paracrine vasodilator factors and also the development of arteriolopathy [25]. Glomerular hemodynamics in these rats is characterized by increased R_E, increased P_{GC} and SNGFR, and unchanged Q_A [24]. Once vasodilador factors are increased in the juxtaglomerular apparatus, renin secretion is increased [25], that makes angiotensin-converting enzyme inhibitor (ACEi) and angiotensin type 1 receptor blockade particularly useful to ameliorate the progression of kidney disease[26, 27]. Fawn-hooded rats have a renal failure locus (Rf-1) indentified on chromosome 1 [28]. This region is located on chromosome 10 in humans. A linkage analysis in African American sib-pairs concordant for end-stage renal disease shows that this locus might be involved in early onset non-diabetic etiologies of end-stage renal disease [29]. Results showing the Rf-1 locus in hypertensive rats and humans suggest that changes that are inherent in the kidney may be responsible for precocious renal injury and fast progression of CKD.

Although the results from animal models of human diseases must be interpreted with caution, they can provide important ways of elucidating the pathophysiology seen in humans. SHR is the most widely used animal model of essential hypertension. The young SHR has increased R_A responsible for unaltered P_{GC}, whereas the old SHR show loss of myogenic tonus in the afferent arteriole and has increased P_{GC} [7]. Mechanisms underlining the elevated R_A in young SHR are: a reduced availability of nitric oxide [30, 31], increased production of thromboxane A_2 [32], and increased endogenous activity of the renin-angiotensin system [7]. The old SHR develops glomerulosclerosis because renal autoregulation is lost after 3 months [33], particularly in the juxtamedullary nephrons [34].

Renal function in hypertensive individuals depends on the stage of hypertension. When arteriolar disease is minimal, arterioles autoregulate appropriately to prevent transmission of systemic hypertension to the glomeruli; GFR then remains relatively preserved and renal disease progresses slowly. However, when significant renal arteriolar disease develops, as in severe hypertension, the autoregulatory response becomes impaired and renal disease progresses much more rapidly [4]. The first stage is most frequently observed in early or borderline hypertension and is characterized by salt-resistance, while in the second stage salt-sensitivity is observed [4].On the other hand, the renovascular hypertension is determined by renal microvascular lesion. In humans with essential hypertension, increased renal arteriolar lesions, reduced RPF and reduced GFR are correlated [4]. Hypertension develops in patients with renovascular ischemia due to activation of the renin-angiotensin system, recruitment of oxidative stress and the sympatho-adrenergic system. A sustained reduction in renal perfusion leads to disturbed microvascular function, vascular rarefaction and ultimately interstitial fibrosis [35]. By infusing angiotensin II into rats and dogs, Anderson and coworkers [36] proposed that hypertension could be induced by structural changes in preglomerular resistant vessel walls.

One experimental model characterized by renal ischemia is 2-kidney, 1-clip Goldblatt hypertension [37, 38]. Sprague-Dawley rats that have one clip installed around the left renal arterial develop increased oxidative stress in the kidney after 3 weeks, hypertension [37, 38] and reduced RPF and GFR [37]. The structural consequences are tubulointerstitial fibrosis, glomerular sclerosis and hyalinosis [39]. Differently, the unclipped kidney in Goldblatt hypertensive rats has increased P_{GC} and unaltered GFR due to reduced K_f as a consequence of increased circulating angiotensin [40].

Renal hemodynamic measurement in a hypertension model dependent on sodium, the Dahl salt-sensitive (Dahl S) rats, shows that these animals develop high renovascular resistance, reduced RBF and reduced GFR in sodium overload [41, 42]. This autoregulation is absent in old rats, but renal injury begins before it has been comprised [41]. Persistent elevated renovascular resistance in Dahl S rats has been correlated with overactivity of NADPH oxidase [42], increased oxidative stress, and also endothelial comprise as observed by reduced renal nitric oxide availability [43] and decreased renal GMPc production [44]. Another experimental model of salt-dependent hypertension is the Milan hypertensive strain

(MHS), in which sodium dependence is partly due to a mutation in the α- and β-adducin genes [45]; this leads to increased expression/activity of renal tubular Na^+K^+ATPase and increased sodium retention [46]. However, these animals develop afferent arteriolar hypertrophy [47], which prevents systemic hypertension transfer to glomerular capillaries. Renal hemodynamics in these animals is characterized by increased RVR that makes them resistant to diabetic nephropathy when they are treated with streptozotocin [48, 49].

Together, these findings cover the pivotal role of renal ischemia or glomerular hypertension in renal injury found in hypertensive individuals, whether hypertension is the cause of renal injury, or renal microvascular alterations are the cause of hypertension.

3. Knowledge of Renal Hemodynamics in Diabetes

Diabetes mellitus is the most common cause of CKD in the USA and other countries [23]. Increased GFR is one of the earliest indications of altered kidney function in diabetic patients [50-52]; it is commonly used as a predictor of the later development of progressive renal dysfunction. The most commonly accepted hypothesis for diabetes-induced glomerular hyperfiltration involves an inactivated TGF mechanism [53-55] and loss of myogenic tonus [3]. One reason for compromised TGF might be increased sodium reabsorption in the proximal tubule throughout the sodium-glucose co-transport that leads to a low sodium in the juxtaglomerular apparatus [56]. Moreover myogenic tonus could also be lost due to a remodeling in afferent arterioles [3]. In the face of renal autoregulation impairment, glomerular hypertension plays a central role on diabetic nephropathy.

Experimental animal models to study diabetic nephropathy are primarily: i) streptozotocin-induced diabetes, a type I diabetes model; ii) obese Zucker rats, a type II diabetes model; iii) spontaneously diabetic rats; and iv) db/db mice, also a type II diabetes model that has mutations in the gene for leptin receptor. Leptin is a cytokine receiving much attention for its role as a regulator of energy balance.

As seen in type I [51] and type II [52] diabetic patients, streptozotocin-induced diabetic rats have increased GFR, due to increased SNGFR in superficial [57, 58] and juxtamedullary nephrons [59], found as soon as 7-10 days after induction. Increased SNGFR is also seen in the type II diabetic model, db/db mice [55] and obese Zucker rats [60]. In contrast, spontaneously diabetic rats do not have glomerular hyperfiltration or glomerular hypertension [61]. Independently from systemic blood pressure, glomerular hyperfiltration and glomerular hypertension have a fundamental role in glomerular injury in diabetic patients. Diabetic American Pima Indians show faster progression of nephropathy than populations with higher BP levels [62].

Exacerbation in vasodilation and compromised vasoconstriction occurs in diabetic impaired renal autoregulation. In db/db mice, increased nitric oxide seems to be involved in TGF impairment [55]. The role of cyclooxygenase products in diabetic hyperperfiltration is also controversial; some reports suggest that they are partially responsible for arteriolar vasodilation and increased GFR [63, 64], while others are contradictory [65, 66]. Furthermore some evidence points to reduced responsiveness to sympatho-adrenergic hormones [59, 67, 68]. Hyperglycemia seems to have a decisive effect on glomerular hyperfiltration [69] and renal injury [70].

4. Influence of Dietary Protein on Renal Hemodynamics

Experimental and clinical studies show that a low protein diet reduces CKD patient morbidity, preserves renal function, relieves uremic symptoms and improves nutritional status [71-73]. Low protein diet for humans means a daily protein intake from 0.58 to 0.6 g/kg [72, 74, 75], compared with a normal diet of around 1.3 g/kg of protein [75]. One mechanism responsible for protection of renal function involves reduction of protein traffic through glomerular capillaries, i.e. reduction in urinary protein [76], partly because increased traffic in podocytes increases production of growth factors, particularly TGF-β, which enhances extracellular matrix production [77], as well as increases infiltration of T lymphocytes [78], impairing glomerular capillary integrity.

However, glomerular hemodynamics measurement in 5/6 nephrectomized rats - an effective model of CKD - indicates that high protein diet leads to increased R_E, increased P_{GC} and elevated GFR [79] in the remnant nephrons, because P_{GC} is influenced by a balance between R_A and R_E. Differently, a low protein diet reduces P_{GC} and SNGFR in the remaining nephrons [80]. Thus reduction in dietary protein ameliorates glomerular hypertension [79] and delays glomerular sclerosis and tubulointerstitial fibrosis index [73] in CKD individuals [71]. It seems that a low protein diet is also beneficial in reducing GFR and protecting renal function in obese hypertensive humans [74].

5. Role of Antihypertensive Drugs on Renal Hemodynamics

On the basis of the above discussion, to protect renal function one drug must not only reduce systemic BP, but also has to reduce P_{GC}. Reduction in P_{GC} results in reduced protein traffic throughout glomerular capillaries, and this protects renal tissue. By measuring glomerular hemodynamics, it can be shown that ACEIs reduce P_{GC} and SNGFR in rats subjected to renal ablation [21, 81]. Comparing effects of different antihypertensive drugs on renal hemodynamics of SHR in cases renal ablation, Kvam and coworkers [81] have shown that ACEIs preferentially reduce R_E, while calcium channel blockers (CCBs) preferentially reduces R_A.

Thus, preferential action of ACEIs on R_E leads to reduction of P_{GC}, while CCB's action in reducing R_A leads to an increase of P_{GC}. In another comparative study between these 2 categories of drugs, using an equihypotensive treatment, CCB did not reduce proteinuria and delayed, but did not prevent, glomerulosclerosis as seen with ACEI. However, CCBs that also act on T-type calcium channel, besides L-type calcium channels can also reduce efferent resistance and effectively ameliorate renal function [82, 83]. In a review, Hayashi and coworkers [84] bring together findings that show how novel calcium antagonists dilate afferent as well as efferent arterioles [84]. Regarding the efficacy of ACEIs and also angiotensin II receptor antagonists, they present - besides their hemodynamic effects - antioxidant and anti-inflammatory actions that protect renal structures [85].

Conclusion

Knowledge of whole renal and glomerular hemodynamics is fundamental to the comprehension of CKD. For the future, it will undoubtedly be crucial to assess the efficacy of new treatments, including drugs, genetic modification or cellular therapy.

Acknowledgments

ADOP, BRMS and LDVF are recipients of CNPq, Fundação Araucária and CAPES fellowships, respectively. We are grateful to BioMedES for editing the manuscript.

References

[1] Cupples, WA; Braam, B. Assessment of renal autoregulation. *Am J Physiol Renal Physiol*, 2007 292, F1105-F1123.

[2] Loutzenhiser, R; Griffin, K; Williamson, G; Bidani, A. Renal autoregulation: new perspectives regarding the protective and regulatory roles of the underlying mechanisms. *Am J Physiol Regul Integr Comp Physiol*, 2006 290, R1153-R1167.

[3] Khavandi, K; Greenstein, AS; Sonoyama, K; Withers, S; Price, A; Malik, RA; Heagerty, AM. Myogenic tone and small artery remodelling: insight into diabetic nephropathy. *Nephrol Dial Transplant*, 2009 24, 361-369.

[4] Johnson, RJ; Segal, MS; Srinivas, T; Ejaz, A; Mu, W; Roncal, C; Sánchez-Lozada, LG; Gersch, M; Rodriguez-Iturbe, B; Kang, DH; Acosta, JH. Essential hypertension, progressive renal disease, and uric acid: a pathogenetic link? *J Am Soc Nephrol*, 2005 16, 1909-1919.

[5] Ochodnický, P; Henning, RH; Buikema, HJ; de Zeeuw, D; Provoost, AP; van Dokkum, RP. Renal vascular dysfunction precedes the development of renal damage in the hypertensive Fawn-Hooded rat. *Am J Physiol Renal Physiol*, 2010 298, F625-F633.

[6] Ren, Y; D'Ambrosio, MA; Liu, R; Pagano, PJ; Garvin, JL; Carretero, OA. Enhanced myogenic response in the afferent arteriole of spontaneously hypertensive rats. *Am J Physiol Heart Circ Physiol*, 2010 298, H1769-H1775.

[7] Tolbert, EM; Weisstuch, J; Feiner, HD; Dworkin, LD. Onset of glomerular hypertension with aging precedes injury in the spontaneously hypertensive rat. *Am J Physiol Renal Physiol*, 2000 278, F839-F846.

[8] Magalhães, JC; da Silveira, AB; Mota, DL; Paixão, AD. Renal function in juvenile rats subjected to prenatal malnutrition and chronic salt overload. *Exp Physiol*, 2006 91, 611-619.

[9] Vieira-Filho, LD; Lucena-Júnior, JM; Barreto, IS; Angelim, JL; Paixão, AD. Repercussion of acetylsalicylic acid during fetal development on later renal hemodynamics of rats. *Fundam Clin Pharmacol*, 2008 22, 379-386.

[10] Silva, LA; Veira-Filho, LD; Barreto, IS; Cabral, EV; Vieyra, A; Paixão, AD. Prenatal undernutrition changes renovascular responses of nimesulide in rat kidneys. *Basic Clin Pharmacol Toxicol*, 2011 108, 115-121.

[11] Maddox, DA; Price, DC; Rector, FC Jr. Effects of surgery on plasma volume and salt and water excretion in rats. *Am J Physiol*, 1977 233, F600-F606.

[12] Fuhr, J; kaczmarczyk, J; kruttgen, CD. A simple colorimetric method of inulin determination in renal clearance studies on metabolically normal subjects and diabetics. Klin Wochenschr, 1955 33, 729-730.

[13] Vallon, V. Micropuncturing the nephron. Pflugers Arch, 2009 458, 189-201.

[14] Brenner, BM; Troy, JL; Daugharty, TM. The dynamics of glomerular ultrafiltration in the rat. *J Clin Invest*, 1971 50, 1776-1780.

[15] Gertz, KH; Mangos, JA; Braun, G; Pagel, HD. Pressure in the glomerular capillaries of the rat kidney and its relation to arterial blood pressure. *Pflugers Arch Gesamte Physiol Menschen Tiere*, 1966 288, 369-374.

[16] Deen, WM; Troy, JL; Robertson, CR; Brenner, BM. Dynamics of glomerular ultrafiltration in the rat. IV. Determination of the ultrafiltration coefficient. *J Clin Invest*, 1973 52, 1500-1508.

[17] Brenner, BM; Troy, JL; Daugharty, TM; Deen, WM; Robertson, CR. Dynamics of glomerular ultrafiltration in the rat. II. Plasma-flow dependence of GFR. *Am J Physiol*, 1972 223, 1184-1190.

[18] Daugharty, TM; Ueki, IF; Mercer, PF; Brenner, BM. Dynamics of glomerular ultrafiltration in the rat. V. Response to ischemic injury. *J Clin Invest*, 1974 53, 105-116.

[19] Dworkin, LD; Hostetter, TH; Rennke, HG; Brenner, BM. Hemodynamic basis for glomerular injury in rats with desoxycorticosterone-salt hypertension. *J Clin Invest*, 1984 73, 1448-1461.

[20] Brenner, BM; Troy, JL; Daugharty, TM; MacInnes, RM. Quantitative importance of changes in postglomerular colloid osmotic pressure in mediating glomerulotubular balance in the rat. *J Clin Invest*, 1973 52, 190-197.

[21] Anderson, S; Meyer, TW; Rennke, HG; Brenner, BM. Control of glomerular hypertension limits glomerular injury in rats with reduced renal mass. *J Clin Invest*, 1985 76, 612-619.

[22] Simons, JL; Provoost, AP; Anderson, S; Rennke, HG; Troy, JL; Brenner, BM. Modulation of glomerular hypertension defines susceptibility to progressive glomerular injury. *Kidney Int*, 1994 46, 396-404.

[23] U.S. Renal Data System. Atlas of Chronic Kidney Disease and End-Stage Renal Disease in the United States. National Institutes of Health, National Institute of Diabetes and Digestive and Kidney Diseases; Bethesda, MD (2008). USRDS 2008 Annual Data Report. *http://www.usrds.org*. 2011.

[24] Simons, JL; Provoost, AP; Anderson, S; Troy, JL; Rennke, HG; Sandstrom, DJ; Brenner, BM. Pathogenesis of glomerular injury in the fawn-hooded rat: early glomerular capillary hypertension predicts glomerular sclerosis. *J Am Soc Nephrol*, 1993 3, 1775-1782.

[25] Weichert, W; Paliege, A; Provoost, AP; Bachmann, S. Upregulation of juxtaglomerular NOS1 and COX-2 precedes glomerulosclerosis in fawn-hooded hypertensive rats. *Am J Physiol Renal Physiol*, 2001 280, F706-F714.

[26] Verseput, GH; Provoost, AP; Braam, BB; Weening, JJ; Koomans, HA. Angiotensin-converting enzyme inhibition in the prevention and treatment of chronic renal damage in the hypertensive fawn-hooded rat. *J Am Soc Nephrol*, 1997 8, 249-259.

[27] Chen, GF; Wagner, L; Sasser, JM; Zharikov, S; Moningka, NC; Baylis, C. Effects of angiotensin type 1 receptor blockade on arginine and ADMA synthesis and metabolic pathways in fawn-hooded hypertensive rats. *Nephrol Dial Transplant*, 2010 25, 3518-3525.

[28] Brown, DM; Provoost, AP; Daly, MJ; Lander, ES; Jacob, HJ. Renal disease susceptibility and hypertension are under independent genetic control in the fawn-hooded rat. *Nat Genet*, 1996 12, 44-51.

[29] Freedman, BI; Rich, SS; Yu, H; Roh, BH; Bowden, DW. Linkage heterogeneity of end-stage renal disease on human chromosome 10. *Kidney Int*, 2002 62, 770-774.

[30] Ono, H; Ono, Y; Frohlich, ED. Nitric oxide synthase inhibition in spontaneously hypertensive rats. Systemic, renal, and glomerular hemodynamics. *Hypertension*. 1995 26, 249-255.

[31] Ichihara, A; Hayashi, M; Hirota, N; Saruta, T. Superoxide inhibits neuronal nitric oxide synthase influences on afferent arterioles in spontaneously hypertensive rats. *Hypertension*, 2001 37, 630-634.

[32] Brännström, K; Arendshorst, WJ. Thromboxane A2 contributes to the enhanced tubuloglomerular feedback activity in young SHR. *Am J Physiol*, 1999 276, F758-F766.

[33] Komatsu, K; Frohlich, ED; Ono, H; Ono, Y; Numabe, A; Willis, GW. Glomerular dynamics and morphology of aged spontaneously hypertensive rats. Effects of angiotensin-converting enzyme inhibition. *Hypertension*, 1995 25, 207-213.

[34] Iversen, BM; Amann, K; Kvam, FI; Wang, X; Ofstad, J. Increased glomerular capillary pressure and size mediate glomerulosclerosis in SHR juxtamedullary cortex. *Am J Physiol*, 1998 274, F365-F373.

[35] Textor, SC; Lerman, L. Renovascular hypertension and ischemic nephropathy. *Am J Hypertens*, 2010 23, 1159-1169.

[36] Anderson, WP; Kett, MM; Stevenson, KM; Edgley, AJ; Denton, KM; Fitzgerald, SM. Renovascular hypertension: structural changes in the renal vasculature. *Hypertension*, 2000 36, 648-652.

[37] Welch, WJ; Mendonca, M; Aslam, S; Wilcox, CS. Roles of oxidative stress and AT1 receptors in renal hemodynamics and oxygenation in the postclipped 2K,1C kidney. *Hypertension*, 2003 41, 692-696.

[38] Palm, F; Onozato, M; Welch, WJ; Wilcox, CS. Blood pressure, blood flow, and oxygenation in the clipped kidney of chronic 2-kidney, 1-clip rats: effects of tempol and Angiotensin blockade. *Hypertension*, 2010 55, 298-304.

[39] Kobayashi, S; Ishida, A; Moriya, H; Mori, N; Fukuda, T; Takamura, T. Angiotensin II receptor blockade limits kidney injury in two-kidney, one-clip Goldblatt hypertensive rats with special reference to phenotypic changes. *J Lab Clin Med*, 1999 133, 134-143.

[40] Steiner, RW; Tucker, BJ; Gushwa, LC; Gifford, J; Wilson, CB; Blantz, RC. Glomerular hemodynamics in moderate Goldblatt hypertension in the rat. *Hypertension*, 1982 4, 51-57.

[41] Karlsen, FM; Andersen, CB; Leyssac, PP; Holstein-Rathlou, NH. Dynamic autoregulation and renal injury in Dahl rats. *Hypertension*, 1997 30, 975-983.

[42] Tian, N; Moore, RS; Phillips, WE; Lin, L; Braddy, S; Pryor, JS; Stockstill, RL; Hughson, MD; Manning, RD Jr. NADPH oxidase contributes to renal damage and dysfunction in Dahl salt-sensitive hypertension. *Am J Physiol Regul Integr Comp Physiol*, 2008 295, R1858-R1865.

[43] Trolliet, MR; Rudd, MA; Loscalzo, J. Oxidative stress and renal dysfunction in salt-sensitive hypertension. *Kidney Blood Press Res*, 2001 24, 116-123.

[44] Manger, WM; Simchon, S; Stokes, MB; Reidy, JJ; Kumar, AR; Baer, L; Gallo, G; Haddy, FJ. Renal functional, not morphological, abnormalities account for salt sensitivity in Dahl rats. *J Hypertens*, 2009 27, 587-598.

[45] Ianchi, G; Tripodi, G; Casari, G; Salardi, S; Barber, BR; Garcia, R; Leoni ,P; Torielli, L; Cusi, D; Ferrandi, M. Two point mutations within the adducin genes are involved in blood pressure variation. *Proc Natl Acad Sci U S A*, 1994 91, 3999-4003.

[46] Ferrandi, M; Tripodi, G; Salardi, S; Florio, M; Modica, R; Barassi, P; Parenti, P; Shainskaya, A; Karlish, S; Bianchi, G; Ferrari, P. Renal Na,K-ATPase in genetic hypertension. *Hypertension*, 1996 28, 1018-1025.

[47] Menini, S; Ricci, C; Iacobini, C; Bianchi, G; Pugliese, G; Pesce, C. Glomerular number and size in Milan hypertensive and normotensive rats: their relationship to susceptibility and resistance to hypertension and renal disease. *J Hypertens*, 2004 22, 2185-2192.

[48] Pugliese, G; Pricci, F; Barsotti, P; Iacobini, C; Ricci, C; Oddi, G; Romeo, G; Leto, G; Marano, G; Sorcini, M; Sabbatini, M; Fuiano, G; Di Mario, U; Pugliese, F; Development of diabetic nephropathy in the Milan normotensive strain, but not in the Milan hypertensive strain: possible permissive role of hemodynamics. *Kidney Int*, 2005 67, 1440-1452.

[49] Pugliese, G; Ricci, C; Iacobini, C; Menini, S; Fioretto, P; Ferrandi ,M; Giardino, LA; Armelloni, S; Mattinzoli, D; Rastaldi, MP; Pugliese, F. Glomerular barrier dysfunction in glomerulosclerosis- resistant Milan rats with experimental diabetes: the role of renal haemodynamics. *J Pathol*, 2007 213, 210-218.

[50] Anderson, S; Brenner, BM. Pathogenesis of diabetic glomerulopathy: hemodynamic considerations. *Diabetes Metab Rev*, 1988 4, 163-177.

[51] Mogensen, CE. Early glomerular hyperfiltration in insulin-dependent diabetics and late nephropathy. *Scand J Clin Lab Invest*, 1986 46, 201-206.

[52] Vora, JP; Dolben, J; Williams, JD; Peters, JR; Owens, DR. Impact of initial treatment on renal function in newly-diagnosed type 2 (non-insulin-dependent) diabetes mellitus. *Diabetologia*, 1993 36, 734-740.

[53] Persson, P; Hansell, P; Palm, F. Tubular reabsorption and diabetes-induced glomerular hyperfiltration. *Acta Physiol* (Oxf), 2010 200, 3-10.

[54] Christensen, PK; Lund, S; Parving, HH. The impact of glycaemic control on autoregulation of glomerular filtration rate in patients with non-insulin dependent diabetes. *Scand J Clin Lab Invest*, 2001 61, 43-50.

[55] Levine, DZ. Hyperfiltration, nitric oxide, and diabetic nephropathy. *Curr Hypertens Rep*, 2006 8, 153-157.

[56] Vallon, V; Richter, K; Blantz, RC; Thomson, S; Osswald, H. Glomerular hyperfiltration in experimental diabetes mellitus: potential role of tubular reabsorption. *J Am Soc Nephrol*, 1999 10, 2569-2576.

[57] Zatz, R; Meyer, TW; Rennke, HG; Brenner, BM. Predominance of hemodynamic rather than metabolic factors in the pathogenesis of diabetic glomerulopathy. *Proc Natl Acad Sci U S A*, 1985 82, 5963-5967.

[58] Bank, N; Lahorra, MA; Aynedjian, HS; Schlondorff, D. Vasoregulatory hormones and the hyperfiltration of diabetes. *Am J Physiol*, 1988 254, F202-F209.

[59] Ohishi, K; Okwueze, MI; Vari, RC; Carmines, PK. Juxtamedullary microvascular dysfunction during the hyperfiltration stage of diabetes mellitus. *Am J Physiol*, 1994 267, F99-F105.

[60] Park, SK; Kang,SK. Renal function and hemodynamic study in obese Zucker rats. Korean *J Intern Med*, 1995 10, 48-53.

[61] Zamlauski-Tucker, MJ; Springate, JE; Van Liew, JB; Noble, B; Feld, LG; Glomerular function in spontaneously diabetic rats. *Proc Soc Exp Biol Med*, 1992 199, 59-64.

[62] Lemley, KV. A basis for accelerated progression of diabetic nephropathy in Pima Indians. *Kidney Int Suppl*, 2003 83, S38-S42.

[63] Viberti, GC; Benigni, A; Bognetti, E; Remuzzi, G; Wiseman, MJ. Glomerular hyperfiltration and urinary prostaglandins in type 1 diabetes mellitus. *Diabet Med*, 1989 6, 219-223.

[64] DeRubertis, FR; Craven, PA. Eicosanoids in the pathogenesis of the functional and structural alterations of the kidney in diabetes. *Am J Kidney Dis*, 1993 22, 727-735.

[65] Linné, T; Körner, A; Rudberg, S; Persson, B; Aperia, A. Renal functional effects of prostaglandin synthesis inhibition in patients with insulin-dependent diabetes mellitus of long duration without nephropathy. *Horm Metab Res*, 1991 23, 383-386.

[66] Jenkins, DA; Craig ,K; Collier, A; Watson, ML; Clarke, BF. Evidence against a role for prostaglandins in sustaining renal hyperfiltration in type 1 diabetes mellitus. *Diabet Med*, 1989 6, 502-505.

[67] Salman, IM; Ameer, OZ; Sattar, MA; Abdullah, NA; Yam, MF; Abdullah, GZ; Abdulkarim, MF; Khan, MA; Johns, EJ. Renal sympathetic nervous system hyperactivity in early streptozotocin-induced diabetic kidney disease. *Neurourol Urodyn*, 2011 30, 438-446.

[68] Kopp, UC; Cicha, MZ; Yorek, MA. Impaired responsiveness of renal sensory nerves in streptozotocin-treated rats and obese Zucker diabetic fatty rats: role of angiotensin. *Am J Physiol Regul Integr Comp Physiol*, 2008 294, R858-R866.

[69] Wiseman, MJ; Viberti, GC; Keen, H. Threshold effect of plasma glucose in the glomerular hyperfiltration of diabetes. *Nephron*, 1984 38, 257-260.

[70] Cherney, DZ; Scholey, JW; Sochett, E; Bradley, TJ; Reich, HN. The acute effect of clamped hyperglycemia on the urinary excretion of inflammatory cytokines/chemokines in uncomplicated type 1 diabetes: a pilot study. *Diabetes Care*, 2011 34, 177-180.

[71] Klahr, S; Buerkert, J; Purkerson, ML. Role of dietary factors in the progression of chronic renal disease. *Kidney Int*, 1983 24, 579-587.

[72] Eyre, S; Attman, PO; Haraldsson, B. Positive effects of protein restriction in patients with chronic kidney disease. *J Ren Nutr*, 2008 18, 269-280.

[73] Gao, X; Wu, J; Dong, Z; Hua, C; Hu, H; Mei, C. A low-protein diet supplemented with ketoacids plays a more protective role against oxidative stress of rat kidney tissue with 5/6 nephrectomy than a low-protein diet alone. *Br J Nutr*, 2010 103, 608-616.

[74] Friedman, AN; Yu, Z; Juliar, BE; Nguyen, JT; Strother, M; Quinney, SK; Li, L; Inman, M; Gomez, G; Shihabi, Z; Moe, S. Independent influence of dietary protein on markers of kidney function and disease in obesity. *Kidney Int*, 2010 78, 693-697.

[75] Menon, V; Kopple ,JD; Wang, X; Beck, GJ; Collins, AJ; Kusek, JW; Greene, T; Levey, AS; Sarnak, MJ. Effect of a very low-protein diet on outcomes: long-term follow-up of

the Modification of Diet in Renal Disease (MDRD) Study. *Am J Kidney Dis*, 2009 53, 208-217.
[76] Remuzzi, G; Benigni, A; Remuzzi, A. Mechanisms of progression and regression of renal lesions of chronic nephropathies and diabetes. *J Clin Invest*, 2006 116, 288-296.
[77] Eddy, AA. Protein restriction reduces transforming growth factor-beta and interstitial fibrosis in nephrotic syndrome. *Am J Physiol*, 1994 266, F884-F893.
[78] De Miguel, C; Lund, H; Mattson, DL. High dietary protein exacerbates hypertension and renal damage in Dahl SS rats by increasing infiltrating immune cells in the kidney. *Hypertension*, 2011 57, 269-274.
[79] Nath, KA; Kren, SM; Hostetter, TH. Dietary protein restriction in established renal injury in the rat. Selective role of glomerular capillary pressure in progressive glomerular dysfunction. *J Clin Invest*, 1986 78, 1199-1205.
[80] Hostetter, TH; Olson, JL; Rennke, HG; Venkatachalam, MA; Brenner, BM; Hyperfiltration in remnant nephrons: a potentially adverse response to renal ablation. *J Am Soc Nephrol*, 2001 12, 1315-1325.
[81] Kvam, FI; Ofstad, J; Iversen, BM. Effects of antihypertensive drugs on autoregulation of RBF and glomerular capillary pressure in SHR. *Am J Physiol*, 1998 275, F576-84.
[82] Takahashi, K; Katoh, T; Fukunaga, M; Badr, KF. Studies on the glomerular microcirculatory actions of manidipine and its modulation of the systemic and renal effects of endothelin. *Am Heart J*, 1993 125, 609-619.
[83] Nakamura, Y; Ono, H; Frohlich, ED. Differential effects of T- and L-type calcium antagonists on glomerular dynamics in spontaneously hypertensive rats. *Hypertension*, 1999 34, 273-278.
[84] Hayashi, K; Ozawa, Y; Fujiwara, K; Wakino, S; Kumagai, H; Saruta, T. Role of actions of calcium antagonists on efferent arterioles--with special references to glomerular hypertension. *Am J Nephrol*, 2003 23, 229-244.
[85] Cravedi, P; Ruggenenti, P; Remuzzi, G. Does remission of renal disease associated with antihypertensive treatment exist? *Curr Hypertens Rep*, 2007 9, 160-165.

Chapter 16

The Hemodynamics of Esophageal Varices

Takahiro Sato[*]
Department of Gastroenterology,
Sapporo Kosei General Hospital, Sapporo, Japan

Keywords: color Doppler, endoscopic ultrasonography, esophageal varices, portal hypertension

Introduction

Esophageal varices are considered to be the most common complication in patients with portal hypertension. Endoscopic injection sclerotherapy (EIS) [1] and endoscopic variceal ligation (EVL) [2] are effective treatments for variceal bleeding. In Japan, there appears to be controversy in deciding which of the two is the best therapy for elective and prophylactic cases. Therefore, it is important to evaluate the hemodynamics of the portal venous system when determining the optimal choice of treatment for patients with portal hypertension. In this chapter, we review the hemodynamics of esophageal varices due to portal hypertension and describe the usefulness of endoscopic color Doppler ultrasonography (ECDUS).

1. Portal Hypertension

Portal hypertension due to increasing intrahepatic and extrahepatic vessel resistance induces hepatofugal flow in collateral veins (left gastric vein, short gastric vein, and posterior gastric vein). Hepatofugal flow in the collateral veins is involved in the formation of

---

[*] Correspondence: Takahiro Sato, Department of Gastroenterology, Sapporo Kosei General Hospital, Kita 3 Higashi 8, Chuo-ku, Sapporo 060-0033, Japan, Tel: 81-11-261-5331, Fax: 81-11-261-6040, E-mail: taka.sato@ja-hokkaidoukouseiren.or.jp.

esophageal varices. The left gastric vein is the major site of esophageal varices in patients with portal hypertension. The morphological changes of the left gastric vein in portal hypertension have been elucidated by angiographic examinations [3-5]. Matsutani et al. reported that hepatofugal blood flow in the left gastric vein increased in direct correlation with enlargement of the size of the varices and a high flow velocity in the left gastric vein was strongly associated with variceal bleeding [6]. It is generally thought that the blood flow in the left gastric vein may change from a hepatopetal direction to the hepatofugal direction in liver cirrhosis.

The palisade zone corresponds to the abdominal esophagus, beginning at the gastro-esophageal junction and extending superiorly for 4-5 cm [7]. The veins in this zone were distributed uniformly, in close proximity to each other and running parallel and longitudinally as a palisade. Palisade veins, which are normally seen in the lamina propria at the lower end of the esophagus, are called sudare like veins. The palisade veins run through the lamina propria and most end draining to the submucosal veins at the critical area. Noda et al. stated that the ruptured veins were situated in the lamina propria and the rupture points were located near the area where the varicosed palisade veins connected to the submucosal varices [8]. Arakawa et al. revealed marked dilatation of the veins in the submucosa more often in patients with well-developed varices than in those without varices via the palisade zone, and they classified these cases into two groups: those with sudare like veins, and those with vascularity in which one or two large dilated vessels run through the submucosa [9]. Hashizume et al. classified the sudare like veins as a palisading type and the dilated vessels as a bar type, and reported that palisading type veins in the lamina propria were dilated introducing into the muscularis mucosae, and were observed circumferentially observed in the submucosa [5, 10].

The routes of esophageal varices are mainly associated with gastric wall blood flow (left gastric vein, short gastric vein, and palisade vein), and perforating veins are recognized as additional passageways. There is little information in the literature on perforating veins [10-12].

On the other hand, the hyperdynamic state from the lower esophagus to the cardiac area also is assoiated with esophageal varices. It is thought that esophageal varices form not only due to hepatofugal flow, but also due to elevation of the venous pressure with the hyperdynamic state in areas of the lower esophagus and the upper part of stomach [13, 14]. The blood flow in the stomach wall supplied from the left gastric artery also participates in variceal blood flow in the early stage [15-17]. The hyperdynamic stage is caused by an increase in the arterio-venous anastomoses in the submucosal layer of esophagus and stomach by which the arterial blood flows in through the left gastric artery and proper esophageal artery. The arterial blood flow in the lower esophagus and the upper part of the stomach may be attributable to the hepatopetal flow in the left gastric vein, and to flow in the opposite direction in the left gastric vein during the venous phase of a selective left gastric arteriogram in esophageal variceal patients. In addition, there have been several reports on the pressure and the oxygen saturation in the portal veins. Nakayama et al. [18] reported that oxygen saturation in the left gastric vein was higher than that in portal veins. The oxygen pressure in esophageal varices also was reported to be higher than in other portal systems [19]. As mentioned in the above literature, the arterial blood flow may have a critical impact on esophageal varices.

2. Diagnosis of Portal Hypertension

Arterioportography has been used to study the portal venous system of patients with esophageal varices. However, this modality has inherent limitations. Percutaneous transhepatic portography can evaluate the detailed hemodynamics of the portal venous system, but with the caveat of it being an invasive method. Computed tomography (CT) and magnetic resonance (MR) angiography are reliable modalities for examining the entire portal venous system [20-22]. Esophageal varices appear on CT scans as well-defined, round, tubular, or serpentine structures that are smooth and have homogeneous attenuation. In particular, 320-row multi-detector CT is useful for the detection and grading of esophageal varices and for evaluating of esophageal varices to predict the risk of hemorrhage [23]. Unfortunately, detailed hemodynamic studies of the vascular anatomy of the lower esophagus and upper stomach are not feasible with CT, MR angiography.

The gold standard in diagnosis of esophageal varices remains esophagogastroduodenoscopy (EGD); this is a useful modality for diagnosing and observing esophageal varices of a certain size and extent, and has a very sensitive predictive value for variceal hemorrhage. The endoscopic findings for esophageal varices were evaluated according to the grading system outlined in 'The General Rules for Recording Endoscopic Findings of Esophago-gastric Varices' prepared by the Japanese Research Committee on Portal Hypertension [24]. The form (F) of the varices is classified as small and straight (F_1), enlarged and tortuous (F_2), large and coil-shaped (F_3), or no varices after treatment (F_0). The fundamental color of the varices was classified as either white (Cw) or blue (Cb). The red color sign (RC) refers to dilated, small vessels or telangiectasia on the variceal surface. RC shows a high risk of variceal bleeding based on endoscopic findings. The following images show blue color and red color-positive enlarged and tortuous esophageal varices (Fig.1).

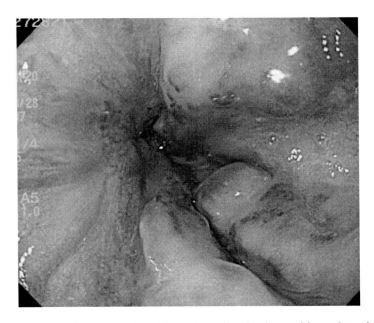

Figure1. Esophagogastroduodenoscopy show blue color and red color-positive enlarged and tortuous esophageal varices.

Endoscopic ultrasonography (EUS) has become a very useful modality for the diagnosis of esophageal varices [25-27]. EUS not only visualizes the surface of the varices but also provides detailed information about their internal structure. It features with a 20 MHz ultrasound catheter probe and has been shown to provide clear images of esophageal collateral veins as well [28, 29], allowing for detailed evaluation of esophageal variceal hemodynamics.

ECDUS is better able to observe the detailed hemodynamics of esophageal varices better than conventional EUS.

3. Evaluation of Esophageal Varices Using Endoscopic Color Doppler Ultrasonography (ECDUS)

Hemodynamic evaluation of the esophago-gastric varices was performed by ECDUS using a PENTAX FG-36UX (forward - oblique viewing), 7.5 MHz, convex type, which provided 100° images (convex type ECDUS) or EG-3630UR (forward viewing), 10 MHz, electronic radial type, which provided 270° images (electronic radial type ECDUS) (Pentax Optical, Tokyo, Japan). The HITACHI EUB565 or EUB8500 was used for the display (Hitachi Medical, Tokyo, Japan).

Exploration of esophago-gastric varices was conducted by introducing deaerated water from an autoinfuser device into the stomach through the working channel. Evaluation of esophago-gastric varices was carried out using ECDUS while the patients remained in a left lateral decubitus position. Velocities were assessed by the pulsed Doppler method, by positioning a sample volume of 1-2 mm in the center of the vessels. The color gain was adjusted so as to eliminate background noise, and the insonation angle was kept below 60° to minimize ambiguity in measurements of blood flow. To begin with, identification of esophago-gastric varices was performed with B-mode scanning and then, color flow mapping was done.

ECDUS is a method for detecting color flow images in blood vessels. The direction of blood flow and the measurement of velocity can be achieved only via ECDUS. This can show graphically esophageal varices, paraesophageal veins, and passageways. Sato et al. have reported previously on the usefulness of convex type ECDUS for evaluating the hemodynamics of esophageal varices [30-32].

Hino et al. analyzed the morphology and hemodynamics of the left gastric vein using ECDUS to evaluate the development of esophageal varices [33]. They reported that hepatofugal blood flow velocity in the left gastric vein trunk increased with the size of the varices. The left gastric vein bifurcates into anterior and posterior branches. As the size of the varices enlarged, the branch pattern was more likely to be anterior branch dominant. EIS is recommended as the better choice of endoscopic treatments for the anterior branch dominant esophageal varices. The image shows anterior branch dominant esophageal varices observed with ECDUS (Fig.2-a).

Vessel images of the palisade veins were discerned with ECDUS running parallel and longitudinally around the gastro-esophageal junction. However, the vessel images of palisade veins produced by ECDUS may show only part of the system of palisade veins. Levovist is an ultrasound echo-enhancing agent that increases the echo signal intensity of the body blood pool following intravenous injection. It is made up of granules that are 99.9% galactose and 0.1% palmitic acid. The sensitivity of ECDUS for the detection of the palisade veins has been raised from 23.9 to 40.3% by incorporating Levovist contrast. Observation of color flow images of palisade veins via ECDUS is difficult because of the fine vessels with low velocity [34]. Sato et al. reported the usefulness of a new electronic radial ECDUS in evaluating the hemodynamics of esophageal varices in comparison with convex type ECDUS, and color flow images of palisade veins were obtained in 12 of 26 (46.2%) cases with electronic radial ECDUS. In addition, the detection rate of palisade veins with electronic radial ECDUS was significantly higher than that with the convex type ECDUS [35]. Endoscopic treatment is very safe and popular, but recurrence of varices is now becoming a serious problem. Intramucosal venous dilatation (IMVD) of esophageal varices has been observed frequently in follow-up endoscopy after endoscopic therapies [36]. IMVD has been evaluated as the regional tortuous dilatation of varices and indicates a risk of bleeding. The palisade veins remaining after endoscopic therapies are related to IMVD.

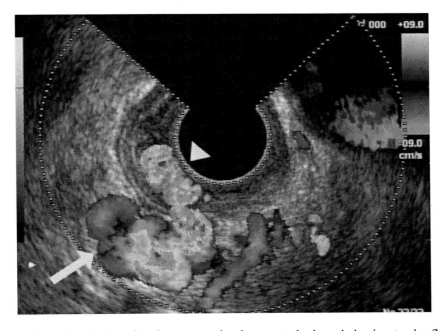

Figure 2a. Endoscopic color Doppler ultrasonography shows anterior branch dominant color flow images of the left gastric vein (arrow) and esophageal varices (arrowhead).

Perforating veins are defined as communicating vessels between esophageal varices and paraesophageal veins. Angiography cannot distinguish between the intramural and extramural vessels of the esophagus. Similarly, it is impossible to discern the perforating veins via CT scans or MR angiography. Perforating veins can be visualized via EUS, but the direction of blood flow in perforating veins cannot be determined by this method. The direction of blood flow in perforating veins can only be shown qualitatively by ECDUS [37]. Choudhuri et al. reported on perforating veins that connect the submucosal and paraesophageal collateral venous channels in the lower esophagus using EUS; these were observed in 15% of patients with small varices and 70% with large varices [26]. The perforating veins detected by

ECDUS were classified into three types according to the flow direction. Type 1 showed inflow from the paraesophageal veins to the esophageal varices [Fig.2-b]. Type 2 showed outflow from the esophageal varices to the paraesophageal veins. Type 3 was a mixed type that revealed both inflow and outflow [35]. In this paper, color flow images of perforating veins were obtained in 18 of 26 (69.2%) cases. The direction of blood flow in perforating veins is an important consideration in the therapeutic management of esophageal varices. Therefore, we should perform EIS on Type 1 for the purpose of obliterating esophageal varices and perforating veins. On the other hand, Type 2 is associated with diversion of esophageal variceal blood flow into the paraesophageal veins and is therefore equivalent to an extra-esophageal shunt [38]. One must use great caution in performing EIS for Type 2 and Type 3 variceal patients and EIS should be performed at the anal site of out-flowing perforating veins. Endoscopic variceal ligation (EVL) may be the optimum treatment for this type of varices [39].

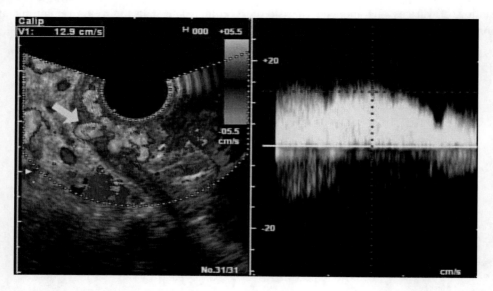

Figure 2b. Endoscopic color Doppler ultrasonography show inflow from the paraesophageal veins to the esophageal varices (arrow).

Hemodynamic evaluation of portal hypertension reveals that hepatofugal flow in the collateral veins is involved in the formation of esophageal varices, and also that a hyperdynamic state from the lower esophagus to the cardiac area is involved in forming esophageal varices. Sato et al. reported the detection of a pulsatile wave (arterial blood flow) in the blood vessels of the esophageal wall using ECDUS and indicated that the sensitivity of convex-type ECDUS in detecting the pulsatile wave was increased from 2.7% to 36.4% with Levovist contrast. ECDUS examinations using Levovist contrast suggest that arterial flow is involved in the formation of esophageal varices [40]. Observation of a pulsatile wave with convex type ECDUS is difficult because of the fine vessels. The detection rate of pulsatile wave with electronic radial ECDUS was significantly higher than using convex type ECDUS. Electronic radial ECDUS provides extended 270° views (convex-type ECDUS provides 100° views), and this advantage provides clearer visualization of pulsatile waves in esophageal varices [35].

4. Hemodynamics of Variceal Recurrence

Although endoscopic treatment is safe and popular, recurrence of esophageal varices has become a serious problem. EUS analysis of gastric cardial vascular structures could be useful for predicting the recurrence of esophageal varices [41-43]. Two publications reported that severe, shallow-type paraesophageal vein and perforating vein detected using an EUS catheter probe after EIS, correlated significantly with variceal recurrence [44, 45]. Other authors have reported previously that the development of a gastro-renal shunt reduces the frequency of variceal relapse [46, 47]. Ito et al. reported that the incidence of variceal relapse was lower in patients with non-variceal systemic portal shunts than in patients without these shunts [48]. ECDUS can be used to evaluate the hemodynamic characteristics of esophageal varices before and after EIS and the data obtained can be used to predict the early recurrence of esophageal varices. In particular, detection of cardiac intramural vein and inflowing perforating vein by ECDUS after EIS showed a strong correlation with early variceal recurrence [49].

Conclusion

In conclusion, it is important to evaluate the hemodynamics of the portal venous system when treating the esophageal varices of patients with portal hypertension. ECDUS is a useful modality for the evaluation of the detailed hemodynamics of esophageal varices.

References

[1] The Veterans Affairs Cooperative Variceal Sclerotherapy Group. Prophylactic sclerotherapy for esophageal varices in men with alcoholic liver disease. *N Engl J Med* 1991, 324, 1779-84.

[2] Goff GV; Reveille RM; Stiegmann GV. Endoscopic sclerotherapy versus endoscopic variceal ligation: esophageal symptoms, complications and motility. *Am J Gastroenterol* 1988, 83, 1240-4.

[3] Widrich WC; Srinivasan M; Semine MC; Robbins AH. Collateral pathways of the left gastric vein in portal hypertension. *AJR* 1984, 142, 375-82.

[4] Takashi M; Igarashi M; Hino S; Musha H; Takayasu K; Arakawa M; et al. Esophageal varices: correlation of left gastric venography and endoscopy in patients with portal hypertension. *Radiology* 1985, 155, 327-31.

[5] Hashizume M; Kitano S; Yamaga H; Higashi H; Sugimachi K. Angioarchitectural classification of varices and paraesophageal veins in selective left gastric venography. *Arch Surg* 1989, 124, 961-6.

[6] Matsutani S; Furuse J; Ishii H; Mizumoto H; Kimura K; Ohto M. Hemodynamics of the left gastric vein in portal hypertension. *Gastroenterology* 1993, 105, 513-8.

[7] Kegaries DL. The venous plexus of the oesophagus. Its clinical significance. *Surg Gynecol Obstet* 1934, 58, 46-5.

[8] Noda T. Angioarchitectural study of esophageal varices. *Virchows Arch* 1984, 404, 381-92.
[9] Arakawa M; Kage M. The anatomy and pathomorphology of esophageal varices. In: Okuda and Benhamou eds. *Portal hypertension.* Springer-Verlag, 1992, 415-28.
[10] Hashizume M; Kitano S; Sugimachi K; Sueishi K. Three-dimensional view of the vascular structure of the lower esophagus in clinical portal hypertension. *Hepatology* 1988, 8, 1482-7.
[11] McCormack TT; Rose JD; Smith PM; Johnson AG. Perforating veins and blood flow in oesophageal varices. *Lancet* 1983, 2, 1442-4.
[12] Vianna A; Hayes PC; Moscoso G; Driver M; Portmann B; Westaby D; et al. Normal venous circulation of the gastroesophageal junction. A route to understanding varices. *Gastroenterology* 1987, 93, 876-89.
[13] Inokuchi K; Kobayashi M; Saku M; Nagasue N; Iwaki A; Nakayama S. Characteristics of splanchnic portal circulation in portal hypertension as analyzed by pressure study in clinical cases (in Japanese with English abstract). *Acta Hepatol.Jpn.* 1977, 18, 891-8.
[14] Aoki H. The hemodynamics and the treatment of esophago-gastric varices (in Japanese with English abstract). *Dig.Surg.Jpn.* 1991, 24, 2309-19.
[15] Reuter SR; Atkin TW. High-dose left gastric angiography for demonstration of esophageal varices. *Radiology* 1972, 105, 573-8.
[16] Hashizume M; Tanaka K; Inokuchi K. Morphology of gastric microcirculation in cirrhosis. *Hepatology* 1983, 3, 1008-12.
[17] Lunderquist A. Pharmacoangiography of the left gastric artery in esophageal varices. *Acta Radiol* 1974, 15, 157-60.
[18] Nakayama S; Beppu K; Sakata H; Saku M; Kobayashi Y; Inoguchi K. Hyperdynamic state of portal area in cirrhotic patients - evaluation of extraction between artery and portal vein-. *Acta Hepatologica Japonica* 1978, 19, 1086. (in Japanese)
[19] Kokubu S. Studies on the pathogenesis of esophago-gastric varices by variceal blood gas analysis. *Kitasato Med* 1989, 19, 208-18. (in Japanese)
[20] Cho KC; Patel YD; Wachsberg RH; Seeff J. Varices in portal hypertension: evaluation with CT. *Radiographics* 1995, 15, 609-22.
[21] Yu NC; Margolis D; Hsu M; Raman SS; Lu DSK. Detection and grading of esophageal varices on liver CT: comparison of standard and thin-section multiplanar reconstructions in diagnostic accuracy. *AJR* 2011, 197, 643-9.
[22] Liu H; Cao H; Wu ZY. Magnetic resonance angiography in the management of patients with portal hypertension. *Hepatobiliary Pancreat Dis Int* 2005, 4, 239-43.
[23] Shen M; Zhu KS; Meng XC; Zhang JS; Liu LY; Shan H. Evaluation of esophageal varices and predicting the risk of esophageal varices bleeding with multi-detector CT in patients with portal hypertension. *Zhonghua Yi Xue Za Zhi* 2010, 90, 2911-5. (in Chinese)
[24] Idezuki Y. General rules for recording endoscopic findings of esophagogastric varices. *World J Surg* 1995, 19, 420-3.
[25] Caletti GC; Brocchi E; Baraldini M; Ferrari A; Gibilara M; Benbara L. Assessment of portal hypertension by endoscopic ultrasonography. *Gastrointest Endosc* 1990, 36, 21-7.

[26] Choudhuri G; Dhiman RK; Agarwal DK. Endosonographic evaluation of the venous anatomy around the gastro - esophageal junction in patients with portal hypertension. *Hepato-Gastroenterol* 1996, 43, 1250-5.

[27] Nakamura H; Inoue H; Kawano T; Goseki N; Endo M; Sugihara K. Selection of the treatment for esophagogastric varices. Analyses of collateral structures by endoscopic ultrasonography. *Surg. Endosc* 1992, 6, 228-34.

[28] Kishimoto H; Sakai M; Kajiyama T; Torii A; Kin G; Tsukada H; et al. Miniature ultrasonic probe evaluation of esophageal varices after endoscopic variceal ligation. *Gastrointest Endosc* 1995, 42, 256-60.

[29] Nagamine N; Ido K; Ueno N; Kimura K; Kawamata T; Kawada H; et al. The usefulness of ultrasonic microprobe imaging for endoscopic variceal ligation. *Am J Gastroenterol* 1996, 91, 523-9.

[30] Sato T; Koito K; Nobuta A; Nagakawa T; Oikawa Y; Watanabe M; et al. Observation of esophageal varices by endoscopic color Doppler ultrasonography (ECDUS) and usefulness of ECDUS for evaluation of endoscopic injection sclerotherapy (in Japanese with English abstract). *Gastroenterol Endosc* 1991, 33, 2379-87.

[31] Sato T; Higashino K; Toyota J; Karino Y; Furukawa T; Murashima Y; et al. Heat-probe coagulation treatment of recurrent intramucosal venous dilatation of the esophagus and endoscopic color Doppler ultrasonographic follow-up. *Dig.Endosc* 1995, 7, 203-7.

[32] Sato T; Yamazaki K; Toyota J; Karino Y; Ohmura T; Suga T. Pulsatile wave in esophageal wall blood vessels after endoscopic therapy for esophageal varices. – evaluation by endoscopic color Doppler ultrasonography-. *Dig.Endosc* 1998, 10, 9-13.

[33] Hino S; Kakutani H; Ikeda K; Uchiyama Y; Sugiyama K; Kuramochi A; et al. Hemodynamic assessment of the left gastric vein in patients with esophageal varices with color Doppler EUS: factors affecting development of esophageal varices. *Gastrointest Endosc* 2002, 55, 512-7.

[34] Sato T; Yamazaki; Toyota J; Karino Y; Ohmura T; Kuwata Y; et al. Visualization of palisade veins in esophageal varices by endoscopic color Doppler ultrasonography. *Dig. Endosc* 2003, 15, 87-92.

[35] Sato T; Yamazaki K; Toyota J; Karino Y; Ohmura T; Kuwata Y; et al. Usefulness of electronic radial endoscopic color Doppler ultrasonography in esophageal varices: comparison with convex type. *J Gastroenterol* 2006, 41, 28-33.

[36] Yazaki Y; Kawashima T; Sekiya C; Ohta H; Ohira M; Kouda H; et al. F0 recurrent esophageal varices - Diagnosis, clinical features, and endoscopic injection sclerotherapy for this new type of varices- (in Japanese with English abstract). *Endoscopia Digestiva* 1992, 4, 1021-9.

[37] Sato T; Higashino K; Toyota J; Karino Y; Ohmura T; Murashima Y; et al. The usefulness of endoscopic color Doppler ultrasonography in the detection of perforating veins of esophageal varices. *Dig.Endosc* 1996, 8, 180-3.

[38] Irisawa A; Obara K; Sakamoto H; Takiguchi F; Tojo J; Saito A; et al. The selection and evaluation of the manipulation for endoscopic injection sclerotherapy against esophageal varices with extra esophageal shunt (in Japanese). *Nihon Monmyakuatsu Koshinsho Gakkai Zasshi* 1997, 3, 147-54.

[39] Saito A; Obara K; Irisawa A; Takiguchi F; Tojo J; Ito M; et al. Experience of endoscopic injection sclerotherapy combined with selective endoscopic variceal

ligation in 3 patients with esophageal varices accompanied by large extra - esophageal shunt (in Japanese). *Nihon Monmyakuatsu Koshinsho Gakkai Zasshi* 1997, 3, 263-8.

[40] Sato T; Yamazaki K; Toyota J; Karino Y; Ohmura T; Akaike J; et al. Evaluation of arterial blood flow in esophageal varices via endoscopic color Doppler ultrasonography with a galactose – based contrast agent. *J Gastroenterol* 2005, 40, 64-69.

[41] Suzuki T; Matsutani S; Umebara K; Sato G; Maruyama H; Mitsuhashi O; et al. EUS changes predictive for recurrence of esophageal varices in patients treated by combined endoscopic ligation and sclerotherapy. *Gastrointest Endosc* 2000, 51, 611-7.

[42] Konishi Y; Nakamura T; Kida H; Seno H; Okazaki K; Chiba T. Catheter US probe EUS evaluation of gastric cardia and perigastric vascular structures to predict esophageal variceal recurrence. *Gastrointest Endosc* 2002, 55, 197-203.

[43] Seno H; Konishi Y; Wada M; Fukui H; Okazaki K; Chiba T. Endoscopic ultrasonograph evaluation of vascular structures in the gastric cardia predicts esophageal variceal recurrence following endoscopic treatment. *J Gastroenterol Hepatol* 2006, 21, 227-31.

[44] Irisawa A; Saito A; Obara K; Shibukawa G; Takagi T; Shishido H; et al. Endoscopic recurrence of esophageal varices is associated with the specific EUS abnormalities: severe periesophageal collateral veins and large perforating veins. *Gastrointest Endosc* 2001, 53, 77-84.

[45] Shibukawa G; Irisawa A; Saito A; Takahashi A; Sato H; Takagi T; et al. Variceal recurrence after endoscopic sclerotherapy associated with the perforating veins in lower esophagus independently. *Hapato-Gastroenterol* 2004, 51, 744-7.

[46] Sakai T; Iwao T; Oho K; Toyonaga A; Tanikawa K. Influence of extravariceal collateral channel pattern on recurrence of esophageal varices after sclerotherapy. *J Gastroenterol* 1997, 32, 715-9.

[47] Dilawari JB; Raju GS; Chawla YK. Development of large spleno-adreno-renal shunt after endoscopic sclerotherapy. *Gastroenterology* 1989, 97, 421-6.

[48] Ito K; Matsutani S; Maruyama H; Akiike T; Nomoto H; Suzuki T; et al. Study of hemodynamic changes in portal systemic shunts and their relation to variceal relapse after endoscopic variceal ligation combined with ethanol sclerotherapy. J Gastroenterol 2006, 41, 119-26.

[49] Sato T; Yamazaki K; Toyota J; Karino Y; Ohmura T; Akaike J. Endoscopic ultrasonographic evaluation of hemodynamics related to variceal relapse in esophageal variceal patients. *Hepatol Res* 2009, 39, 126-33.

Chapter 17

The Modulation of Portal Venous Hemodynamics in Living Donor Liver Transplantation

Hiroshi Sadamori[*], *Yuzo Umeda, Takahito Yagi and Toshiyoshi Fujiwara*

Department of Gastroenterological Surgery, Okayama University Graduate School of Medicine, Dentistry and Pharmaceutical Sciences, Okayama, Japan

Keywords: Living donor liver transplantation, portal venous hemodynamics, portosystemic shunt, small-for-size, splenic artery, embolization, liver regeneration

1. Introduction

The management of portal venous hemodynamics has a pivotal role in achieving good outcome of living donor liver transplantation (LDLT). Two issues related to portal venous hemodynamics are important in LDLT.

One issue is the management of prior large portosystemic shunts. Central portosystemic shunts, such as the surgical portacaval shunt, should be closed immediately after graft implantation to avoid diversion of portal venous flow from the liver graft. On the other hand, regarding splenorenal shunts, controversy exists as to whether the occlusion of these shunts during the transplant procedure is warranted. Because a sufficient restoration of the liver vascular bed cannot be achieved in the early postoperative period after adult LDLT, any preserved portosystemic shunts can easily steal graft portal venous flow in LDLT. Thus, we propose a strategy for surgical prophylactic management of spontaneous large portosystemic shunts during the adult LDLT procedure. In this chapter, we review previous studies about the

---

[*] Corresponding author: Hiroshi Sadamori, MD, PhD. Department of Gastroenterological Surgery, Okayama University Graduate School of Medicine, Dentistry and Pharmaceutical Sciences, 2-5-1 Shikata, Okayama 700-8558, Japan. Tel: +81-86-235-7257 Fax: +81-86-221-8775; e-mail: sada@md.okayama-u.ac.jp.

management of portosystemic shunts in liver transplantation, and describe our results with prophylactic surgical management of portosystemic shunts in LDLT.

The second issue related to portal venous hemodynamics in LDLT is a treatment strategy for preventing small-for-size syndrome. In partial liver transplantation, adequate portal venous flow and portal shear stress are closely related to the regeneration of the transplanted liver graft. Conversely, excessive portal venous inflow causes tissue injury of the liver graft, and also inhibits post-transplant liver regeneration. In small-for-size grafts with severe portal hypertension, we have conducted prophylactic embolization or ligation of the splenic artery to relieve hyperperfusion injury and to improve the outcome. In this chapter, we present our data on the effects of prophylactic splenic artery modulation to optimize the outcome of small-for-size grafts in LDLT.

2. Effects of Large Portosystemic Shunts on Liver Transplantation Outcomes

The outcomes of patients with spontaneous or surgical portosystemic shunts in deceased donor liver transplantation (DDLT) have been reported [1-12]. There is general agreement that central portosystemic shunts, such as the surgical portacaval shunt and the spontaneous shunt derived from the main portal vein (PV) inflowing directly to the systemic venous circulation, should be closed to avoid diversion of portal venous flow from the graft. On the other hand, the management of prior spontaneous splenorenal shunts is a controversial issue. In fact, some spontaneous splenorenal shunts virtually disappear after removal of the cirrhotic liver and transplantation of the liver graft. However, some post-transplant conditions, such as acute rejection and severe ischemic damage, might cause increased intra-hepatic vascular resistance that enhances the post-transplant development of preserved or residual splenorenal shunts. In these circumstances, the graft portal venous flow could be easily stolen by the developed splenorenal shunts, leading to serious graft dysfunction. Thus, several authors have reported that spontaneous large splenorenal shunts should be occluded during the transplant procedure to achieve a similar patient and graft survival as in patients without such shunts [2,3,5,6,10].

LDLT is an established treatment modality for end-stage liver disease and serves to alleviate the shortage of cadaveric donor organs. There have been noticeable improvements in LDLT [13-17]. However, there is little information about the outcome of LDLT in the presence of prior spontaneous large portosystemic shunts. It has been generally accepted that adequate portal venous flow is essential for postoperative liver regeneration after liver resection and partial liver transplantation [18-20]. Because sufficient restoration of the liver vascular bed cannot be achieved in the early postoperative period in adult LDLT, post-transplant portal hypertension caused by acute rejection or severe ischemic damage might appear more strongly in LDLT than in DDLT. Therefore, the steal of graft portal venous flow by the preserved portosystemic shunt might be more prone to occur in LDLT than in DDLT.

3. Assessment of Portal Venous Hemodynamics

There are inter-individual differences regarding portal venous hemodynamics, including blood flow direction of the main PV and the degree of steal of the superior mesenteric vein (SMV) blood flow by portosystemic shunts. In addition, portosystemic shunts enhance the likelihood of portal vein phlebosclerosis, which makes subsequent vascular anastomosis difficult. Those pre-transplant situations of portal venous hemodynamics affect the management of portosystemic shunts and the options for PV reconstruction. Therefore, pre-transplant assessment of portal venous hemodynamics is important for improving the outcome of LDLT.

We carried out Doppler ultrasonography (US), computed tomography (CT) and/or magnetic resonance angiography before LDLT in 155 patients with chronic end-stage liver disease to evaluate the anatomy and hemodynamics of portal venous and hepatic arterial circulation. A large portosystemic shunt was defined as a shunt with a diameter of more than 10 mm and portal venous flow of more than 400 ml/min. As a result of these evaluations, 33 patients (21.2%) were found to have spontaneous large portosystemic shunts. These 33 patients were classified into four types of large portosystemic shunts: 11 had splenorenal shunts (SRS), 6 had shunts derived from coronary veins (CVS) inflowing directly to the systemic venous circulation, 15 had umbilical vein shunts (UVS), and 1 had a shunt from an inferior mesenteric vein. Of these shunts, we retrospectively investigated and compared portal venous hemodynamics, surgical procedures for shunts, and morbidity and mortality after LDLT in three types of spontaneous large portosystemic shunts: splenorenal shunt (SRS group; n=11), coronary vein shunt (CVS group; n=6) and umbilical vein shunt (UVS group; n=15) [21].

Table 1. Preoperative blood flow direction and patency of main portal vein (PV)

Shunt Type	Hepatopetal	Hepatofugal	Patent	Narrowed	Total
SRS	10	1	9	2	11
CVS	2	4	4	2	6
UVS	15	0	15	0	15
Total	27	5	28	4	

Hepatofugal: SRS vs UVS $P<0.01$; Narrowed: CVS vs UVS $P<0.05$; SRS/CVS $P<0.05$.

SRS, splenorenal shunt; CVS, coronary vein shunt; UVS, umbilical vein shunt.

We assessed the patency and flow direction of the main PV and the splenic vein (SPV), and also detected the grade of preoperative steal of SMV blood flow by spontaneous portosystemic shunts. Table 1 shows the preoperative blood flow direction and patency of the main PV. The preoperative blood flow direction of the main PV as assessed by Doppler US was hepatopetal in 10 patients and hepatofugal in 1 of 11 patients of the SRS group. In the UVS group, there was no patient with hepatofugal blood flow of the main PV. In contrast, 4 of 6 patients of the CVS group showed hepatofugal blood flow of the main PV. Narrowing of the main PV was observed in 2 of 11 patients of the SRS group and in 2 of 6 patients of the CVS group. The grade of preoperative steal of SMV blood flow by portosystemic shunt is demonstrated in Table 2. The steal of SMV blood flow by shunt was significantly higher in the CVS group than in the SRS and CVS groups. The grade of steal of SMV blood flow in the CVS group was partial in 2 and complete in 4 of 6 patients.

Table 2. Preoperative blood flow direction of proximal SPV and grade of steal of SMV blood flow by shunt

Shunt Type	Flow direction of proximal SPV Hepatopetal	Hepatofugal	Steal of SMV flow by shunt None	Partial	Complete	Total
SRS	7	4	6	4	1	11
CVS	1	5	0	2	4	6
UVS	14	1	0	14	1	15
Total	22	10	6	20	6	

Hepatofugal: CVS vs UVS $P < 0.01$; Complete steal: SRS vs CVS $P < 0.01$, CVS vs UVS $P < 0.05$

SPV, splenic vein; SMV, superior mesenteric vein; SRS, splenorenal shunt; CVS, coronary vein shunt; UVS, umbilical vein shunt.

4. Surgical Management of Spontaneous Large Portosystemic Shunts

Table 3 summarizes the surgical procedures for the large portosystemic shunts and for PV reconstruction in our series. The splenorenal shunts were ligated at the inflow site to the left renal vein without splenectomy in 7 patients, and were transected by splenectomy in 2 patients. The SMV and SPV blood flows were diverted by ligation at the root of the SPV in 1 patient, in whom the SMV blood flow had been completely stolen by the splenorenal shunt preoperatively. In the CVS group, coronary vein shunts were ligated at the root in 5 patients, and diversion of blood flow in the SMV and SPV by ligation at the root of the SPV was performed in 1 patient. In all patients of the UVS group, the umbilical vein shunt was dissected at the beginning of the hepatectomy. In the SRS group, the portal inflow was reconstructed by direct anastomosis to the native PV in 9 patients, and with an interposed vein graft to the splenoportal junction in 2 patients. In the CVS group, PV reconstruction with the native PV was performed in 3 patients, with the native PV after thrombectomy in 1 patient, and with an interposed vein graft in 2 patients. In all patients of the UVS group, PV reconstruction with the native PV was performed.

Table 3. Surgical procedures for shunts and portal vein (PV) reconstruction

	Procedures for Shunts	PV Reconstruction
SRS (n=11)	Ligation of shunts at the inflow site to LRV (7)	Native PV (9)
	Diversion of SMV and SPV flow (1)	Interposed vein graft (2)
	Splenectomy (2)	
	No procedure (1)	
CVS (n=6)	Ligation of coronary vein at the root (5)	Native PV (3)
		Native PV after thrombectomy (1)
	Diversion of SMV and SPV flow (1)	Interposed vein graft (2)
UVS (n=15)	Ligation of UVS (15)	Native PV (15)

SRS, splenorenal shunt; CVS, coronary vein shunt; UVS, umbilical vein shunt; LRV, left renal vein; SPV, splenic vein; SMV, superior mesenteric vein.

5. Outcome of Prophylactic Surgical Procedures for Large Portosystemic Shunts

Table 4 shows the morbidity and mortality after LDLT in recipients with spontaneous large portosystemic shunts. The mean portal venous flow of the grafts before occlusion of the portosystemic shunts was 621 ± 47 ml/min in the SRS group, and 739 ± 116 ml/min in the CVS group. The mean portal venous flow of the grafts after occlusion of the portosystemic shunts increased significantly to 1278 ± 134 ml/min in the SRS group and 1661 ± 159 ml/min in the CVS group, compared with the portal venous flow before shunt occlusion. There were no significant differences between the three groups with respect to operative time, blood loss, intensive care unit stay, hospital stay, and postoperative mortality. With regard to postoperative complications, the number of portal complications in the CVS group was significantly higher than in the SRS and UVS groups. The steal of graft portal venous flow was detected postoperatively in the preserved or remaining splenorenal shunt in 2 of 11 patients in the SRS group. In contrast, none of the patients of the CVS group had postoperative steal of graft portal venous flow by the residual portosystemic shunt. There was no significant difference in the actuarial survival rate between patients with SRS/CVS/UVS (n=32) and those without these portosystemic shunts (n=122) (84.3 % vs. 88.2 % at 1 year, respectively; P=0.083). Furthermore, there was no significant difference in the actuarial survival rate between the three groups of SRS, CVS and UVS (81.8% vs. 83.3% vs. 86.6 % at 1 year, respectively).

Two cases experienced postoperative steal of graft portal venous flow by a spontaneous portosystemic shunt after LDLT. In one patient, in whom the splenorenal shunt was not occluded during the transplant procedure, the graft portal venous flow was completely stolen by the preserved splenorenal shunt on postoperative day (POD) 9 due to steroid-resistant acute rejection. Although the splenorenal shunt was occluded during an emergency laparotomy on POD 9, together with commencement of infusion of OKT3, the liver graft function deteriorated rapidly and the patient died on POD 39. In the other patient, who underwent occlusion of the main splenorenal shunt during the transplant procedure, the graft portal venous flow was completely stolen by the residual splenorenal shunt on POD2, probably due to severe ischemic graft injury. We diverted the SMV and SPV blood flow by ligation at the root of the SPV on POD2 to prevent the steal of the graft portal venous flow, leading to recovery of the liver graft function.

6. Controversy in LDLT Using Small-for-Size Grafts

Previous studies have indicated that the size of the liver graft correlates with clinical outcome [22-24]. The clinical manifestations, referred to as small-for-size syndrome, consist of delayed synthetic function, prolonged hyperbilirubinemia and intractable ascites, leading to higher mortality. Although various recipient and donor factors are involved in the development of small-for-size syndrome, severe portal hypertension and excessive portal venous flow have been suggested as important mechanisms of small-for-size graft injury [25-30]. Accordingly, several surgeons have reported that small-for-size grafts could be successfully treated by the reduction of portal venous pressure with the construction of a surgical portosystemic shunt or a temporary transjugular intrahepatic portosystemic shunt [31-34]. On the other hand, Yagi et al. [20] investigated optimal portal venous circulation for liver graft function after LDLT in adult recipients. These authors endeavored to maintain the portal venous pressure below 20 mmHg and keep the graft portal venous flow above 800 ml/min by either occluding or preserving the prior portosystemic shunt in their 28 patients, resulting in better liver graft function. In our series, the mean graft portal venous flow before occlusion of the portosystemic shunt was below 800 ml/min in both the SRS and CVS groups, and increased significantly after surgical repair of these shunts. Furthermore, neither intractable ascites nor prolonged hyperbilirubinemia were seen in the SRS and CVS groups except in one patient with portal vein thrombosis, while 6 patients, with graft-to-recipient body weight ratio of less than 0.8%, were included in the SRS and CVS groups.

The outcome of LDLT with prior spontaneous large portosystemic shunts in our series is satisfactory despite the complexity of the transplant procedures for repair of these shunts. However, postoperative steal of the graft portal venous flow by a residual splenorenal shunt is still a potential cause of graft dysfunction. With regard to patients with small-for-size grafts, further investigations are necessary to assess the optimal portal venous circulation for small-for-size grafts and to determine the precise management strategy for portosystemic shunt.

Table 4. Morbidity and mortality after LDLT among the three groups

	SRS group (n=11)	CVS group (n=6)	UVS group (n=15)	P value
Operation				
Operative time (min)	595 ± 23	712 ± 65	596 ± 36	NS
Blood loss (g)	6920 ± 1440	13820 ± 8460	5867 ± 1610	NS
Graft PVF (ml/min)				
Shunt open	621 ± 47 ⎤ P<0.01	739 ± 116 ⎤ P<0.01		NS
Shunt occluded	1278 ± 134 ⎦	1661 ± 159 ⎦		NS
Hospitalization				
ICU stay (d)	13 ± 2.9	16 ± 8.8	9.9 ± 1.0	NS
Hospital stay (d)	61 ± 8.9	77 ± 17	65 ± 6.9	NS
Postoperative complication				
Intra-abdominal hemorrhage	2 / 11	2 / 6	1 / 15	NS
Arterial complications	0 / 11	0 / 6	0 / 15	NS
Portal complications	0 / 11	2 / 6	0 / 15	< 0.05 *
Biliary complications	4 / 11	2 / 6	2 / 15	NS
Intractable ascites	0 / 11	0 / 6	2 / 15	NS
Prolonged hyperbilirubinemia	0 / 11	1 / 6	2 / 15	NS
Steal of graft PVF by shunt	2 / 11	0 / 6	0 / 15	NS
Postoperative mortality	1 / 11	1 / 6	2 / 15	NS
1Y patient survival rate (%)	81.8	83.3	86.6	NS

SRS, splenorenal shunt; CVS, coronary vein shunt; UVS, umbilical vein shunt; PVF: Portal venous flow; LDLT, living donor liver transplantation.
0.048 (CVS versus SRS); 0.022 (CVS versus UVS).

7. Mechanisms of Small-for-size Syndrome

Patients scheduled for liver transplantation frequently have portal hypertension and, consequently, the transplanted liver graft receives a high portal venous flow. When the graft volume is small, particularly in adult LDLT, various problems affecting the prognosis often occur because the partial graft cannot sustain excessive portal venous perfusion. It is widely known that liver transplant recipients can potentially develop a specific syndrome known as "small-for-size syndrome" in the presence of portal hypertension [25-30]. Small-for-size syndrome can result in large-volume ascites, hyperbilirubinemia, and coagulopathy. The pathologic mechanism of this syndrome is associated with graft injury caused by excessive portal inflow into the small-for-size graft. Previous studies examining post-transplant biopsies have revealed progressive damage of the graft due to irreversible endothelial injury after reperfusion [35-36]. In addition, other studies analyzing intra-graft gene expression have provided evidence for sinusoidal damage due to portal hyperperfusion in the small-for-size graft [37-38]. Patients with small-for-size syndrome have shown the up-regulation of endothelin-1 and down-regulation of heme-oxigenase-1 and heat shock protein-70 in the liver graft.

Previous studies have indicated that liver regeneration begins in the early period after partial liver transplantation [39-41]. Although the detailed mechanism remains unknown, both high portal venous flow and pressure are considered as important triggers of liver regeneration. In partial liver transplantation, a high level of liver regeneration is observed when the graft size is small, or when portal pressure is high. On the other hand, liver graft injury caused by high portal pressure results in serious interference with the process of liver regeneration. Interestingly, interleukin (IL)-6 and tumor necrosis factor (TNF)-alpha play key roles in liver regeneration, although they are also considered as markers of acute-phase tissue damage. Local activation and excessive production of these cytokines is associated with poor liver regeneration, since they can act as negative regulators of cell proliferation. In fact, TNF-alpha could trigger the cell death pathway after binding to the TNF-receptor [42]. Thus, although the role of these cytokines remains controversial, they are considered to function as inflammatory cytokines, rather than as liver regenerative factors, in patients with small-for-size syndrome.

7. Treatment Strategies for Prevention of Small-for-size Syndrome

Treatment strategies for the prevention of small-for-size syndrome include approaches aimed at reducing excessive portal inflow and lowering the graft perfusion pressure. For the decompression of portal venous inflow into a small-for-size graft, the construction of a surgical portosystemic shunt has been used [31-34]. However, the separation of the graft portal venous flow may result in the steal of portal venous flow by the surgical portosystemic shunt. This steal phenomenon sometimes leads to fatal events, especially in cases with decreased vascular compliance of the liver graft, such as a steatotic liver graft and acute cellular rejection. Based on this potential complication, some centers have adopted precautionary measures using a modified technique for closure of the surgical portosystemic shunt after LDLT [43].

The level of spleen-derived blood flow is an important factor in determining the portal inflow volume and pressure, thus highlighting the benefits of splenectomy and ligation of the splenic artery [25, 27, 44-45]. However, patients with end-stage liver disease exhibit a hyperdynamic state of splanchnic blood flow, and are at increased risk of hemorrhage associated with invasive surgical procedures. Thus, careful attention should be paid to the expansion of surgical dissection during transplantation, especially in patients with collateral circulation around the splenic artery, such as gastric coronary vein and splenorenal shunts. Recently, the development of surgical techniques and devices has allowed the reduction of blood loss during splenectomy [46]. Although the invasiveness of splenectomy could be diminished, adverse events, such as increased susceptibility to infection and portal vein thrombosis, may occur after splenectomy.

Splenic artery embolization could be an effective procedure for portal decompression instead of the conventional treatment. In this regard, we previously reported that preoperative portal decompression by splenic artery embolization reduced blood loss during surgery and shortened the operating time, resulting in favorable prognosis without serious complications related to the procedure [47]. In our institution, preoperative splenic artery embolization is selected for patients who developed collaterals around the peri-celiac trunk. In patients scheduled for preoperative splenic artery embolization, abdominal angiography was performed 12 to 18 hours before transplantation, and metallic coils were placed at the root of the splenic artery for achieving embolization of the splenic artery (Figure 1). Evaluation of post-transplant graft hemodynamics by Doppler US showed a significant reduction in the level of graft portal venous flow after splenic artery embolization in the portal modulation group, compared with the non-portal modulation group (Figure 2). In the portal modulation group, the efficacy of portal decompression following splenic artery embolization was equivalent to that after splenic artery ligation. Furthermore, hepatic arterial flow in the graft was significantly higher during the postoperative phase in the portal modulation group, reflecting an arterial flow shift from the spleen to the hepatic artery or a hepatic arterial buffer response. In our series, no complications were observed after splenic artery embolization (e.g., splenic infarction, septic complication associated with immune compromise, or portal thrombosis). The rate of small-for-size syndrome has been significantly reduced by preoperative portal decompression using splenic artery embolization, resulting in a significant reduction of the mortality rate [48].

Regarding the decision on treatment strategies for small-for-size syndrome, flexible countermeasures are necessary. While surgical portosystemic shunts have been used for preventing small-for-size syndrome, there is no doubt that both splenectomy and splenic artery ligation are also effective for achieving portal decompression. Furthermore, splenic artery embolization prior to transplantation could be an alternative treatment modality, especially in patients with developed collateral circulation in the peri-celiac trunk, which makes it difficult to carry out splenic artery ligation or splenectomy safely. When sufficient portal decompression cannot be achieved through a single technique, a combination of those procedures should be applied. The treatment strategies for portal decompression can inhibit portal overperfusion injury in the liver graft, leading to prevention of small-for-size syndrome. Also, these strategies have beneficial effects on liver generation, as well as post-transplant prognosis of small-for-size grafts, leading to good outcomes and cost benefits in liver transplantation.

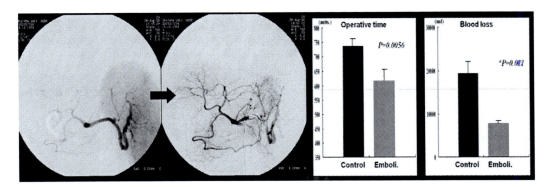

Figure 1. Preoperative splenic artery embolization as a prophylactic procedure for the prevention of small-for-size syndrome. The splenic artery was totally embolized adjacent to the root of the celiac artery 12-18 hours before liver transplantation. Splenic artery embolization reduced portal flow and increased hepatic arterial flow. Preoperative portal decompression also decreased blood loss and shortened the operative time.

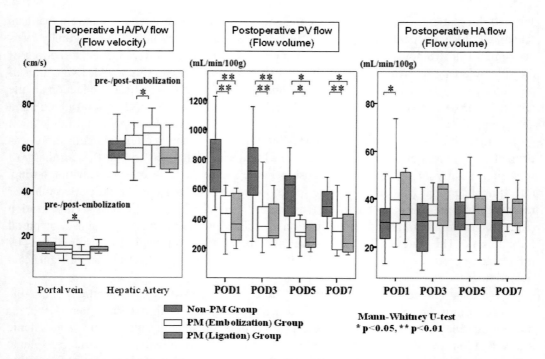

Figure 2. Box-and-whisker plots of portal vein flow and hepatic artery flow in patients of the non-portal modulation (PM) and PM groups during postoperative days (POD) 1, 3, 5 and 7.

Conclusion

The effects of portal venous hemodynamics on liver transplantation outcomes are complex and diverse, depending on the status of the liver graft and the postoperative course in each case. In LDLT, a small-for-size graft and events affecting vascular resistance in the graft are problematic and deteriorate the complications related to preserved large portosystemic shunts and portal hypertension. Prophylactic surgical modulations for prior large portosystemic shunts and excessive portal hypertension can contribute to improving the prognosis of LDLT by preventing the fatal events due to preserved large portosystemic shunts and by minimizing the deleterious effects of portal hypertension on small-for-size grafts. Further investigations are needed to assess the optimal portal venous circulation for small-for-size grafts and to determine the precise management strategy for preventing small-for-size syndrome.

Acknowledgments

This work was supported by a Grant-in-Aid for scientific research from the Ministry of Education, Culture, Sports, Science and Technology of Japan.

References

[1] Esquivel CO, Klintmaln G, Iwatsuki S, et al. Liver transplantation in patients with patent splenorenal shunt. *Surgery* 1986;101:430-432.

[2] Mazzafero V, Todo S, Tzakis AG, et al. Liver transplantation in patients with previous portasystemic shunt. *Am J Surg 1990*;160:111-116.

[3] Boillot O, Houssin D, Santoni P, et al. Liver transplantation in patients with a surgical portasystemic shunt. *Gastroenterol Clin Biol* 1991;15:876-880.

[4] AbouJaoude MM, Grant DR, Ghent CN, et al. Effect of portasystemic shunts on subsequent transplantation of the liver. *Surg Gynecol Obstet* 1991;172:215-219.

[5] Langnas AN, Marujo WC, Stratta RJ, et al. Influence of a prior porta-systemic shunt on outcome after liver transplantation. *Am J of Gastroenterol* 1992;87:714-718.

[6] Ploeg RJ, D'Alessandro AM, Stegall M, et al. Effect of surgical and spontaneous portasystemic shunts on liver transplantation. *Transplant Proc* 1993;25:1946-1948.

[7] Dell'Era A, Grande L, Barros-Schelotto P, et al. Impact of prior portosystemic shunt procedures on outcome of liver transplantation. *Surgery* 2005;137:620-625.

[8] Menegaux F, Emmet BK, Baker E, et al. Comparison of transjugular and surgical portosystemic shunts on the outcome of liver transplantation. *Arch Surg* 1994;129:1018-1024.

[9] Brems JJ, Hiatt JR, Klein AS, et al. Effect of a prior portasystemic shunt on subsequent liver transplantation. *Ann Surg* 1989;209:51-56.

[10] Carlis LD, Favero ED, Rondinara G, et al. The role of spontaneous portosystemic shunts in the course of orthotopic liver transplantation. *Transplant Int* 1992;5:9-14.

[11] Shapiro RS, Varma CVR, Schwartz ME, et al. Splenorenal shunt closure after liver transplantation: Intraoperative Doppler assessment of portal hemodynamics. *Liver Transpl* 1997;3:641-642.

[12] Margarit C, Lazaro JL, Charco R, et al. Liver transplantation in patients with splenorenal shunts: Intraoperative flow measurements to indicate shunt occlusion. *Liver Transpl* 1999;5:35-39.

[13] Broelsch CE, Whitington PE, Emond JC, et al. Liver transplantation in children from living related donors: surgical techniques and results. *Ann Surg* 1991;214:428-437.

[14] Tanaka K, Uemoto S, Tokunaga Y, et al. Surgical techniques and innovations in living related liver transplantation. *Ann Surg* 1993;217:82-91.

[15] Kawasaki S, Makuuchi M, Matsunami H, et al. Living related liver transplantation in adults. *Ann Surg* 1998;227:269-274.

[16] Takayama T, Makuuchi M, Kubota K, et al. Living-related transplantation of left liver plus caudate lobe. *J Am Coll Surg.* 2000;190:635-638.

[17] Fan ST, Lo CM, Liu CL. Technical refinement in adult-to-adult living donor liver transplantation using right lobe grafts. *Ann Surg* 2000;231:126-131.

[18] Kawasaki T, Moriyasu F, Kimura T, Someda H, Fukuda Y, Ozawa K. Changes in portal blood flow consequent to partial hepatectomy: Doppler estimation. *Radiology* 1991;180:373-377.

[19] Marcos A, Olzinski AT, Ham JM, Fisher RA, Posner M. The interrelationship between portal and arterial blood flow after adult to adult living donor liver transplantation. *Transplantation* 2000;70:1697-1703.

[20] Yagi S, Iida T, Hori T, et al. Optimal portal venous circulation for liver graft function after living-donor liver transplantation. *Transplantation* 2006;81:373-378.
[21] Sadamori H, Yagi T, Matsukawa H, et al. The outcome of living donor liver transplantation with prior spontaneous large portasystemic shunts. *Transpl Int* 2008;21:156-162.
[22] Emond J, Renz JF, Ferrell LD, et al. Functional analysis of grafts from living donors. *Ann Surg* 1996;224:544-554.
[23] Kiuchi T, Kasahara M, Uryuhara K, et al. Impact of graft size mismatching on graft prognosis in liver transplantation from living donors. *Transplantation* 1999;67:321-327.
[24] Sugawara Y, Makuuchi M, Takayama T, et al. Small-for-size grafts in living-related liver transplantation. *J Am Coll Surg* 2001;192:510-513.
[25] Lo CM, Liu CL, Fan ST. Portal hyperperfusion injury as the cause of primary nonfunction in a small-for-size liver graft-successful treatment with splenic artery ligation. *Liver Transpl* 2003;9:626-628.
[26] Kiuchi T, Tanaka K, Ito T, et al. Small-for-size graft in living donor liver transplantation: How far should we go? *Liver Transpl* 2003;9:29-35.
[27] Troisi R, Cammu G, Militerno G, et al. Modulation of portal graft inflow: A necessity in adult living-donor liver transplantation? *Ann Surg* 2003;237:429-436.
[28] Dahm F, Georgiev P, Clavien PA, et al. Small for size syndrome after partial liver transplantation: Definition, mechanism of disease and clinical implications. *Am J Transpl* 2005;5:2605-2610.
[29] Ogura Y, Hori T, EL Moghazy WM, et al. Portal pressure <15 mm Hg is a key for successful adult living donor liver transplantation utilizing smaller grafts than before. *Liver Transpl* 2010,16:718-728.
[30] Hessheimer AJ, Fondevila C, Taura P, et al. Decompression of the portal bed and twice-baseline portal inflow are necessary for the functional recovery of a "small for size" graft. *Ann Surg* 2011,253:1201-1210.
[31] Boillot O, Delafosse B, Mechet I, et al. Small-for-size partial liver graft in an adult recipient; a new transplant technique. *Lancet* 2002;359:406-407.
[32] Takada Y, Ueda M, Ishikawa Y, et al. End-to-side portocaval shunting for a small-for-size graft in living donor liver transplantation. *Liver Transpl* 2004;10:807-810.
[33] Troisi R, Ricciardi S, Smeets P, et al. Effects of hemi-portocaval shunts for inflow modulation on the outcome of small-for-size grafts in living donor liver transplantation. *Am J Transpl* 2005;5:1397-1404.
[34] Sampietro R, Ciccarelli O, Wittebolle X, et al. Temporary transjugular intrahepatic portosystemic shunt to overcome small-for-size syndrome after right lobe adult split liver transplantation. *Transpl Int* 2006,19:1032-1034.
[35] Man K, Lo CM, Ng IO, et al. Liver transplantation in rats using small-for-size grafts: A study of hemodynamic and morphological changes. *Arch Surg* 2001;136:280-285.
[36] Demetris AJ, Kelly DM, Eghtead B, et al. Pathophysiologic observation and histopathologic recognition of the portal hyperfusion or small-for-size syndrome. *Am J Surg Pathol* 2006;30:986-993.
[37] Man K, Lo CM, Lee TK, et al. Intragraft gene expression profiles by cDNA microarray in small-for-size liver grafts. *Liver Transpl* 2003;9:425-432.

[38] Man K, Fan ST, Lo CM, et al. Graft injury in relation to graft size in right lobe live donor liver transplantation: A study of hepatic sinusoidal injury in correlation with portal hemodynamics and intragraft gene expression. *Ann Surg* 2003;237:256-264.

[39] Eguchi S, Yanaga K, Sugiyama N, et al. Relationship between portal venous flow and liver regeneration in patients after living donor right-lobe liver transplantation. *Liver Transpl* 2003;9:547-551.

[40] Yagi S, Iida T, Taniguchi K, et al. Impact of portal venous pressure on regeneration and graft damage after living-donor liver transplantation. *Liver Transpl* 2005;11:68-75.

[41] Marcos A, Fisher RA, Ham JM, et al. Liver regeneration and function in donor and recipient after right lobe adult to adult living donor liver transplantation. *Transplantation* 2000;69:1375-1379.

[42] Park A, Baichwal VR. Systemic mutational analysis of the death domain of the tumor necrosis factor receptor 1-associated protein TRADD. *J Biol Chem* 1996;271:9858-9862.

[43] Botha JF, Campos BD, Johanning J, et al. Endovascular closure of a hemiportocaval shunt after small for size adult-to-adult left lobe living donor liver transplantation. *Liver Transpl* 2009;15:1671-1675.

[44] Sato Y, Yamamoto S, Oya H, et al. Splenectomy for reduction of excessive portal hypertension after adult living-related donor liver transplantation. *Hepatogastroenterology* 2002;49:1652-1655.

[45] Shimada M, Ijichi H, Yonemura Y, et al. The impact of splenectomy or splenic artery ligation on the outcome of a living donor adult liver transplantation using a left lobe graft. *Hepatogastroenterology* 2004;51:625-629.

[46] Ikegami T, Toshima T, Takeishi K, et al. Bloodless splenectomy during liver transplantation for terminal liver diseases with portal hypertension. *J Am Coll Surg* 2009;51:e1-4.

[47] Umeda Y, Yagi T, Sadamori H, et al. Preoperative proximal splenic artery embolization: A safe and efficacious portal decompression technique that improves the outcome of live donor liver transplantation. *Transpl Int* 2007;20:947-955.

[48] Umeda Y, Yagi T, Sadamori H, et al. Effects of prophylactic splenic artery modulation on portal overperfusion and liver regeneration in small for size graft. *Transplantation* 2008;86:673-680.

Chapter 18

Optimizing Hemodynamic Performance after Heart Surgery, the Role of Cardiac Resynchronization Therapy

F. Straka[1]* and D. Schornik[2]

[1]Department of Cardiovascular Surgery, Institute for Clinical and Experimental Medicine, Prague, Czech Republic
[2]Institute of Physiology, Academy of Sciences, Prague, Czech Republic

Introduction

Congestive heart failure (CHF) is a constellation of symptoms and signs resulting from a low cardiac output state. The prevalence of CHF in the general population ranges from 1 to 5%. The proportion of patients with chronic heart failure in the general population increases with age.

The number of patients with New York Heart Association (NYHA) III-IV heart failure possessing a dilated and dysfunctional left ventricle (LV) and coronary artery disease in combination with valvular heart disease that are indicated for heart surgery is increasing. These patients have an increased operative risk that is possible to predict using various scoring systems (i.e. APACHE, EuroSCORE, Thoracoscore). The causes of heart failure are multiple ranging from myocardial ischemia, heart valve malformations, to genetically or environmentally acquired defects of myocardium. Cardiac surgery and cardiology have evolved as the main approaches of therapy of these conditions. Operative myocardial revascularization, heart valve replacement and heart transplantation represent accepted standards of therapy, saving lives and improving quality of life. It is known that the prognosis of patients indicated for heart surgery deteriorates in proportion to the degree of LV

---

*Correspondence: Frantisek Straka, MD, Department of Cardiac Surgery, Institute for Clinical and Experimental Medicine, Videnska 1958/9, 140 21 Prague, Czech Republic. Telephone 420-26136 5198, fax 420-26136 2799, e-mail frst@ikem.cz.

dysfunction and a history of clinically overt heart failure. [1] Optimal postoperative pharmacotherapy and inotropic support therapy cannot always accomplish an adequate cardiac output postoperatively. The most critical period for these patients is the early postoperative period (first 3 days) which in some cases requires the institution of an intraaortic balloon pump (IABP) or some other mode of mechanical circulatory support involving external continuous or pulsatile pumps to maintain adequate cardiac output (CO). These devices augment cardiac output and can permit patients to live a near normal life for an extended period while awaiting heart transplantation or myocardial recovery. However, these devices are also associated with complications such as infection, thrombosis and device failure. Therefore, along with improved operative techniques, pharmacotherapy and mechanical circulatory augmentation have evolved new ways of improving cardiac hemodynamic performance and clinical outcome in patients with heart failure. Postoperative cardiac resynchronization therapy (CRT) using biventricular (BIV) pacing is a new method which can improve the hemodynamic performance and clinical outcome of heart failure patients undergoing heart surgery avoiding the use of more invasive operative techniques.

In indicated cases, CRT using BIV pacing modifies the adverse pathophysiological mechanisms caused by cardiac contraction dyssynchrony, improves functional classification and stress tolerance, and positively influences the overall morbidity and mortality of NYHA III and IV heart failure patients (CARE-HF study, COMPANION trial). [2,3] The REVERSE trial [4] and the MADIT-CRT trial [5] confirm that CRT reduces the risk of death or heart failure even in mildly symptomatic patients and both trials demonstrated the positive effect of CRT on left ventricular (LV) remodeling leading to an improvement in left ventricular ejection fraction (LVEF) and left ventricular end systolic volume index (LVESVI). CRT is also associated with a reduction of mitral regurgitation grade. [6]

Postoperative Monitoring after Heart Surgery

Standard monitoring approaches in patients after open heart surgery involve monitorig the basic physiological functions of the human body including electrocardiographic monitoring of heart rhythm, pulse oximetry (arterial oxygen saturation), arterial gas analysis, temperature, fluid balance, central venous pressure and arterial blood pressure. Transesophageal echocardiography (TEE) is routinely used to improve perioperative patient care. These methods serve not only as important diagnostic tools for the detection of complications, but also help to balance circulatory volume therapy and establish optimal catecholamine dosing. Information gained from TEE has an influence on perioperative therapy in 10 to 52% of patients. [7] TEE plays a key role in the postoperative evaluation of heart valve surgery, left ventricular and right ventricular function and the detection of postoperative complications such as cardiac tamponade. In high risk patients with LV dysfunction, LVEF below 35%, low CO syndrome and pulmonary hypertension it is also useful to monitor CO, cardiac index (CI), systemic (SVRI) and peripheral vascular resistance index (PVRI) using a Swan-Ganz catheter. [8] Based on the measurement of mixed venous oxygen saturation (SvO2) it is possible to evaluate the ratio between global oxygen supply and consumption which can influence the morbidity in heart surgery patients. [9] An alternative to this measurement is transpulmonary thermodilution and calibrated pulse contour analysis.

Postoperative monitoring guides postoperative fluid management, inotropic support therapy and vasoactive therapy to maintain adequate tissue perfusion and oxidative metabolism. Recommended values for critically ill patients include a central venous oxygen saturation (ScvO$_2$) > 70% , SvO$_2$ > 65%, mean arterial pressure (MAP) > 65 mmHg, CI > 2.0 l/min/m^2, central venous pressure 8-12 mmHg (which can be influenced by the ventilation mode), pulmonary capillary wedge pressure (PCWP) 12-15 mmHg, diuresis > 0.5 ml/kg BW/h and a serum lactate < 2.0 mmol/l. Patients with a low cardiac output after heart surgery are characterized by peripheral vasoconstriction, centralization of the circulation, ScvO$_2$ < 60% , MAP < 60 mmHg, urine output < 0.5 ml/kg BW/h and a serum lactate > 2.0 mmol/l.

A low CO state in the early postoperative period after heart surgery can be caused by volume depletion from postoperative blood loss, reduced left ventricular function and can be worsened by dyssynchrony of ventricular contraction, significant valvular regurgitation or cardiac tamponade. Treatment consists of strengthening the work of the failing myocardium using inotropic support therapy (i.e. dobutamine, epinephrine), reducing preload and afterload with vasodilators such as sodium nitroprusside and performing pericardiocentesis or emergent surgical reexploratiion to remove pericardial fluid or blood. Phosphodiesterase inhibitors such as milrinone and amrinone play a very important role because they have a combined inotropic and vasodilatory effect, unlike alpha mimetics that increase peripheral vascular resistance and afterload. [10] Levosimendan is a calcium sensitiser that increases CO and lowers preload and afterload, but it is not approved for clinical use in several countries. Mechanical circulatory support is indicated in patients with refractory heart failure after heart surgery despite optimal inotropic support therapy and vasodilator administration.

The Significance of Mechanical Ventricular Dyssynchrony

Patients with a dilated and dysfunctional LV with an EF below 35%, a reduced functional capacity and a history of repeated hospital stay due to heart failure represent a high risk group of patients indicated for heart surgery. The postoperative period in these patients is prolonged with the need of extended administration of catecholamines, prolonged mechanical ventilation or stay in the postoperative ward. [6] In addition to left ventricular dysfunction, one of the contributing factors to poor outcome in these patients involves dyssynchrony of myocardial ventricular contraction that reduces the pumping efficacy of the heart, in many cases compounded by progressive mitral regurgitation leading to a reduced CO and CI. This pathophysiological effect is often difficult to treat with catecholamine administration alone or mechanical circulatory support such as intraaortic balloon counterpulsation. Mechanical dyssynchrony may also be worsened in the immediate postoperative period by pacing. The standard procedure of using only right sided ventricular epicardial pacing after heart surgery results in a slow spread of depolarization through the working myocardium instead of a fast spread by the specialized conduction system of the heart. The best way to improve electrical and thus mechanical resynchronization of the cardiac cycle in such a situation is by using BIV or LV pacing optimized by echocardiographic imaging. CRT reduces the energy requirement of the heart by improving the efficiency of cardiac pump function because the amount of stroke work generated by a unit of oxygen consumed is approximately 30% lower during mechanical ventricular dyssynchrony. [11] Despite the described benefits of CRT, BIV pacing has not been commonly used in patients after heart surgery and there is an ongoing discussion concerning the most appropriate location of pacing electrodes and the best pacing mode. [12,13]

Real-time Three-Dimensional Echocardiography (RT3DE) and Doppler tissue imaging (DTI) in the Assessment of LV Mechanical Dyssynchrony

CRT is at present time an established therapy for patients with heart failure who have a wide QRS complex and LV mechanical dyssynchrony. [14] The presence of a wide QRS complex ($\geq$ 120 ms) has been used as an indicator of ventricular dyssynchrony. However, a wide QRS value is poor in predicting the response to CRT. [15] Several echocardiographic techniques are presently used for detecting LV dyssynchrony, but most of them are also weak in predicting the response to CRT. [16, 17, 18] The parasternal short axis view is used to determine the M-Mode septal to posterior wall motion delay (SPWMD). This delay is measured as the shortest interval between the maximal posterior deflection of the anterior septal wall segment and the maximal inward deflection of the posterior LV wall segment after the QRS complex.

Real-time three-dimensional echocardiography (RT3DE) is a new method for detecting LV dyssynchrony that can also accurately measure LV volume (ESV- end systolic volume, EDV- end diastolic volume) and LVEF. [19] RT3DE acquisitions are made using a matrix-array transducer. Several consecutive heart cycles and a constant RR interval is used to create a full volume data acquisition of the LV from the apical window. Analyses of the RT3DE data sets can be performed using specific software which creates a 3D model of the LV. The papillary muscles are usually included in the LV cavity calculations. Cardiac output by RT3DE (RT3DE CO) can be calculated as (LVEDV – LVESV) times heart rate. Cardiac index by RT3DE (RT3DE CI) is RT3DE CO divided by body surface area. A 16 segment LV model (6 basal segments, 6 mid segments, 4 apical segments) is used for the evaluation of ventricular mechanical dyssynchrony as described by the American Society of Echocardiography. [20] Time-volume data are recorded for the entire LV and for each volumetric segment during the cardiac cycle and the time to minimal systolic volume (Tmsv) is obtained. LV systolic dyssynchrony index (SDI, Figure 1) is calculated as the standard deviation of the Tmsv for all 16 segments (Tmsv16-SD) expressed as a percentage of the RR interval (thus eliminating the effect of heart rate variability). Although there is currently no uniformity in the accepted cut-off value of SDI by RT3DE in determining LV mechanical dyssynchrony, a cut-off value of SDI $\geq$ 6.0% is predictive of hemodynamic response to CRT as was shown by clinical trials. The latest activated segment of the LV can be established using "timing bull's eye parametric imaging" (Figure 2). By preoperatively detecting the latest activated segment of the LV it is possible to locate the best site for epicardial LV lead placement for postoperative BIV pacing. [21]

Doppler tissue imaging (DTI) is a standard echocardiographic technique for quantifying LV mechanical dyssynchrony. [17] DTI recordings are made using standard 4, 2 and 3 chamber image planes, care being taken to store 3 consecutive heart beats at a frame rate over 150/sec. The time interval from the onset of QRS to the peak systolic velocity of each curve is measured. Dyssynchrony is defined as a time difference between the contraction of the opposite walls of the LV greater than 65 msec. Septal flash can identify dyssynchronous contraction induced by left bundle branch block (LBBB) by detecting early activation of the septum as shown by early septal thickening within the isovolumic contraction period. [22]

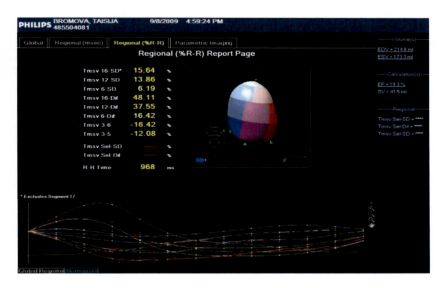

Figure 1. RT3DE – LV volumetric regional curves of 16 segments in a patient with severe intraventricular dyssynchrony. Systolic dyssynchrony index - SDI (Tmsv16SD) = 15.64%.

Burgess et al. [23] compared RT3DE and DTI for the assessment of LV dyssynchrony in 100 patients with ischemic cardiomyopathy. They found a poor correlation between these two techniques for evaluating the magnitude of intraventricular dyssynchrony (r = 0.11, p = NS) and the site of maximal mechanical delay. Concordance between DTI and RT3DE in identifying the site of maximal mechanical delay was observed in only 12 (16%) patients. The authors explained that this could be due to longitudinal versus radial timing of LV contraction, each method measuring something different. Some authors have tried to improve the accuracy of DTI measurements. Fornwald et al. [24] found that using a 30 x 6 mm region of interest (ROI) instead of the generally used 6 x 6 mm ROI default size to quantify DTI dyssynchrony reduces variability by 47% and diagnostic inconsistency by 44%. A novel method for displaying LV function and dyssynchrony using DTI and its application to patients with dilated cardiomyopathy with wide and narrow QRS complexes was described by Ito et al. [25] The time to peak velocities (TPVs) obtained from 6 basal segments were assumed to be vectors and aligned radially to the corresponding LV segment. The resulting hexagonal graph reflected global LV function, net-delay magnitude of mechanical contraction and the delayed contraction site of the LV. With this method (net-delay magnitude > 90 ms) LV mechanical dyssynchrony was detectable in 68% of patients with wide QRS complexes and in 39% of patients with narrow QRS complexes. The percentages were similar to those obtained using conventional DTI derived indices (standard deviation and dispersion of TPVs in the 12 myocardial segments). Patients with a wide QRS complex had delayed contraction sites more often located between lateral and inferior LV wall segments than controls (68% vs. 35%; p < 0.001). This new DTI method can be extended to more advanced modalities such as strain and two-dimensional speckle-tracking imaging. [26]

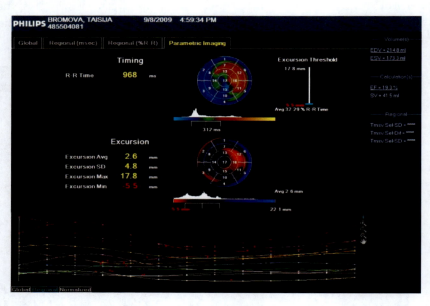

Figure 2. Example of left ventricular (LV) dyssynchrony analysis using RT3DE parametric imaging before CRT. The latest LV activated segment is mid anterolateral – coded in red.

The Role of CRT after Heart Surgery

Myocardial dysfunction and dilation of the cardiac chambers is frequently associated with cardiac conduction disorders in both the atria and the ventricles resulting in cardiac dyssynchrony, a common scenario after heart surgery. The adverse effects of ventricular dyssynchrony include suboptimal diastolic filling, paradoxical movement of the interventricular septum, reduced LV contractility and progression of mitral regurgitation. It is known that about 9% of patients after coronary artery bypass grafting (CABG) require pacing for atrioventricular block or sinus bradydardia. [27] At present time, postsurgical therapy routinely involves right ventricular (RV) pacing which is not physiological. Isolated RV pacing requires conduction of electrical depolarization through the myocardium from the right ventricle to the left ventricle, which is slower than through the specialized conduction system of the heart (His-Purkinje system). This results in dyssynchrony of contraction between the two ventricles. [28] Optimized CRT using BIV pacing corrects ventricular contraction dyssynchrony by initiating the contraction of the LV directly.

It has been published that BIV pacing in patients with poor LV function and bundle branch block is associated with improved CO, coronary flow and diastolic function. [29, 30] This mode of pacing may improve volumetric and functional echocardiographic parameters and may lead to LV reverse remodeling with a reduction of mitral regurgitation grade. [18]

By improving CO, BIV pacing may be an effective way to avoid the use of more invasive approaches in the treatment of postoperative heart failure, lowering postoperative inotrope requirements and ICU stay. [21] The feasibility and safety of temporary BIV pacing have been previously demonstrated in the study by Eberhard and colleagues [31] and similar positive results were reported by Dzemali et al. [13] and Hanke et al. [32]

CRT has been extensively studied in patients with ischemic or dilated cardiomyopathy. Boriani et al. [33] found that CRT also appears to be effective in patients with valvular heart disease. In this group of patients, they found an improvement in LVEF and a reduction in ventricular volumes at 6-12 months. A favorable clinical response was observed at 12 months with improvement of the clinical composite score similar to that observed in patients with dilated cardiomyopathy. This was even more pronounced in patients with ischemic heart disease. In clinical practice, many patients with ischemic heart disease that undergo heart surgery also have concomitant heart valve disease, but only limited CRT experience is available for this group of patients. In such patients, reverse remodeling of the LV as well as response to BIV pacing may be the result of a combination of factors including LV electrode positioning, myocardial revascularization and by the physiological changes that occur after the surgical correction of heart valve disease. It is difficult to assess which of these factors has the greatest impact and probably all have an additive positive hemodynamic effect in the early postoperative period.

BIV pacing can be performed after heart surgery using epicardial leads. The LV electrode should be placed on the LV at the location of the latest activated segment. This can be determined by several methods including RT3DE. Electrode impedance, sensing and pacing thresholds should be measured during surgery. A satisfactory pacing threshold is ≤ 3 V/0.5 ms. Correct lead placement is guided by intraoperative TEE and confirmed postoperatively by chest X-ray (AP view, LAO 40, RAO 30). Atrioventricular delay (AVD) should be optimized in the early postoperative period using pacemaker programming. An accepted method for AVD optimization is measuring the velocity time integral (VTI) of the transmitral flow using Doppler ultrasound. Optimal AVD is defined as the AVD resulting in the highest VTI when the A wave of transmitral flow is not truncated. AVD optimization is also important for lowering the grade of mitral valve regurgitation. Interventricular delay (VVD) optimization corrects interventricular dyssynchrony and is done by adjusting the VVD to achieve the highest VTI in the LV outflow tract. The recommended pacing rate is between 80-90 bpm.

The Hemodynamic Effect of CRT after Heart Surgery

Hemodynamic measurements are recommended in high risk group of patients undergoing heart surgery who have LV dysfunction and an EF below 35%. It is routinely performed using a Swan-Ganz thermodilution catheter. Using this catheter it is possible to measure the mean pulmonary artery pressure (MPAP), cardiac output (CO), cardiac index (CI), pulmonary vascular resistance index (PVRI), systemic vascular resistance index (SVRI), left ventricular stroke work index (LVSWI) and right ventricular stroke work index (RVSWI). A radial artery catheter is usually used for measuring the mean arterial pressure (MAP). The feasibility and safety of temporary BIV pacing in patients after cardiac surgery has been demonstrated in our study. [21] We have shown that LV pacing in patients with CHF in the early period after heart surgery is less effective than BIV pacing and that both of these pacing modes are significantly better than isolated RV pacing which worsens LV dyssynchrony. Our study included 21 patients with ischemic heart disease or valvular heart disease (16 men, 5 women, average age 69 years) with LV dysfunction after cardiac surgery. Patients undergoing BIV (CO 6.7 ± 1.7 l/min, CI 3.5 ± 0.8 l/min/m²) and LV (CO 6.2 ± 1.5 l/min, CI 3.2 ± 0.7 l/min/m²) pacing had a statistically significantly higher CO and CI than patients undergoing RV (CO 5.4 ± 1.4 l/min, CI 2.8 ± 0.6 l/min/m²) pacing (BIV vs. RV p ≤ 0.001; LV vs. RV p ≤ 0.05; BIV vs. LV p ≤ 0.05). A decrease in the SVRI is another benefit of BIV pacing in patients with CHF. The PVRI was also lower during LV and BIV pacing than during RV pacing, but these differences were not statistically significant. There was also an increase in LVSWI and RVSWI during LV and BIV pacing which reflect an improved function of the left and right ventricle. Similar results were shown by Hanke and colleagues [32] where there was an average 12-14% improvement in stroke work during DDD-BIV or DDD-LV pacing relative to DDD-RVOT pacing. It has been published that BIV pacing in patients with poor LV function and bundle branch block is associated with improved CO, coronary flow [29] and diastolic function. [30] The results of our study have shown that the improved hemodynamic parameters achieved by early postoperative LV or BIV pacing can be a survival advantage for patients with low EF (≤ 35%) and LV dyssynchrony undergoing heart surgery. Such an improvement in hemodynamic performance can lower postoperative inotrope requirements and reduce ICU stay. [21]

The negative influence of isolated RV pacing on LV mechanical dyssynchrony was also described by the study performed by Liu et al. [34] in patients with sick sinus syndrome and right ventricular apical pacing (RVA). RVA pacing worsened the myocardial performance index (RVA pacing 0.42 ± 0.18 vs. without RVA pacing 0.31 ± 14) and LVEF derived by RT3DE was significantly lower (p = 0.013) (with RVA 54.4 ± 7.7% vs. without RVA 56.7 ± 7.9%). RVA pacing also worsened the parameters of LV dyssynchrony measured using SDI by RT3DE (with RVA 7.0 ± 2.54% vs. without RVA 5.36 ± 2.17%, p=0.003).

RT3DE SDI in Predicting the Hemodynamic Response to CRT

SDI by RT3DE is not only a way to detect LV dyssynchrony and the optimal site for LV lead placement for postoperative BIV pacing in patients scheduled for heart surgery, but is also a means of predicting which patients may benefit from this therapy and to what extent. Various echocardiographic parameters and techniques were tested for the detection of LV dyssynchrony and response to BIV pacing. Some echocardiographic parameters previously used for evaluating LV dyssynchrony proved to be nonspecific on the basis of the multicenter PROSPECT trial. [35] There was no correlation between LV dyssynchrony and parameters such as SPWMD or septal flash. The evaluation of SPWMD is problematic in patients with ischemic heart disease and this parameter cannot be used for the detection of LV dyssynchrony in patients with myocardial infarction of the posterior LV wall or anterior septum. The limitations of DTI parameters in determining LV dyssynchrony include minimal base-apex motion in patients with LV dysfunction, translational and tethering effects, inadequate setting of the sample volume and asymmetric arrangement of the myocardial muscle fibers which change the shape of the LV to spherical in long-standing heart failure. All these factors explain the difficulty in assessing DTI curves in echocardiography where the parameters of LV dyssynchrony rely primarily on identifying peak contraction. In patients who have myocardial dysfunction the speed of the DTI velocity curve flattens which also makes it difficult to assess LV dyssynchrony. Interobserver variability of DTI dyssynchrony parameter measurements was over 30% in the PROSPECT Trial. [35]

Another factor making it very difficult to accurately determine and predict LV dyssynchrony and the response to BIV pacing using DTI is the finding of postsystolic contraction as a nonspecific marker of myocardial dysfunction. This may arise on the basis of scars, fibrosis, or even viable stunned myocardium and may be further complicated by excessive chamber filling based on the Starling law. Some authors have recently recommended investigating myocardial viability and contractile reserve as a complement to DTI parameters for better prediction of the response to CRT. [5]

There is currently no uniformity in the accepted value of SDI by RT3DE for defining LV dyssynchrony. Harkel et al. [36] found that normal values of SDI in a group of healthy adolescents are 1.26 ± 0.53% and confirmed that this measurement could be performed with good interobserver (0.3 ± 0.2%) and intraobserver variability (0.0 ± 0.27%). Gimenes et al. [37] found normal values of SDI in a normal population (EF 50-80%) to be 0.2 to 3.8% for a 6-segment model, 0.22 to 4.01% for a 12-segment model, and 0.29 to 4.88% for a 16-segment model. Kleijn and colleagues [19] reported that an optimal cut-off value of 6.7% for SDI by RT3DE (16-segment model) yielded a sensitivity of 90% and specificity of 87% in predicting a clinical response to CRT, and a sensitivity of 88% and specificity of 70% in predicting LV reverse remodeling. Marshan and colleagues [38] found a lower cut-off value of SDI $\geq$ 5.6% as evidence of intraventricular dyssynchrony which yielded a sensitivity of 88% and specificity of 86% in predicting an acute response to CRT.

We used an intermediate cut-off value of SDI by RT3DE $\geq$ 6.0% for determining LV dyssynchrony and for enrolling patients into our study. [21] The average SDI by RT3DE in our group of patients was 10.4 ± 4.9% and this yielded a positive correlation between SDI and BIV pacing response. We found that preoperatively measured SDI by RT3DE is predictive of BIV pacing response after heart surgery in a high risk group of patients with ischemic heart disease with or without heart valve disease, with LV dysfunction (LVEF $\leq$ 35%) and dyssynchrony, undergoing CABG with or without a valve procedure. The severity of ventricular dyssynchrony measured using SDI by RT3DE positively correlates with postoperative CO during BIV pacing. Higher values of SDI before pacing yielded a higher CO and CI during BIV pacing (in press). Conversely, higher SDI values before pacing were associated with a lower CI measured by RT3DE before pacing (in press). Postoperative BIV pacing was also shown to produce significantly better hemodynamic results than standardly used RV pacing. We found no correlation between DTI dyssynchrony parameters, SPWMD, septal flash and hemodynamic values during RV or BIV pacing. Other studies have used magnetic resonance imaging and gated myocardial perfusion single photon emission computed tomography (GMPS) for assessing LV dyssynchrony and for predicting the response to CRT. [39,40] Marsan et al. [41] found a good correlation between LV dyssynchrony assessed with RT3DE and GMPS (r = 0.76-0.8, p < 0.0001). This further supports the use of RT3DE as a reliable means of assessing not only LV function but also LV dyssynchrony. [42]

LV mechanical dyssynchrony also can be defined by QRS complex duration. However, some authors have demonstrated the deterioration in SDI (Tmsv16SD) with progression of LV dysfunction independent of QRS duration or type of cardiomyopathy. [43] Futhermore, it has been reported that LV mechanical dyssynchrony may also be present in patients with normal QRS length. [44] Soliman et al. [45] found only a weak correlation ($r2= 0.07$, $p < 0.05$) between QRS duration and SDI by RT3DE for the 16-segment LV model. Patients with heart failure had a higher SDI ($13.4\% \pm 8.1\%$) in comparison to controls ($4.1\% \pm 2.2\%$) and volumetric responders who underwent CRT had a significant reduction in SDI ($16.3\% \pm 3.3\%$ to $7.7\% \pm 2.4\%$, $p < 0.001$) at 12 months follow-up.

A recently published study by Kuppahally et al. [46] showed that dyssynchrony assessment using DTI and regional volumetric analysis by 3D echocardiography did not predict long-term response to CRT. The possible explanation for this may be the following. First, the basic clinical diagnosis in their study was dilated cardiomyopathy, whereas the patients we studied had ischemic heart disease with or without heart valve disease. The type of heart disease can influence the degree of response to CRT, a diseased dilated myocardium may not be able to respond to BIV pacing to such an extent as ischemic viable myocardium after revascularization. Second, the average SDI was higher in our study group before pacing ($10.4 \pm 4.9\%$) compared to $7.0 \pm 4.1\%$ in their study. A SDI of 7.0% represents a borderline cut-off value defining LV dyssynchrony which is 6-7%. [19] This borderline value of SDI may not be as predictive of response to CRT as are higher values. Finally, LV electrode positioning in their study was not optimized using RT3DE or other similar methods (e.g. magnetic resonance imaging). Such positioning may not be as effective for CRT as targeted intraoperative LV epicardial lead placement using RT3DE which we have shown to be an accurate way of determining the latest activated segment of the LV for LV lead placement and postoperative BIV pacing. [21]

The Significance of LV epicardial Electrode Positioning and Optimization of Pacing Parameters during CRT

There is much controversy regarding the optimal lead placement site for heart failure patients. There is also great individual variability in the best site for LV pacing. [47] Several studies used paraseptal pacing for both RV and LV leads, although this was not as effective as LV lateral wall pacing. [48] Berger et al. [49] used noninvasive imaging of cardiac electrophysiology (NICE) for visualizing both epicardial and endocardial ventricular electrical activation. They confirmed that during RV pacing the septal, endocardial and epicardial activation times of the LV are markedly delayed as compared to those seen with native sinus rhythm. This resulted in an increase in the total RV and LV activation duration. This increase in ventricular activation time may be due to cell-to-cell coupled propagation of the activation waveform with delayed connection to the intrinsic conduction system (Purkinje system). BIV pacing did not affect the direction of transseptal activation and the timing of LV septal breakthrough. This suggests that the major effect of CRT is direct LV stimulation which is not mediated by the intrinsic conduction system. Therefore, the optimal placement of the LV lead is very important. This lead should be placed at the site of latest LV activation during native sinus rhythm. This results in a significant decrease in LV total activation duration during CRT. By reducing the additional dyssynchrony of papillary muscle contraction, mitral regurgitation is reduced which also compromises patients with CHF. The latest activated segment of the LV was found to lie epicardially in the LV lateral wall and its inhomogeneity reflects the individual differences in patients with heart failure. The identification of target sites for optimal LV lead placement can be accomplished using NICE and this may also be helpful in determining responders to CRT. Spragg et al. [50] showed that endocardial pacing of the LV is more effective than coronary sinus lead pacing, but there is a disconnection between electrical and mechanical activation observed in patients with ischemic cardiomyopathy that may be caused by regions of slow conduction or conduction block.

Several studies have used paraseptal placement for both RV and LV leads. [48] However, published works suggest that the inferolateral and anterolateral aspect of the LV are the optimal sites for BIV pacing. [47] In our study we used a new approach where the LV lead was surgically positioned at the site of the latest activated segment of the LV detected by RT3DE. [21] In 33% of our patients the latest activated segment of the LV was mid-anterolateral (Figure 3) which was the most frequent site of delayed LV activation in our study. A surgical approach to lead placement allows, in comparison to the transvenous approach, accurate positioning of the pacing leads without the limitations imposed by the anatomy of the cardiac veins. This allows the surgeon to avoid areas such as scarred myocardium. [31] Positioning the LV lead at the site of the latest activated segment allows optimal pacing of the LV by activating the site of greatest contraction delay, improving cardiac hemodynamic performance. The mid and basal anterolateral segments of the LV represent the segments that are the furthest away from the interventricular septum.

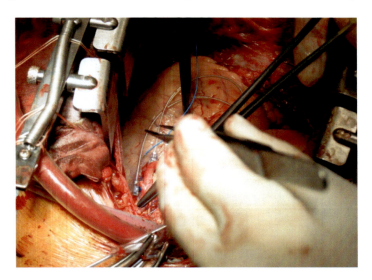

Figure 3. Intraoperative LV electrode placement onto the latest activated segment of the left ventricle.

Positioning the LV lead in the baseline/midventricle segments may improve the clinical outcome and apical LV placement is conversely associated with worse CRT outcomes as was shown by the study published by Merchant et al. [51] In their study they compared apical LV lead placement to basal/midventricle lead placement. The event free survival (primary outcome was heart failure hospitalization, cardiac transplantation, or all-cause mortality) was better in the basal/midventricle lead placement group (79%) compared to the apical lead placement group (52%), hazard ratio [HR] 2.7 (95% CI: 1.5-5.5, p = 0,006). The apical lead placement group also had less improvement in NYHA functional class and less LV reverse remodeling. The explanation for this finding is that pacing in the region of less delayed electrical and mechanical activation cannot adequately correct LV electrical and mechanical dyssynchrony. Ansalone et al. [52] published that in 43% of patients indicated for CRT the latest activated segment was not in the free lateral or posterolateral wall, which is the common position used during transvenous LV lead placement. Murphy et al. [53] found that placing the LV electrode in the site of maximal delay is in concordance with LV reverse remodeling and improvement in NYHA class.

Epicardial RV lead site position paraseptally in the lower third of the exposed anterior wall of the RV is similar to what is presently used for endoventricular BIV pacing. This position is better than endoventricular apical lead placement because it results in a more rapid spread of the RV depolarization wave. [48] This RV positioning has been confirmed to be the best location to achieve maximal electrical separation (MES) and a better correction of electrical and mechanical dyssynchrony. [54] *The extent of LV reverse remodeling following CRT is not related to the RV lead position, but it is significantly higher in patients with concordant LV lead placement in the latest contracting area.* Differences exist in the method that is used for the detection of the latest activated segment of the LV. In our study we used RT3DE, but similar results were described using two-dimensional speckle tracking radial strain imaging. [55]

An optimal combination of AVD and VVD during BIV pacing is also very important in patients with heart failure and it is known to correlate with an improvement in clinical performance status and LV reverse remodeling. [56] Optimal LV filling and atrial emptying reduce diastolic mitral regurgitation and VVD optimization improves ventricular dyssynchrony leading to a more effective ventricular output. Jansen and colleagues [57] confirmed that Doppler echocardiography is a reliable tool for optimizing AVD compared to the invasive measurement of $LvdP/dt_{max}$. In our study we found that AVD and VVD optimization is very important for patients with heart failure and LV dysfunction undergoing BIV pacing after heart surgery and can improve hemodynamic parameters such as CO and CI. [21] Similar results were published in a recent study by Wang et al. [58] where temporary BIV pacing increased intraoperative CO in patients with LV dysfunction undergoing heart surgery. The authors reported that AVD and VVD optimization improves this benefit.

Conclusion

Postoperative CRT using BIV pacing is way of optimizing the cardiac hemodynamic performance in indicated patients who have undergone heart surgery. SDI by RT3DE and RT3DE targeted epicardial LV lead positioning are new ways to treat patients with LV dysfunction (LVEF ≤ 35%) and ventricular dyssynchrony (SDI by RT3DE ≥ 6%), with ischemic heart disease with or without valvular heart disease, who have undergone CABG with or without a valve procedure. BIV or LV pacing in the early postoperative period after heart surgery is beneficial in this high risk group of patients and BIV pacing produces significantly better hemodynamic results than standardly used RV pacing. RT3DE also allows the preoperative detection of the latest activated segment of the LV for optimal positioning of the LV epicardial pacing lead. Patients undergoing BIV pacing after heart surgery have a shorter ICU stay and lower time on inotropic support than patients undergoing isolated RV pacing.

Preoperative SDI by RT3DE correlates with improved hemodynamic response during CRT in the early postoperative period after heart surgery- higher values of SDI before pacing yield a higher CO and CI during BIV pacing. Conversely, higher SDI values before pacing are associated with a lower CI measured by RT3DE before pacing. This suggests that more severe LV dyssynchrony is more likely to be corrected by CRT postoperatively and that ventricular resynchronization plays an important role in determining cardiac hemodynamic function.

A positive response to CRT may be predicted in CABG patients with salvageable ischemic myocardium after revascularization. Patients with irreversible large areas of infarcted myocardium, especially involving the inferolateral LV, may not respond to such an extent as patients with smaller areas of salvageable ischemic myocardium. Concomitant heart valve disease may also influence the response to CRT and poorer response rates may be expected with long-standing heart valve pathology and myocardial remodelling. This may suggest the importance of early surgical correction of significant heart valve pathology or myocardial ischemia in patients with LV dysfunction and dyssynchrony in order to preserve viable myocardium needed for CRT response. Finally, proper adjustment of AVD and VVD during BIV pacing and accurate LV lead placement will improve the hemodynamic response of patients indicated for postoperative CRT. Myocardial viability and localization of myocardial scarring can be assessed before surgery using MRI [59] or Dobutamine stress echocardiography [60] to select patients who will respond to postoperative CRT.

Based on accepted guidelines [61], patients who are indicated for heart surgery and who fulfill the criteria for CRT (LV dysfunction, EF $\leq$ 35%, QRS $\geq$ 120 ms, with signs of LV dyssynchrony - SDI by RT3DE $\geq$ 6%) should undergo LV epicardial electrode implantation at the time of surgery for postoperative BIV pacing, with the possiblilty of long-term DDD BIV or DDD BIV/ICD therapy. Another application of CRT using a surgically implanted epicardial LV lead may be in patien

References

[1] Nalysnyk L, Fahrbach K, Reynolds MW, Zhao SZ, Ross S. Averse events in coronary artery bypass graft (CABG) trials: a systematic review and analysis. *Heart.* 2003;89:767-72.

[2] Cleland JGF, Daubert JC, Erdmann E, Freemantle N, Gras D, Kappenberger L, Klein W, et al. The CARE-HF study (Cardiac Resynchronization in Heart Failure study): Rationale, design, and endpoints. *Eur J Card Fail* 2001; 3:481-489.

[3] Saxon LA, Bristol MR, Boehmer J, Krueger S, Kass DA, DeMarco T, Carson P, et al. Predictors of sudden cardiac death and appropriate shock in the Comparison of Medical Therapy, Pacing, and Defibrillation in Heart Failure (COMPANION) Trial. *Circulation* 2006; 114:2766-2772.

[4] Linde C, Abraham WT, Gold MR, St. John Sutton M, Ghio S, Daubert C; REVERSE (REsynchronization reVErses Remodeling in Systolic left vEntricular dysfunction) Study Group. *J Am Coll Cardiol.*2008; 52: 1834-43.

[5] Moss AJ, Hall WJ, Cannom DS, Klein H, Brown MW, Daubert JP, Esters NA 3rd et al. Cardiac-resynchronization therapy for prevention of heart-failure events. *N Engl J Med* 2009; 361: 1329-38.

[6] Senechal M, Lancellotti P, Magne J, Garceau P, Champagne J, Philippon F, O´Hara G et al. Impact of mitral regurgitation and myocardial viability on left ventricular reverse remodeling after cardiac resynchronization therapy in patients with ischemic cardiomyopathy. *Am J Cardiol.* 2010; 106:31-7.

[7] Click RL, Abel MD, Schaff HV. Intraoperative transesophageal echocardiography: 5-year prospective review of impact on surgical management. *Mayo Clin Proc.*2000;75:241-7.

[8] Pulmonary Artery Catheter Consensus Conference: consensus statement. Crit Care Med. 1997;25:910-25.

[9] Pölönen P, Ruokonen E, Hippeläinen M et al. A prospective randomized study of goal-oriented hemodynamic therapy in cardiac surgical patients. *Anesth Anag.* 2000;90:1052-9.

[10] Vroom MB. Pharmacologic management of acute heart failure: A review. *Seminars in Cardiothorac and Vascular Anesthesia* 1998;2:191-203.

[11] Prinzen F, Vernooy K, DeBoeck BWL et al.: Mechano-energetics of the asynchronous and resynchronized heart. *Heart Fail Rev.* 2011;16:215-24.

[12] Jessup M., Abraham WT, Cassey DE, Feldman AM, Francis GS, Ganiats TG, Konstam MA et all. 2009 focused update: ACCF/AHA Guidelines for the Diagnostics and Management of Heart Failure in Adults: a report of the American College of Cardiology Foundation/American Heart Association Task Force on Practice Guidelines: deloped in collaboration with the International Society for Heart and Lung Transplantation. *Circulation* 2009; 119: 1977-2016.

[13] Dzemali O, Bakhtiary F, Dogan S, Wittlinger T, Moritz A, Kleine P. Perioperative biventricular pacing leads to improvement of hemodynamics in patients with reduced left-ventricular function-interim results. *Pacing Clin Electrophysiol.* 2006; 29:1341-5.

[14] Abraham WT, Fisher WG, Smith AL, et al.: Cardiac resynchronization in chronic heart failure. *N Engl J Med* 2002; 346:1845-53.

[15] Ghio S, Constantin C, Klersy C, et al.: Interventricular and intraventricular dyssynchrony are common in heart failure patients, regardless of QRS duration. *Eur Heart J* 2004; 25:571-578.

[16] Bax JJ, Bleeker GB, Marwick TH, et al.: Left ventricular dyssynchrony predicts response and prognosis after cardiac resynchronization therapy. *J Am Coll Cardiol* 2004; 44:1834-1840.

[17] Yu CM, Chau E, Sanderson JE, et al.: Tissue Doppler echocardiographic evidence of reverse remodeling and improved synchronicity by simultaneously delaying regional contraction after biventricular pacing therapy in heart failure. *Circulation* 2002; 105:438–445.

[18] Sogaard P, Egeblad H, Kim WY, et al.: Tissue Doppler imaging predicts improved systolic performance and reversed left ventricular remodeling during long-term cardiac resynchronization therapy. *J Am Coll Cardiol* 2002; 40:723-730.

[19] Kleijn SA, van Dijk J, de Cock CC, et al.: Assessment of intraventricular mechanical dyssynchrony and prediction of response to cardiac resynchronization therapy: comparison between tissue Doppler imaging and real-time three-dimensional echocardiography. *J Am Soc Echocardiogr* 2009; 22:1047-54.

[20] Lang RM, Bierig M, Devereux RB, et al.: Recommendations for chamber quantification: a report from the American Society of Echocardiography's Guidelines and Standards Committee and the Chamber Quantification Writing Group, developed in conjunction with the European Association of Echocardiography, a branch of the European Society of Cardiology. *J Am Soc Echocardiogr* 2005; 18:1440-63.

[21] Straka F, Pirk J. Pindak M et al. The hemodynamic effect of right ventricle (RV), RT3DE targeted left ventricle (LV) and biventricular (BIV) pacing in the early postoperative period after cardiac surgery. *PACE* 2011; 34:1231-40.

[22] Pavlopoulos H, Nihoyannopoulos P.: Recent advances in cardiac resynchronization therapy: echocardiographic modalities, patient selection, optimization, non-responders - all you need to know for more efficient CRT. *Int J Cardiovasc Imaging* 2010; 26:177–191.

[23] Burgess MI, Jenkins C, Chan J, et al.: Measurement of left ventricular dyssynchrony in patients with ischemic cardiomyopathy - a comparison of real-time three-dimensional and tissue Dopper echocardiography. *Heart* 2007; 93:1191-6.

[24] Fornwalt BK, Sprague WW, Carew JD, et al.: Variability in tissue Doppler echocardiographic measures of dyssynchrony is reduced with use of a larger region of interest. *J Am Soc Echocardiogr* 2009; 22:478-85.

[25] Ito T, Kawanishi Y, Tsukada B, Futai R, et al.: Novel method for displaying left ventricular function and dyssynchrony using tissue Doppler imaging: evaluation of its applicability in dilated cardiomyopathy with wide and narrow QRS complexes. *J Am Soc Echocardiogr* 2008; 21:1236-43.

[26] Donal E, Tournoux F, Leclercq C, et al.: Assessment of longitudinal and radial ventricular dyssynchrony in ischemic and nonischemic chronic systolic heart failure a two-dimensional echocardiographic speckle-tracking strain study. *J Am Soc Echocardiogr* 2008; 21:58-65.

[27] Bethea BT, Salazar JD, Grega MA, Doty JR, Fitton TP, Alejo DE, Borowicz LM Jr, et al. Determining the utility of temporary pacing wires after coronary artery bypass surgery. *Ann Thorac Surg.* 2005; 79:104-7.

[28] Healy DG, Hargrove M, Doddakulla K, Hinchion J, O'Donnell A, Aherne T. Impact of pacing modality and biventricular pacing on cardiac output and coronary conduit flow in the post-cardiotomy patient. *Interact Cardiovasc Thorac Surg.* 2008; 7:805-8.

[29] Yildirim A, Soylu O, Dagdeviren B, Ergelen M, Celik S, Zencirci E, Tezel T. Cardiac resynchronization improves coronary blood flow. *Tohoku J Exp Med* 2007; 211:43-47.

[30] Muehlschlegel JD, Peng YG, Lobato EB, Hess PJ Jr, Martin TD, Klodell CT Jr.: Temporary biventricular pacing postcardiopulmonary bypass in patients with reduced ejection fraction. *J Card Surg.* 2008; 23:324-30.

[31] Eberhardt F, Hanke T, Heringlake M, et al.: Feasibility of temporary biventricular pacing in patients with reduced left ventricular function after coronary artery bypass grafting. *Pacing Clin Electrophysiol.* 2007; 30:S50-3.

[32] Hanke T, Misfeld M, Heringlake M, Schreuder JJ, Wiegand UK, Eberhardt F. The effect of biventricular pacing on cardiac function after weaning from cardiopulmonary

bypass in patients with reduced left ventricular function: a pressure-volume loop analysis. *J Thorac Cardiovasc Surg.* 2009; 138:148-56.

[33] Boriani G, Gasparini M, Landolina M, et al.: Effectiveness of cardiac resynchronization therapy in heart failure patients with valvular heart disease: comparison with patients affected by ischaemic heart disease or dilated cardiomyopathy. The InSync/InSync ICD Italian Registry. *Eur Heart J* 2009; 30:2275-83.

[34] Liu WH, Chen MC, Chen YL, et al.: Right ventricular apical pacing acutely impairs left ventricular function and induces mechanical dyssynchrony in patients with sick sinus syndrome: a real-time three-dimensional echocardiographic study. *J Am Soc Echocardiogr* 2008; 21:224-9.

[35] Chung ES, Leon AR, Tavazzi L, et al.: Results of the Predictors of Response to CRT (PROSPECT) trial. *Circulation* 2008; 117:2608-16.

[36] Ten Harkel AD, Van Osch-Gevers M, Helbing WA: Real-time transthoracic three dimensional echocardiography: normal reference data for left ventricular dyssynchrony in adolescents. *J Am Soc Echocardiogr* 2009; 22:933-8.

[37] Gimenes VM, Vieira ML, Andrade MM, et al.: Standard values for real-time transthoracic three-dimensional echocardiographic dyssynchrony indexes in a normal population. *J Am Soc Echocardiogr* 2008; 21:1229-35.

[38] Marsan NA, Bleeker GB, Ypenburg C, et al.: Real-time threedimensional echocardiography permits quantification of left ventricular mechanical dyssynchrony and predicts acute response to cardiac resynchronization therapy. *J Cardiovasc Electrophysiol* 2008; 4:392–399.

[39] Westenberg JJ, Lamb HJ, van der Geest RJ, et al.: Assessement of left ventricular dyssynchrony in patients with conduction delay and idiopathic dilated cardiomypathy: head-to-head comparison between tissue Doppler imaging and velocity-encoded magnetic resonance imaging. *J Am Coll Cardiol* 2006; 47:2042-8.

[40] Henneman MM, Chen J, Dibbets P, et al.: Can LV dyssynchrony as assessed with phase analysis on gated myocardial perfusion SPECT predict response to CRT? *J Nucl Med* 2007; 48:1104-11.

[41] Marsan NA, Henneman MM, Chen J, et al.: Real-time three-dimensional echocardiography as a novel approach to quantify left ventricular dyssynchrony: a comparison study with phase analysis of gated myocardial perfusion single photon emission computed tomography. *J Am Soc Echocardiogr* 2008; 21:801-7.

[42] Monaghan MJ: Role of real time 3D echocardiography in evaluating the left ventricle. *Heart* 2006; 92:131-136.

[43] Park SM, Kim KC, Jeon MJ, et al.: Assessment of left ventricular asynchrony using volume-time curves of 16 segments by real-time 3 dimensional echocardiography: comparison with tissue Doppler imaging. *Eur J Heart Fail* 2007; 9:62-7.

[44] Achilli A, Sassara M, Ficili S, et al.: Long-term effectiveness of cardiac resynchronization therapy in patients with refractory heart failure and "narrow" QRS. *J Am Coll Cardiol* 2003; 42:2117-24.

[45] Soliman OI, van Dalen BM, Nemes A, et al.: Quantification of left ventricular systolic dyssynchrony by real-time three-dimensional echocardiography. *J Am Soc Echocardiogr* 2009; 22:232-9.

[46] Kuppahally SS, Fowler MB, Vagelos R et al: Dyssynchrony assessment with tissue Doppler imaging and regional volumetric analysis by 3D echocardiography do not

predict long-term response to cardiac resynchronization therapy. *Cardiol Res Pract* 2011; 568918.

[47] Dekker A, Phelps B, Dijkman B, van Der Nagel T, van Der Veen F, Geskes G, Maessen J. Epicardial left ventricular lead placement for cardiac resynchronization therapy: optimal pace site selection with pressure-volume loops. *J Thorac Cardiovasc Surg* 2004; 127:1641-1647.

[48] Butter C, Auricchio A, Stellbrink C, Fleck E, Ding J, Yu Y, Huvelle E et al. Effect of resynchronization therapy stimulation site on the systolic function of heart failure patients. *Circulation*. 2001; 104:3026-9.

[49] Berger T, Pfeifer B, Hanser FF, Hintringer F, Fischer G, Netzer M, Trieb T et al. Single-beat noninvasive imaging of ventricular endocardial and epicardial activation in patients undergoing CRT. *PLoSOne*. 2011; 27:e16255.

[50] Spragg DD, Dong J, Fetics BJ, Helm R, Marine JE, Cheng A, Henrikson CA et al. Optimal left ventricular endocardial pacing sites for cardiac resynchronization therapy in patients with ichemic cardiomyopathy. *J Am Coll Cardiol*. 2010; 56:774-81.

[51] Merchant FM, Heist EK, McCarty D, Kumar P, Das S, Blendea D, Ellinor PT et al: Impact of segmental left ventricle lead position on cardiac resynchronization therapy outcomes. *Heart Rhythm*. 2010; 7:639-44.

[52] Ansalone G, Giannantoni P, Ricci R et al.: Doppler myocardial imaging to evaluate the effectiveness of pacing sites in patients receiving biventricular pacing. *J Am Coll Cardiol*. 2002; 39: 489-99.

[53] Murphy RT, Sigurdsson G, Mulamalla S et al.: Tissue synchronization imaging and optimal left ventricular pacing site in cardiac resynchronization therapy. *Am J Cardiol*. 2006; 97: 1615-21.

[54] Miranda RI, Nault M, Simpson CS et al: The right ventricular septum presents the optimum site for maximal electrical separation during left ventricular pacing. *J Cardivasc Electrophysiol* 2011;doi:10.1111/ j.1540-8167[Epub ahead of print].

[55] Khan FZ, Salahshouri P, Duehmke R, et al.: The impact of the right ventricular lead positron on response to cardiac resynchronization therapy. *Pacing Clin Electrophysiol* 2011;34:467-74.

[56] Sutton MG, Plappert T, Hilpisch KE, et al.: Sustained reverse left ventricular structural remodeling with cardiac resynchronization at one year is a function of etiology: quantitative Doppler echocardiographic evidence from the Multicenter InSync Randomized Clinical Evaluation (MIRACLE). *Circulation* 2006;113:266-72.

[57] Jansen AH, Bracke FA, van Dantzig JM et al.: Correlation of Echo-Doppler Optimization of Atrioventricular Delay in Cardiac Resynchronization Therapy with Invasive Hemodynamics in Patients With Heart Failure Secondary to Ischemic or Idiopathic Dilated Cardiomyopathy. *Am J Cardiol* 2006;97:552–557.

[58] Wang DY, Richmond ME, Quinn TA et al.: Optimized temporary biventricular pacing acutely improves intraoperative cardiac output after weaning from cardiopulmonary bypass: a substudy of randomized clinical trial. *J Thorac Cardiovasc Surg*. 2011; 141:1002-1008.

[59] Leyva F, Foley PWX: Current and future role of cardiovascular magnetic resonance in cardiac resynchronization therapy. *Heart Fail Rev*. 2011;16:251-62.

[60] Iacopino S, Gasparini M, Zanon F et al.: Low-dose dobutamine stress echocardiography to assess left ventricular contractile reserve for cardiac resynchronization therapy: data

from the low-dose dobutamine stress echocardiography to predict cardiac resynchronization therapy response(LODO-CRT) Trial. *Congestive Heart Failure.* 2010;16:104-10.

[61] Diskstein K, Vargas PE, Auricchio A et al.: 2010 focused update of ESC guidelines on device therapy in heart failure. An update of the 2008 ESC guidelines for the diagnosis and treatment of acute and chronic heart failure and the 2007 ESC guidelines for cardiac resynchronization therapy. 2010; *EHJ* 31: 2677-87.

Index

A

Abraham, 95, 98, 244
acid, 125, 133, 135, 193, 201, 211
acquisitions, 37, 234
adaptation, 84, 91, 96
adhesion, 133
adipose, 128
adiposity, 45
adjustment, 16, 87, 243
adolescents, 133, 239, 246
adulthood, 97
adults, vii, 14, 55, 64, 65, 83, 85, 124, 126, 173, 182, 185, 189, 227
adventitia, 58
adverse effects, 236
adverse event, 224
aerobic capacity, 65
aerobic exercise, 67
afebrile, 129
age, 28, 31, 36, 38, 59, 60, 64, 65, 66, 82, 87, 90, 91, 93, 124, 128, 138, 139, 154, 192, 231, 238
agonist, 73, 74
albumin, 63, 67
albuminuria, 197
alcoholic liver disease, 213
aldosterone, 64, 102, 122, 124, 127, 133
allergic asthma, 46
alters, 137, 168
American Heart Association, 244
amino, 134
amniotic fluid, 181
amplitude, 2, 74, 75, 79, 81, 82, 144
amyloidosis, 109
anastomosis, 219, 220
anatomy, 1, 36, 37, 41, 149, 150, 209, 214, 215, 219, 241
anemia, 137, 138, 140, 142

anesthetics, 109
aneurysm, 55, 130, 153, 154, 155, 157, 159, 160, 163, 165, 168, 171, 172, 173, 174, 175, 176, 177
angiography, 44, 83, 153, 159, 162, 175, 176, 209, 211, 214, 219, 225
angioplasty, 118
angiotensin II, 24, 53, 111, 122, 200
angiotensin II receptor antagonist, 200
angiotensin receptor blockers, 64
anisocytosis, 138, 140
antibody, 125
antihypertensive drugs, 200, 206
antioxidant, 200
aorta, 4, 5, 6, 10, 23, 29, 31, 49, 50, 52, 55, 57, 58, 63, 64, 68, 71, 72, 73, 74, 76, 108, 118, 128, 148, 154, 155, 156, 157, 158, 159, 162, 164, 168, 169, 176, 180, 181, 183, 186
aortic regurgitation, 82, 93
aortic stenosis, 97, 128, 129, 185
aortic valve, 10, 28, 50, 61, 76, 108, 110, 112, 134, 147, 191
apex, 37, 81, 82, 88, 91, 102, 238
apoptosis, 125, 127, 131
arginine, 203
arterial hypertension, 67, 118
arteries, 3, 50, 52, 53, 57, 58, 60, 62, 63, 64, 65, 66, 69, 76, 91, 148, 154, 156, 157, 158, 159, 160, 161, 162, 165, 167, 168, 169, 170, 171, 173, 174, 175, 176, 177
arteriogram, 208
arterioles, 50, 197, 198, 199, 200, 203, 206
arteriosclerosis, 63
artery, 5, 16, 29, 52, 55, 62, 63, 64, 65, 66, 70, 76, 110, 118, 129, 130, 131, 148, 154, 155, 156, 159, 162, 165, 167, 168, 173, 174, 175, 177, 180, 182, 183, 186, 187, 188, 189, 192,

193, 196, 201, 208, 214, 217, 218, 224, 225, 226, 228, 229, 237, 245
ascites, 222, 223
assessment, vii, 13, 15, 21, 22, 42, 43, 46, 49, 50, 53, 58, 65, 66, 76, 77, 80, 83, 84, 86, 87, 89, 90, 92, 93, 94, 95, 97, 101, 103, 104, 110, 111, 112, 115, 118, 131, 162, 172, 174, 177, 185, 189, 190, 191, 193, 215, 219, 227, 235, 240, 246
asymmetry, 38
asymptomatic, 66, 82, 93, 154
atherosclerosis, 55, 66, 67, 154, 168
athletes, 84, 95, 108, 112
ATP, 127
atria, 40, 102, 103, 110, 236
atrial fibrillation, 101, 105, 109, 112, 125
atrial septal defect, 126, 128
atrioventricular block, 101, 236
atrium, 14, 37, 81, 91, 92, 101, 102, 103, 105, 107, 108, 109, 110, 180, 182, 186, 188
attachment, 156
auscultation, 77
autoimmune disease, 128
autoimmune diseases, 128
autonomic nervous system, 148
awareness, 167

B

background noise, 210
baroreceptor, 64, 68, 122
base, 193, 238
BBB, 235
beneficial effect, 225
benefits, 34, 224, 234
biochemistry, 132
biomarkers, 121, 122, 123, 125, 130, 131, 135, 139
biomechanics, 97
birth weight, 190
BJA, 43
bleeding, 207, 208, 209, 211, 214
blood circulation, 71, 101, 168, 195
blood flow, 1, 5, 27, 39, 41, 49, 50, 55, 57, 63, 71, 77, 79, 102, 105, 107, 108, 127, 145, 146, 150, 151, 156, 157, 159, 163, 164, 165, 168, 172, 173, 174, 175, 176, 179, 184, 188, 190, 191, 193, 195, 203, 208, 210, 211, 212, 214, 216, 219, 220, 222, 224, 227, 245
blood gas analysis, 214
blood plasma, 127

blood pressure, 1, 17, 18, 19, 21, 57, 60, 62, 63, 64, 65, 66, 68, 126, 127, 146, 148, 176, 195, 199, 202, 204, 232
blood pressure reduction, 64
blood stream, 10, 79, 180
blood transfusion, 140
blood vessels, 39, 55, 57, 58, 60, 63, 129, 210, 212, 215
BMA, 42
body size, 15, 16, 82, 90
body weight, 182, 222
bone, 138, 140
bone marrow, 138, 140
brain, 123, 132, 135, 180, 184, 186, 190
branching, 110, 148
Brazil, 195
breakdown, 129, 130, 131
breathing, 116
bundle branch block, 235, 236, 238
bypass graft, 168

C

Ca^{2+}, 35, 45
cables, 27, 28
calcium, 23, 35, 53, 64, 125, 182, 200, 206, 233
calcium channel blocker, 200
caliber, 57, 69
calibration, 26, 27, 28, 30, 31, 41, 44
cancer, 172
candidates, 171
capillary, 102, 195, 200, 202, 203, 206
cardiac catheterization, 26, 41, 43, 51, 53, 65, 94
cardiac muscle, 44, 125, 128
cardiac output, 1, 35, 52, 77, 83, 92, 108, 109, 122, 180, 181, 182, 183, 184, 185, 186, 189, 190, 191, 193, 231, 232, 233, 237, 245, 247
cardiac reserve, 35, 84
cardiac structure, 45
cardiac surgery, 93, 237, 245
cardiac tamponade, 232, 233
cardiomyopathy, 24, 91, 95, 98, 109, 122, 131, 235, 237, 240, 241, 244, 245, 247
cardiopulmonary bypass, 246, 247
cardiovascular disease, vii, 3, 49, 64, 112, 113, 118, 121, 128, 130, 132, 134, 135, 137, 138, 139, 141, 143
cardiovascular morbidity, 55
cardiovascular physiology, 41, 148, 179
cardiovascular risk, 6, 66
cardiovascular system, vii, 9, 143, 145, 149, 150, 151
carotid sinus, 148

cartilage, 128
catecholamines, 19, 97, 124, 233
catheter, 9, 14, 23, 26, 27, 28, 29, 30, 31, 34, 36, 37, 38, 39, 40, 41, 42, 43, 44, 45, 46, 83, 113, 155, 210, 213, 237
catheterizations, 28, 30
cDNA, 228
cell death, 224
central nervous system, 102, 123
challenges, 26, 29, 35, 36, 103, 173
chemical, 156
chemokines, 205
chest radiography, 21, 121
CHF, 124, 231, 238, 241
childhood, 91
children, viii, 6, 14, 15, 51, 52, 55, 64, 65, 67, 68, 77, 82, 83, 84, 87, 88, 90, 92, 93, 96, 98, 99, 112, 116, 118, 124, 126, 127, 128, 129, 132, 133, 185, 227
cholesterol, 173
chromosome, 198, 203
chromosome 10, 198, 203
chronic heart failure, 6, 79, 98, 109, 122, 125, 126, 127, 130, 132, 135, 139, 231, 244, 248
chronic kidney kidney disease (CKD), 67, 196, 197, 199, 200, 201, 205
circulation, 6, 17, 29, 40, 73, 84, 90, 101, 118, 124, 125, 127, 131, 143, 149, 150, 155, 179, 181, 183, 185, 189, 191, 214, 218, 219, 222, 224, 225, 226, 228, 233
cirrhosis, 214
classification, 40, 78, 124, 127, 172, 213, 232
clinical application, 23, 49, 66, 79, 111, 159
clinical diagnosis, 240
clinical symptoms, 21
clinical trials, 132, 234
closure, 50, 76, 102, 105, 224, 227, 229
CO2, 14
coagulopathy, 223
coarctation, 23, 64, 68, 128
coefficient of variation, 137
collaboration, 42, 244
collagen, 58, 67, 127, 128, 133
collateral, 52, 177, 207, 210, 211, 212, 215, 216, 224, 225
commercial, 27, 34, 37, 40, 139
communication, 183
community, 24, 93, 119
compaction, 99
compensation, 106, 110
complement, 239
complete blood count, 139
complex interactions, 9, 69, 141

complexity, 32, 40, 222
compliance, 1, 3, 5, 6, 20, 49, 50, 67, 102, 103, 105, 107, 109, 110, 111, 119, 146, 147, 148, 224
complications, 113, 130, 153, 154, 155, 171, 173, 213, 221, 224, 226, 232
composition, 156, 197
comprehension, 201
compression, 69, 71, 73, 74, 75, 76
computational fluid dynamics, 163, 165
computational modeling, 41
computed tomography, 104, 157, 219, 239, 246
computer, 143, 162, 193
computer simulations, 143
computing, 52, 147
concordance, 242
conductance, 14, 23, 26, 27, 28, 29, 30, 31, 32, 33, 34, 36, 38, 39, 40, 41, 42, 43, 44, 45, 46
conduction, 44, 99, 146, 150, 233, 236, 240, 246
conductivity, 33, 37, 39, 45
conductors, 38
configuration, 117, 118, 165
congenital heart disease, 1, 22, 51, 52, 64, 79, 82, 83, 84, 92, 98, 116, 118, 124, 133, 134, 141, 143, 149, 150, 193
congestive heart failure, 5, 22, 108, 118, 124, 132, 186
Consensus, 244
conservation, 70, 149
construction, 37, 41, 149, 222, 224
consumption, 232
contour, 233
control condition, 73, 74
control group, 65
controlled trials, 171
controversial, 148, 185, 199, 218, 224
coordination, 65, 101, 109
coronary angioplasty, 94
coronary arteries, 130, 177
coronary artery aneurysms, 64, 134
coronary artery bypass graft, 236, 243, 245
coronary artery disease, 122, 130, 135, 231
coronary heart disease, 55
correction factors, 32
correlation, 35, 58, 60, 63, 82, 83, 84, 93, 94, 114, 115, 116, 125, 126, 127, 130, 132, 185, 188, 193, 197, 208, 213, 229, 235, 238, 239, 240
correlations, 35, 82, 116, 117
cortex, 127, 203
cost, 17, 57, 139, 225
cost benefits, 225
covering, 175

CPI, 40
creatine, 125
creatinine, 64, 196
critical period, 232
CRP, 128, 129
crystals, 14
CT scan, 172, 209, 211
CTA, 159
cyanosis, 127, 128
cycles, 164, 165, 234
cycling, 35, 67
cyclooxygenase, 199
Cyprus, 25
cytokines, 127, 131, 140, 205, 224
cytoplasm, 125
Czech Republic, 231

D

damping, 50, 92
data analysis, 80
data distribution, 34
data set, 234
deaths, 129
decay, 36, 72
decoupling, 35
defects, 77, 84, 90, 231
defibrillation, 98, 109
deficiency, 60, 140
deformation, 84, 85, 88, 89, 90, 94, 95, 96, 97
degradation, 130
dehydration, 118
depolarization, 103, 233, 236, 242
derivatives, 69
destruction, 138, 140
detachment, 35
detectable, 128, 235
detection, 32, 103, 110, 121, 125, 127, 129, 130, 172, 209, 211, 212, 213, 215, 232, 238, 242, 243
detection techniques, 32
diabetes, 66, 199, 204, 205, 206
diabetic kidney disease, 205
diabetic nephropathy, 64, 195, 199, 201, 204, 205
diabetic patients, 199
dialysis, 63
diastole, 10, 20, 40, 46, 80, 85, 87, 91, 93, 102, 103, 105, 106, 107, 117, 186, 187, 188
diastolic blood pressure, 60, 62
diastolic pressure, 3, 11, 12, 13, 20, 21, 22, 24, 35, 44, 50, 53, 82, 83, 84, 102, 107, 112, 125, 144
diet, 45, 200, 205

differential diagnosis, 137, 138, 140
dilated cardiomyopathy, 44, 91, 97, 98, 109, 112, 133, 235, 237, 240, 245, 246
dilation, 6, 17, 18, 67, 96, 107, 129, 130, 236
direct measure, 197
discordance, 24, 83
diseases, vii, 5, 55, 63, 64, 67, 85, 139, 141, 149, 190, 198
dislocation, 177
disorder, 91
dispersion, 162, 168, 236
displacement, 30, 61, 84, 85, 87, 88, 93
disposition, 85, 88, 91
distribution, 137, 141, 142, 147, 148, 180, 184, 186, 190
diuretic, 124
diversity, 1
dogs, 11, 15, 22, 23, 24, 42, 44, 53, 174, 198
dominance, 35, 108, 109
donors, 227, 228
doppler, 190, 191, 192, 193
dosing, 232
Down syndrome, 118
down-regulation, 223
drawing, 60, 121
drug treatment, 127
drugs, 14, 64, 108, 200, 201
ductus arteriosus, 180, 181, 182, 183
durability, 159
dynamism, 150
dyspnea, 21

E

ECM, 129
EIS, 207, 210, 212, 213
elastin, 58
elderly population, 153
electric field, 26, 30, 34, 36, 37, 39, 41
electrical resistance, 42
electrocardiogram, 72, 86, 117
electrodes, 27, 30, 37, 38, 234
electrolyte, 127, 183
e-mail, 217, 231
emboli, 162, 168, 217, 218, 224, 225, 229
embolization, 217, 218, 224, 225, 229
emergency, 121, 222
emission, 27, 30, 36, 37, 38, 239, 246
emission field, 27, 36
endocardium, 38, 85, 91
endocrine, 111
endoscopy, 159, 162, 175, 176, 211, 213
endothelial dysfunction, 55

endothelium, 63, 130
end-stage renal disease, 6, 198, 203
energy, 12, 16, 17, 23, 47, 55, 69, 108, 110, 127, 199, 233
energy efficiency, 12
energy transfer, 23
engineering, 26, 41, 92
enlargement, 109, 110, 154, 208
environment, 30, 37, 42, 163, 186
enzyme, 64, 127, 130, 197, 202, 203
enzyme inhibitors, 64
enzymes, 129
epicardium, 85, 91
epidemic, 24, 93
epidemiologic, 58
epinephrine, 150, 233
epithelial cells, 128
equipment, 42, 121
erythrocytes, 137, 138
erythropoietin, 140
esophageal varices, 207, 208, 209, 210, 211, 212, 213, 214, 215, 216
esophagus, 208, 209, 211, 212, 214, 215, 216
estrogen, 60
ethanol, 216
etiology, 247
Europe, 58
evidence, 6, 33, 36, 46, 66, 77, 141, 172, 196, 199, 223, 239, 244, 247
evolution, 172, 191
examinations, 21, 77, 121, 208, 212
excitation, 26, 27, 39, 41
exclusion, 156, 157, 174, 177
excretion, 63, 67, 124, 202, 205
exercise, 17, 18, 23, 63, 66, 109, 121
experimental condition, 113
expertise, 31
exposure, 29, 35, 58, 121, 172, 177
extracellular matrix, 34, 129, 133, 200
extraction, 37, 214

F

fat, 45
fatty acids, 127
fetal development, 201
fetal growth, 185, 186
fetus, 179, 180, 181, 182, 183, 184, 185, 187, 188, 190, 191, 192, 193
fibers, 84, 125, 185, 239
fibrillation, 101, 109
fibrinolysis, 66
fibrinolytic, 130

fibroblasts, 128, 133
fibrosis, 122, 127, 128, 133, 198, 200, 206, 239
fibrous cap, 129, 130
filtration, 63, 124, 140, 195, 196, 197, 204
fixation, 156, 165, 174, 175, 176
flank, 155
fluctuations, 141
fluid, 153, 163, 164, 172, 176, 195, 197, 232, 233
fluid balance, 232
folate, 140
foramen, 180, 181, 187, 188, 190, 193
foramen ovale, 180, 181, 187, 188, 190, 193
force, 35, 43, 49, 75, 93, 108, 110, 112, 145
Ford, 141
formation, 130, 168, 207, 212
formula, 108
foundations, 25
Fourier analysis, 1, 2
Frank-Starling mechanism, 182
friction, 146
functional changes, 192

G

gadolinium, 42
gastroesophageal reflux, 118
gastrointestinal tract, 184
gene expression, 133, 223, 228, 229
general anesthesia, 155
genes, 199, 204
genetic background, 45
genomics, 26
geometry, 46
gestation, 180, 181, 182, 184, 185, 186, 190, 193
gestational age, 182, 184, 190, 192
global scale, 63
glucose, 66, 199, 205
grades, 124
grading, 209, 214
graft healing, 175
graft technique, 156
grants, 42
granules, 211
graph, 79, 235
growth, 93, 96, 124, 127, 184, 185, 188, 189, 192, 193, 200
growth factor, 127, 200
guidance, 14, 173, 176
guidelines, 125, 132, 243, 248

H

half-life, 124
health, 24, 139
heart disease, 1, 9, 23, 64, 79, 85, 89, 91, 92, 109, 111, 139, 141, 149, 150, 237, 238, 239, 240, 242
heart failure, 17, 23, 24, 43, 55, 82, 83, 85, 86, 89, 92, 93, 94, 95, 101, 105, 109, 110, 122, 123, 124, 125, 127, 129, 130, 131, 132, 133, 134, 135, 139, 140, 141, 142, 187, 193, 231, 232, 233, 234, 237, 239, 240, 242, 244, 245, 246, 247, 248
heart rate, 2, 9, 17, 35, 43, 49, 53, 60, 64, 77, 80, 82, 83, 85, 87, 93, 106, 107, 122, 144, 148, 150, 182, 191, 234
heart rate (HR), 35, 49, 60
heart transplantation, 94, 231
heart valves, 150
heat shock protein, 223
height, 61, 73, 76
hematocrit, 196
heme, 223
hemodialysis, 67
hemoglobin, 140, 182
hemoglobinopathies, 140
hemorrhage, 209, 224
heterogeneity, 138, 203
high blood pressure, 131
high risk patients, 232
history, 22, 64, 68, 154, 232, 233
homeostasis, vii, 32, 122, 123, 190
hormone, 102, 140, 190
hormones, 199, 204
hospital death, 154
hospitalization, 139, 242
human, vii, 1, 14, 24, 26, 35, 46, 52, 65, 66, 95, 112, 140, 144, 151, 153, 159, 163, 164, 177, 179, 180, 181, 183, 184, 190, 191, 192, 198, 203, 232
human body, vii, 164, 232
human genome, 26
human right, 46
human subjects, 159
hydrops, 189
hyperactivity, 205
hyperbilirubinemia, 222, 223
hyperfiltration, 199, 204, 205
hyperglycemia, 205
hyperplasia, 118, 168, 177
hypertension, 6, 19, 20, 23, 63, 64, 65, 66, 67, 95, 97, 101, 128, 134, 139, 154, 195, 197, 198, 199, 200, 201, 202, 203, 204, 206, 207, 214, 223, 226
hypertonic saline, 29, 32, 33, 34, 41
hypertrophic cardiomyopathy, 21, 24, 84, 91, 95, 97, 133
hypertrophy, 84, 91, 95, 97, 109, 122, 123, 124, 127, 133, 199
hypotension, 17
hypotensive, 17, 64
hypothesis, 60, 199
hypoxemia, 128, 187
hypoxia, 126, 128

I

ID, 177
ideal, 58, 62
identification, 210, 241
idiopathic, 24, 95, 133, 246
ILAR, 28, 32, 35, 41, 43
image, 26, 35, 37, 40, 41, 154, 157, 158, 159, 160, 162, 173, 176, 188, 193, 210, 235
imaging modalities, 28, 29, 41, 90
immersion, 30
impairments, vii, 179
improvements, 92, 98, 109, 171, 172, 218
in utero, 179, 180, 186, 189, 191
in vitro, 95, 177
in vivo, 23, 46, 53, 76, 95, 111, 143, 163, 189
incidence, 130, 154, 213
independence, 82, 92, 150, 197
independent variable, 128
Indians, 199, 205
individual differences, 219, 241
individuals, 130, 195, 198, 199, 200
inducer, 140
induction, 28, 30, 199
inequality, 39
inertia, 49, 57, 71, 72, 75, 146
infancy, 97
infants, 6, 67
infarction, 122, 139
infection, 128, 224, 232
inferences, 25
inferior vena cava, 13, 23, 29, 103, 113, 114, 118, 119, 179, 180, 181, 182, 186, 187, 188, 190, 192
inflammation, 123, 126, 128, 129, 130, 138, 140, 142, 177
inflation, 14
inhibition, 67, 202, 203, 205
inhibitor, 67, 128, 134, 197
inhomogeneity, 241

Index

innate immunity, 134
insertion, 82, 113, 155, 168
insulin, 204, 205
integration, 32, 89, 108
integrity, 195, 200
intensive care unit, 118, 126, 221
interaction effect, 176
interaction effects, 176
interface, 159
interference, 87, 156, 165, 168, 173, 224
intervention, 65, 110, 177, 191
intima, 58, 59, 66
intrauterine growth retardation, 192
inversion, 193
iron, 138, 140
IRT, 186
ischaemic heart disease, 246
ischemia, 85, 91, 110, 126, 131, 197, 198, 199
isolation, 28
issues, vii, 1, 14, 41, 55, 90, 92, 156, 217

J

Japan, 1, 9, 49, 55, 57, 58, 60, 63, 69, 77, 101, 113, 121, 137, 143, 179, 207, 210, 217, 226

K

K^+, 199
Kawasaki disease, 5, 64, 65, 129, 130
kidney, vii, 67, 102, 124, 195, 196, 197, 198, 199, 202, 203, 205, 206
kidneys, 161, 195
kinetics, 35, 45

L

laminar, 163, 164
laparotomy, 155, 222
LDL, 173
lead, vii, 2, 34, 52, 98, 110, 122, 132, 162, 168, 196, 234, 236, 237, 238, 240, 241, 242, 243, 247
leakage, 26, 38, 43
left atrium, 11, 20, 102, 103, 105, 107, 108, 109, 110, 111, 147, 150, 180, 181, 187
left ventricle, 11, 17, 22, 23, 24, 44, 49, 53, 72, 88, 91, 95, 97, 102, 103, 107, 108, 110, 118, 144, 147, 149, 150, 180, 181, 182, 183, 185, 191, 231, 236, 241, 245, 246, 247
leptin, 199
lesions, 1, 64, 65, 80, 129, 130, 135, 198, 206

leukocytes, 130
life expectancy, 155
lifetime, 173
light, 14, 125
linear dependence, 33
lipids, 130
liver, vii, 128, 208, 214, 217, 218, 219, 222, 223, 224, 225, 226, 227, 228, 229
liver cirrhosis, 208
liver disease, 218, 219, 224, 229
liver transplant, 217, 218, 223, 224, 225, 226, 227, 228, 229
liver transplantation, 217, 218, 223, 224, 225, 226, 227, 228, 229
local anesthesia, 155
localization, 243
locus, 197
lumen, 4, 114, 131, 159, 168, 172
lymph, 65
lymphoid, 68

M

macrophages, 130
magnetic resonance (MR), 15, 24, 40, 43, 78, 94, 95, 96, 97, 104, 133, 193, 209, 219, 239, 240, 246, 247
magnetic resonance imaging (MRI), 15, 28, 32, 35, 36, 37, 40, 41, 44, 45, 46, 47, 78, 83, 84, 88, 91, 94, 95, 96, 97, 104, 133, 189, 193, 239, 240, 243, 246
magnitude, 4, 5, 69, 71, 74, 235
majority, 65, 171
malnutrition, 140, 201
mammals, 40
man, 7, 23, 53, 95
management, 9, 113, 141, 175, 212, 214, 217, 218, 219, 222, 226, 244
manganese, 43
manipulation, 215
mapping, 210
Marx, 53, 191
mass, 45, 70, 108, 149, 202
mast cells, 133
materials, 38, 163, 167
matrix, 134, 234
matrix metalloproteinase, 134
matter, iv
mean arterial pressure, 196, 233, 237
measurement, 1, 4, 5, 9, 14, 15, 22, 26, 29, 42, 44, 46, 57, 58, 62, 63, 65, 66, 70, 79, 93, 95, 103, 112, 114, 116, 118, 125, 126, 128, 130,

132, 154, 160, 164, 189, 194, 197, 198, 200, 210, 232, 239, 242
mechanical properties, 50, 69, 90
mechanical ventilation, 116, 117, 119, 233
media, 58, 59, 66, 124
median, 126, 187
medical, 9, 92, 111, 155, 159, 173
medicine, 23, 24, 67, 111, 132, 190, 193, 194
mellitus, 199, 205
membrane permeability, 125
menopause, 60
MES, 242
mesentery, 162
meta-analysis, 133
metabolic pathways, 203
metabolism, 17, 47, 127, 128, 140, 233
metalloproteinase, 53, 129, 134
methodology, 5, 14, 15, 30, 41
mice, 26, 28, 31, 34, 36, 42, 43, 44, 45, 46, 47, 199
microcirculation, 214
microscopy, 42
migration, 153, 156, 159, 172, 174
miniature, 26, 27, 28
Ministry of Education, 226
MIP, 155, 161
misunderstanding, 86
mitochondria, 127
mitral regurgitation, 51, 76, 77, 103, 107, 110, 232, 233, 236, 241, 242, 244
mitral valve, 10, 21, 76, 91, 102, 105, 108, 109, 147, 191, 237
mixing, 179
MMP, 129
MMP-9, 129
models, 27, 36, 37, 41, 43, 46, 89, 143, 147, 148, 149, 151, 153, 166, 167, 168, 169, 172, 176, 196, 198, 199
modifications, 28, 86, 144, 156
modulus, 2, 57
molecular biology, 34
molecular structure, 124
molecular weight, 127
momentum, 70, 76, 149
morbidity, 155, 173, 200, 219, 221, 232
morphological abnormalities, 52
morphology, 34, 47, 49, 51, 84, 172, 174, 185, 203, 210
mortality, 6, 55, 132, 133, 135, 139, 140, 141, 154, 155, 159, 171, 173, 177, 219, 221, 222, 223, 225, 232, 242
mortality rate, 135, 139, 154, 155, 225
MPI, 185, 186

MSW, 15
multiple regression, 128
multiple regression analysis, 128
multiples, 2
muscle contraction, 125, 241
muscles, 102, 125, 234
mutation, 199
mutational analysis, 229
mutations, 199
myocardial infarction, 43, 45, 46, 84, 94, 97, 101, 110, 111, 125, 128, 130, 131, 133, 134, 139, 141, 238
myocardial ischemia, 66, 84, 96, 104, 105, 126, 131, 231, 243
myocardial necrosis, 125, 130, 131
myocardium, 34, 37, 38, 39, 45, 77, 78, 79, 80, 84, 85, 87, 88, 89, 91, 92, 94, 122, 125, 127, 128, 131, 179, 182, 187, 190, 231, 233, 236, 239, 240, 241, 243
myocyte, 35, 37, 135
myoglobin, 125, 133
myosin, 35, 47, 125

N

Na^+, 199
NaCl, 183
National Institutes of Health, 202
necrosis, 125, 127, 131
neonates, 116, 138, 192
nephrectomy, 205
nephron, 197, 202
nephropathy, 199, 203, 204, 205
nephrotic syndrome, 118, 206
nerve, 108, 122, 182, 190
nervous system, 131
New England, 24
nitric oxide, 67, 111, 198, 199, 203, 204
nitric oxide synthase, 67, 203
NMR, 46
non-insulin dependent diabetes, 204
normal children, 112
normal distribution, 137
North America, 174
numerical analysis, 150
nutritional status, 140, 200

O

obesity, 205
objective symptoms, 130
obstruction, 51, 131, 187

occlusion, 13, 14, 15, 21, 23, 29, 44, 63, 162, 183, 217, 221, 222, 227
oesophageal, 214
open heart surgery, 232
optimization, 44, 156, 237, 242, 245
ordinary differential equations, 149
organ, vii, 64, 193, 196
organism, 195
organs, vii, 17, 26, 107, 122, 184, 191, 218
oscillation, 4
osmotic pressure, 202
ostium, 154, 156, 157, 158, 159, 162, 165, 168, 176
ox, 179, 181
oxidation, 130
oxidative stress, 66, 198, 203, 205
oxygen, 29, 35, 182, 187, 189, 191, 192, 194, 208, 232, 233, 234

P

pacing, 44, 79, 82, 86, 92, 95, 98, 99, 232, 233, 234, 236, 237, 238, 239, 240, 241, 242, 243, 244, 245, 246, 247
pain, 133
palpation, 77
parallel, 26, 27, 29, 30, 33, 34, 36, 40, 41, 43, 44, 45, 46, 55, 186, 208, 210
partial differential equations, 149
patent ductus arteriosus, 52
pathogenesis, 123, 204, 205, 214
pathology, 26, 42, 122, 243
pathophysiological, 55, 65, 123, 137, 232, 233
pathophysiology, vii, 9, 18, 23, 49, 85, 92, 101, 110, 111, 134, 143, 189, 198
pathways, 213
patient care, 232
penetrance, 45
peptide, 102, 111, 123, 124, 131, 132, 133, 134, 135, 139, 140, 141
peptides, 132, 134
perfusion, 55, 118, 122, 156, 161, 184, 187, 198, 223, 224, 239, 246
pericardiocentesis, 233
pericardium, 21
perinatal, 193
peripheral blood, 124, 186
permeability, 37, 38, 102, 125
permit, 232
permittivity, 37, 38, 39, 45
Perth, 153, 174
pharmacology, 34
pharmacotherapy, 232

phase diagram, 104
phenotypes, 45
Philadelphia, 44
phosphorylation, 36, 44, 45
physicians, 85, 117
physics, 4
Physiological, 22, 163
physiology, 2, 5, 22, 23, 24, 26, 34, 42, 49, 67, 77, 85, 96, 111, 112, 132, 179, 182, 185, 191
pilot study, 205
placenta, 179, 181, 182, 184
plaque, 129, 130, 168, 177
platelets, 66
platform, 156
plexus, 213
point mutation, 204
population, 17, 52, 83, 84, 96, 189, 231, 239, 246
porosity, 156
portal hypertension, 207, 208, 212, 213, 214, 215, 218, 222, 223, 226, 229
portal vein, 181, 208, 214, 218, 219, 221, 222, 224, 226
portal venous system, vii, 207, 209, 213
positive correlation, 239
positive relationship, 183
positron, 247
post-transplant, 83, 218, 223, 225
pre-ejection period, 72
pregnancy, 182, 190
preparation, iv, 32
preservation, 156, 158
pressure gradient, 91, 145, 172
prevention, 98, 130, 155, 156, 202, 224, 225, 244
principles, 159
probe, 80, 81, 196, 210, 213, 215, 216
procurement, 130
prognosis, 65, 92, 95, 129, 130, 131, 133, 134, 140, 185, 223, 224, 225, 226, 228, 231, 244
programming, 237
project, viii
proliferation, 57, 156, 177, 224
propagation, 61, 148, 240
prophylactic, 207, 217, 218, 225, 229
proposition, 36
propranolol, 73
prostaglandins, 205
prosthesis, 155
protection, 200
protective role, 205
protein kinase C, 44
proteins, 125
proteinuria, 200
prototype, 27

pulmonary arteries, 180
pulmonary artery pressure, 237
pulmonary capillary wedge pressure, 94, 233
pulmonary circulation, 40, 101, 102, 179, 190
pulmonary edema, 109
pulmonary embolism, 126, 133
pulmonary hypertension, 23, 109, 139, 232
pulmonary stenosis, 128
pulmonary vascular resistance, 126, 237
pumps, 16, 232
PVA, 12, 16, 17, 107

Q

QRS complex, 10, 86, 99, 234, 235, 240, 245
quality control, 65
quality of life, 155, 231
quantification, 26, 29, 33, 35, 36, 41, 45, 97, 245, 246

R

radiation, 121, 172, 177
radioisotope, 121
radiopaque, 91
radius, 4, 60, 146
rat kidneys, 201
reactive oxygen, 126
reading, 196
real time, 246
receptors, 127, 128, 148, 203
recognition, 228
recommendations, iv, 95
reconstruction, 38, 219, 220, 221
recovery, 14, 222, 228, 232
recurrence, 211, 213, 216
red blood cells, 140
regeneration, 217, 218, 224, 229
Registry, 246
regression, 32, 52, 206
rejection, 218, 222, 224
relaxation, 10, 19, 20, 24, 35, 43, 44, 72, 73, 75, 76, 77, 78, 82, 83, 91, 97, 102, 103, 107, 109, 111, 112, 144, 182, 185, 186
relaxation rate, 24
relevance, 35, 39
reliability, 80
remission, 206
remodelling, 97, 134, 201, 243
renal dysfunction, 63, 125, 140, 153, 159, 199, 204
renal failure, 63, 197

renin, 64, 102, 122, 127, 133, 197, 198
repair, 6, 64, 68, 77, 84, 96, 133, 153, 154, 155, 156, 159, 168, 171, 172, 173, 174, 175, 176, 177, 222
reproduction, 39
requirements, 237, 238
researchers, vii, 149, 163
resection, 218
resilience, 57
resistance, 1, 2, 5, 17, 22, 26, 27, 49, 50, 109, 122, 143, 146, 147, 148, 180, 181, 183, 186, 192, 196, 198, 200, 204, 207, 218, 226, 232, 233, 237
resolution, 35, 37, 43, 78, 84, 85, 86, 88, 92, 98, 159
resources, 148
respiration, 29, 80, 113, 191
response, 9, 15, 17, 18, 41, 95, 96, 103, 122, 126, 127, 128, 129, 137, 143, 148, 150, 156, 182, 196, 198, 201, 206, 225, 234, 237, 238, 239, 240, 243, 244, 245, 246, 247, 248
responsiveness, 190, 199, 205
restoration, 217, 218
retardation, 185
reticulum, 35
rhythm, 232, 241
right atrium, 14, 103, 147, 150, 181, 187
right ventricle, 21, 83, 95, 98, 147, 180, 183, 185, 189, 236, 238, 245
risk, 64, 67, 113, 121, 132, 135, 139, 154, 155, 163, 168, 172, 173, 176, 209, 211, 214, 224, 231, 232, 233, 237, 239, 242
risk factors, 154
risks, 131
ROI, 79, 80, 87, 235
root, 150, 220, 222, 225
Rouleau, 132
routes, 208
routines, 30
rules, 214

S

safety, 14, 156, 159, 165, 168, 169, 237
saturation, 182, 189, 194, 208, 232, 233
saving lives, 231
scaling, 30
schema, 88
science, 111
sclerosis, 198, 200, 202
sclerotherapy, 207, 213, 215, 216
scope, 24, 32, 93
secretion, 102, 111, 140, 197

self-repair, 122
sensing, 27, 38, 237
sensitivity, 24, 64, 68, 85, 115, 116, 117, 127, 183, 198, 204, 211, 212, 239
sensors, 27, 28
sepsis, 133
septum, 21, 180, 185, 188, 235, 236, 238, 241
serum, 64, 124, 125, 128, 133, 134, 135, 173, 196, 233
sex, 28, 31, 38, 125
shape, 20, 50, 103, 239
shear, 145, 165, 167, 168, 171, 177, 218
sheep, 179, 182, 189, 190, 191, 194
shock, 243
shortage, 218
showing, 27, 31, 36, 38, 39, 40, 51, 90, 103, 164, 167, 187, 188, 198
sick sinus syndrome, 238, 246
signals, 27, 28, 29, 39, 77, 79, 80, 128
signs, 28, 95, 186, 231, 243
simulation, vii, 37, 38, 143, 146, 150, 167, 170, 171, 176
simulations, 37, 38, 39, 42, 163
sinus rhythm, 240
skeletal muscle, 127
smoking, 154
smooth muscle, 58, 63
sodium, 124, 196, 198, 199, 233
software, 28, 29, 30, 32, 37, 234
solution, 70, 183
somatic cell, 128
specialists, 173
species, 35, 126, 196
speculation, 127
spleen, 224, 225
splenic infarction, 225
Sprague-Dawley rats, 197, 198
stability, vii, 157, 159, 172
standard deviation, 137, 234, 236
standardization, 126
state, 14, 16, 23, 41, 53, 95, 105, 117, 128, 130, 131, 142, 144, 185, 208, 212, 214, 224, 231, 233
steel, 156
stenosis, 63, 91, 96, 109, 110, 112, 118, 134, 162, 169, 191
stent, 153, 155, 156, 157, 158, 159, 161, 162, 163, 164, 165, 166, 167, 168, 169, 170, 171, 172, 173, 174, 175, 176, 177
stimulant, 122
stimulation, 45, 108, 122, 125, 127, 131, 240, 247
stomach, 208, 209, 210
storage, 124

stratification, 121, 131, 135, 139
stress, 23, 110, 122, 123, 130, 131, 165, 167, 168, 171, 176, 177, 182, 204, 218, 232, 243, 247
stressors, 124
stroke, 11, 12, 15, 18, 19, 21, 22, 26, 29, 30, 31, 32, 35, 52, 77, 82, 102, 104, 105, 108, 110, 111, 150, 183, 184, 189, 191, 234, 237
stroke volume, 11, 18, 19, 21, 26, 29, 30, 31, 32, 35, 52, 77, 102, 111, 150, 183, 184, 189, 191
structural changes, 196, 198, 203
structural protein, 125
structure, 44, 58, 63, 78, 87, 88, 91, 129, 150, 156, 163, 172, 176, 187, 210, 214
style, 90
submucosa, 208
substrates, 98
success rate, 172
Sun, vi, 98, 151, 153, 174, 175, 176, 177
superior vena cava, 103, 180, 181, 182
suppression, 124, 128
surface area, 15, 93, 234
surgical technique, 224, 227
surveillance, 156, 172
survival, 6, 132, 218, 221, 238, 241
survival rate, 221
susceptibility, 197, 202, 203, 204, 224
Swan-Ganz catheter, 232
Sweden, 14
sympathetic denervation, 133
sympathetic nervous system, 122, 131, 205
symptoms, 92, 121, 122, 125, 154, 200, 213, 231
synchronization, 117, 247
syndrome, 17, 65, 68, 90, 96, 109, 125, 126, 185, 187, 188, 191, 192, 193, 218, 222, 223, 224, 225, 226, 228, 232
synthesis, 124, 203, 205
systolic blood pressure, 60, 62, 64
systolic pressure, 5, 11, 12, 13, 15, 21, 32, 35, 50, 67, 77, 102, 105, 106, 144, 150

T

T lymphocytes, 200
tachycardia, 24
target, 17, 64, 141, 148, 159, 241
Task Force, 244
tau, 97
TDI, 79, 80, 82, 83, 84, 85, 86, 87, 89, 92, 98, 189
technical support, 42
techniques, 37, 55, 58, 96, 121, 163, 173, 227, 232, 234, 235, 238
technological developments, 156

technology, 28, 36, 92, 159, 171, 173
telangiectasia, 209
temperature, 232
temporal variation, 39, 40
temporal window, 28, 32
tension, 60, 192
testing, 121, 132
tetralogy, 6, 64, 67, 68, 90, 94, 96, 128
TGF, 195, 199, 200
thalassemia, 140
therapy, vii, 9, 16, 17, 22, 24, 58, 64, 79, 86, 95, 96, 98, 99, 109, 129, 130, 155, 201, 207, 215, 231, 232, 233, 234, 236, 238, 243, 244, 245, 246, 247, 248
thermoregulation, 28
thinning, 129, 130
three-dimensional model, 148, 176
thrombosis, 66, 67, 131, 168, 222, 224, 225, 232
thrombus, 176
thymus, 118
thyroid, 190
time periods, 31
TIMP, 130
tissue, 21, 26, 27, 37, 38, 39, 40, 77, 79, 80, 81, 82, 84, 85, 86, 91, 92, 93, 94, 96, 97, 98, 103, 105, 127, 129, 134, 189, 191, 193, 200, 205, 218, 224, 233, 234, 235, 245, 246
tissue perfusion, 233
TNF, 123, 125, 126, 128, 131, 140, 224
TNF-alpha, 224
tonometry, 57
torsion, 88, 91, 92, 97
total cholesterol, 140
Toyota, 215, 216
trajectory, 3, 13, 16, 50, 52
transducer, 27, 28, 38, 40, 197, 234
transformation, 1, 172
transforming growth factor, 206
transfusion, 185, 187, 192, 193
translation, 82, 87, 118
translocation, 86
transmission, 3, 27, 50, 57, 65, 143, 198
transplant, 217, 218, 219, 222, 223, 228
transplant recipients, 223
transplantation, 218, 224, 225, 227, 228, 232, 242
transport, 111, 127, 199
transthoracic echocardiography, 103
trauma, 130
treatment, 19, 90, 98, 110, 121, 122, 123, 125, 126, 128, 130, 153, 155, 168, 171, 172, 173, 174, 175, 177, 200, 202, 204, 206, 207, 209, 211, 212, 213, 214, 215, 216, 218, 224, 225, 228, 237, 248
trial, 65, 92, 98, 110, 130, 132, 171, 174, 177, 232, 238, 246, 247
tricuspid valve, 82, 83, 147, 180, 185, 192
triggers, 130, 224
tumor, 123, 140, 224, 229
tumor necrosis factor, 123, 140, 224, 229
turnover, 133
twist, 96, 97
type 1 diabetes, 205
type 2 diabetes, 66, 67

U

UK, 154, 245
ultrasonography, 119, 188, 207, 210, 211, 212, 214, 215, 216, 219
ultrasound, 35, 44, 95, 97, 112, 113, 118, 154, 172, 177, 190, 191, 193, 210, 211, 237
underlying mechanisms, 91, 201
undernutrition, 201
uniform, 39, 89, 144, 148
United States (USA), 37, 58, 197, 199, 202
unmasking, 82
urban, 119
ureter, 196
uric acid, 201
urine, 233
uterus, 181

V

validation, 23, 37, 93, 94, 95, 96
valuation, 214
valve, 10, 62, 77, 81, 97, 102, 105, 107, 108, 109, 110, 145, 147, 231, 232, 237, 239, 240, 242, 243
valvular heart disease, 231, 237, 238, 242, 246
variables, 45, 83
varieties, 87, 90
vascular surgeon, 172
vascular system, 49, 69, 153, 163
vascular wall, 130
vasculature, 32, 203
vasculitis, 64, 130
vasoconstriction, 14, 102, 131, 186, 195, 199, 233
vasodilation, 17, 122, 131, 184, 199
vasodilator, 19, 24, 123, 124, 197, 233
vasomotor, 76
vein, 14, 102, 107, 109, 118, 179, 180, 187, 188, 193, 196, 207, 208, 210, 211, 213, 215, 219, 220, 221, 223, 224

Index

velocity, 3, 4, 5, 6, 21, 55, 57, 62, 63, 65, 66, 67, 68, 69, 70, 71, 72, 73, 74, 76, 77, 78, 79, 80, 81, 82, 83, 84, 85, 86, 87, 89, 91, 93, 94, 95, 98, 106, 107, 108, 111, 112, 151, 163, 164, 165, 168, 170, 180, 182, 185, 186, 187, 188, 191, 192, 193, 208, 210, 211, 235, 237, 239, 246
venography, 213
ventilation, 45, 46, 116, 191, 233
ventricle, 1, 4, 5, 6, 12, 16, 17, 21, 22, 46, 72, 73, 81, 83, 84, 88, 90, 91, 92, 94, 99, 101, 108, 110, 118, 126, 144, 180, 182, 183, 189, 193
ventricular septal defect, 92, 126, 128
ventricular septum, 247
vessels, 9, 23, 27, 39, 40, 50, 55, 58, 92, 128, 146, 148, 149, 159, 164, 168, 172, 173, 174, 184, 186, 208, 209, 210, 211, 212
viscosity, 49, 57, 164
visualization, 28, 153, 162, 173, 175, 176, 212

vitamin B1, 138
vitamin B12, 138
vitamin B12 deficiency, 138
VLDL, 173
VSD, 92, 126, 128

W

water, 70, 102, 127, 202, 210
wave propagation, 148, 149
weakness, 80
Western Australia, 153, 177
wires, 157, 165, 166, 167, 168, 173, 176, 245

Y

yield, 5, 30, 34, 38, 243